NATIONAL UNIVERSITY LIBRARY

D0787630

Contributions to Psychology and Medicine

Contributions to Psychology and Medicine

1

Medical Thinking: An Introduction

As soon as questions of will or decision or reason or choice of action arise, human science is at a loss.

Noam Chomsky

What a piece of work is man! How noble in reason! How infinite in faculty!

William Shakespeare

To those who are medically naive, the complexity of modern medicine can sometimes appear overwhelming. Consider, for example, the case of Mrs. K.*

It is the 23rd of September; Mrs. K. has just arrived at the emergency room of a large city hospital. She is having difficulty breathing, her heartbeat is irregular, and she has a moderately high fever. To the admitting physician, she looks very sick indeed. The emergency room doctors begin their workup, ordering blood tests and a set of abdominal x-rays and a chest x-ray. In addition, Mrs. K. begins to receive several different medications and is transferred to the Intensive Care Unit (ICU). The cause of her illness remains unclear.

On her second day in the ICU Mrs. K. has 15 different blood tests, a urinalysis, and a second chest x-ray, and, septicemia apparently being suspected, she is placed on additional antibiotics. Her condition continues to be grave, prompting her doctors to place her on a blood-gas monitor, a device that measures the amount of oxygen in her blood.

On the following day Mrs. K. undergoes additional laboratory tests as her doctors continue to search for the source of her illness. In addition, she has an electrocardiogram, and more x-rays.

On the fourth day Mrs. K. is still gravely ill. She is placed on intravenous medicines, receives a second electrocardiogram, another chest x-ray, and more laboratory tests.

On her fifth day in the hospital Mrs. K. develops serious breathing difficulties and is put on a respirator. On the 28th of September, Mrs.

---

* The story of Mrs. K.'s hospitalization is adapted from Hellerstein (1984) and is summarized here with the permission of *Harper's* Magazine.

K.'s sixth day in the hospital, she undergoes additional tests, another chest x-ray, and a brief surgical procedure.

On the seventh hospital day additional blood tests are performed, including five repeats of a test called the Chem-8—a test that measures sodium, potassium, and six other blood chemical levels. She also has a chest x-ray and another abdominal x-ray. She continues to deteriorate. Because her kidneys begin to fail, she is placed on peritoneal dialysis.

During Mrs. K.'s second week in the hospital, lack of sleep, noise, pain, fear, and drugs make her disoriented and she must be restrained (tied down) to keep her from pulling the tubes out of her arms. No specific pathogen has been isolated. On October 2 a tracheotomy is performed to help her breathe and, because she is now bleeding internally, she receives blood plasma and other blood products.

Mrs. K.'s third week in the hospital is fairly similar to her second. A gated blood-pool study (in which radioactive tagging allows her doctors to observe blood passing through her heart), confirms their clinical judgment that her heart is failing. In her fourth week Mrs. K. receives a lumbar puncture along with further blood tests and chest x-rays. There now appears to be a specific diagnosis, but she is too far gone to save. On October 18th Mrs. K.'s heart fails and she dies.

During her 25 days in the hospital, Mrs. K. was x-rayed 31 times, received pharmacy drugs 136 times (not counting intravenous drips), and underwent $11,000 of laboratory tests. The total bill came to $47,311.20.

Mrs. K.'s case is certainly not typical; most patients seen by doctors do not present anywhere near such a diagnostic puzzle. Also, while it is true that, despite receiving the best technical care available, Krs. K. died, her story is certainly not presented here as an indictment of modern medicine. Only a few years ago, she probably would not have lasted four days let alone almost four weeks. Each additional day she survived increased her chance of long-term survival. On the other hand, Mrs. K.'s hospital stay was not entirely a success story either. Her treatment caused her some suffering and cost her (actually, her insurance company) a great deal of money. It is worthwhile, therefore, asking whether some things could have been handled differently. For organizational purposes, the relevant questions may be divided into six topic areas (each topic is discussed in more detail in one or more of the later chapters of this book).

1. *Identifying causes.* How did Mrs. K.'s doctors decide which tests to perform? Did they first set out the most likely hypothesis on the basis of her symptoms and then order tests in an attempt to confirm their theory? Or, did they withhold judgment, viewing the test results as a data base from which a diagnosis would emerge? In other words, did their hypothesis determine the tests they chose or vice versa?

Contents

there anything special about how expert clinicians think that distinguishes them from less experienced doctors? Can medical judgment be improved through training? Can it be automated? We attempt to answer these questions by systematically describing and interpreting psychological research concerned with medical judgment and decision making. Although applied decision making is the major focus of this book, the present volume is not meant to be a "how to do it" guide to decision making. The main goal of the book is to provide insight into the cognitive operations underlying medical thinking. In other words, this is a book about cognitive psychology.

The book has been written with several audiences in mind: as a textbook for physicians with an interest in understanding and improving medical judgment, medical students, medical educators, and psychologists interested in cognitive psychology in general and in medical decision making in particular. We have attempted to keep the focus on problems and procedures; theories and mathematical tools are brought into the discussion only as they are needed to answer a clinically relevant question. Although we expect most readers to be familiar with basic psychological concepts and terminology, all new terms and concepts are explained as they arise and the details of the specific studies are given when necessary. Because the book is meant to appeal to a variety of readerships, no specific psychological or medical knowledge is assumed.

The book consists of six chapters. The first chapter is introductory. It sets the stage for what follows by reviewing the major questions psychologists and others have raised about medical judgment and decision making. The remaining chapters deal with research on several important topics in the psychology of medical decision making: how information is gathered and evaluated, how choices are made, learning to make better decisions, the nature of expertise, and the influence of social forces. While it is always dangerous to try to predict the future, in the final chapter, we make a conservative attempt to extrapolate from current work to future trends, pointing out research areas that seem likely to yield fruitful results.

Because of the nature of their work, authors are generally indebted to many people for their support, advice, criticisms, and help. The first author's research has been generously supported by the Australian Research Grants Scheme for many years. In addition, many people helped us prepare this book. We would like to acknowledge the helpful advice of Arthur Elstein, Jack Dowie, Paul Glasziou, and Dick Eiser. If faults and errors remain in the book, the responsibility is entirely ours—and may the judgment be not too heavy upon us.

Steven Schwartz
Timothy Griffin

Preface

Decision making is the physician's major activity. Every day, in doctors' offices throughout the world, patients describe their symptoms and complaints while doctors perform examinations, order tests, and, on the basis of these data, decide what is wrong and what should be done. Although the process may appear routine—even to the physicians involved—each step in the sequence requires skilled clinical judgment. Physicians must decide: which symptoms are important, whether any laboratory tests should be done, how the various items of clinical data should be combined, and, finally, which of several treatments (including doing nothing) is indicated. Although much of the information used in clinical decision making is objective, the physician's values (a belief that pain relief is more important than potential addiction to pain-killing drugs, for example) and subjectivity are as much a part of the clinical process as the objective findings of laboratory tests.

In recent years, both physicians and psychologists have come to realize that patient management decisions are not only subjective but also probabilistic (although this is not always acknowledged overtly). When doctors argue that an operation is fairly safe because it has a mortality rate of only 1%, they are at least implicitly admitting that the outcome of their decision is based on probability.

Understanding how doctors reach patient management decisions (and the role that subjective values play in clinical judgment) has been the subject of intensive psychological research over the past ten years. The present book contains a critical review of this research; its major focus is on the cognitive strategies doctors use to make everyday clinical judgments. The book is intended to answer several related questions: Can the thought processes underlying medical judgment be understood? Is

Medicine is a science of uncertainty and an art of probability.

Sir William Osler

Who shall decide, when doctors disagree,
And soundest casuists doubt, like you and me?

Alexander Pope

to our wives Carolyn and Helen

Steven Schwartz
Department of Psychology
University of Queensland
St. Lucia, Queensland 4067
Australia

Timothy Griffin
Department of Psychology
University of Queensland
St. Lucia, Queensland 4067
Australia

Advisor
J. Richard Eiser
Department of Psychology
University of Exeter
Exeter EX4 40G
England

Library of Congress Cataloging in Publication Data
Schwartz, Steven.
    Medical thinking.
    (Contributions to psychology and medicine)
    Bibliography: p.
    Includes indexes.
    1. Medicine—Decision making—Evaluation. 2. Medical
logic—Evaluation. 3. Cognition. I. Griffin,
Timothy. II. Title. III. Series. [DNLM: 1. Decision
Making. 2. Diagnosis. WB 141 S399m]
    R723.5.S38   1986   610'.68   86-6475

© 1986 by Springer-Verlag New York Inc.
All rights reserved. No part of this book may be translated or reproduced in
any form without written permission from Springer-Verlag, 175 Fifth Avenue,
New York, New York 10010, U.S.A.
The use of general descriptive names, trade names, trademarks, etc., in this
publication, even if the former are not especially identified, is not to be taken
as a sign that such names, as understood by the Trade Marks and
Merchandise Marks Act, may accordingly be used freely by anyone.

While the advice and information in this book are believed to be true and accurate
at the date of going to press, neither the authors nor the editors nor the publisher
can accept any legal responsibility for any errors or omissions that may be made.
The publisher makes no warranty, express or implied, with respect to the
material contained herein.

Typeset by TC Systems, Shippensburg, Pennsylvania.
Printed and bound by R.R. Donnelley & Sons, Harrisonburg, Virginia.
Printed in the United States of America.

9 8 7 6 5 4 3 2 1

ISBN 0-387-96315-4 Springer-Verlag New York Berlin Heidelberg
ISBN 3-540-96315-4 Springer-Verlag Berlin Heidelberg New York

Steven Schwartz   Timothy Griffin

Medical Thinking
The Psychology of
Medical Judgment
and Decision Making

With 28 Figures

Springer-Verlag
New York Berlin Heidelberg
London Paris Tokyo

Assuming hypotheses were generated first, was there any rationale for the sequence in which laboratory tests were ordered? For example, Mrs. K. received a laboratory test for parasites on her third day in ICU. Was this test left for the third day because Mrs. K.'s symptoms were unlikely to be caused by a parasitic disease or because no one thought of this earlier (or both)? Could the sequence of tests have been altered so that the results of each built on the results of the previous one(s)?

2. *Choosing actions.* How did Mrs. K.'s doctors intend to use the information they gathered? Assuming that her doctors were using chest x-rays to help monitor her heart–lung functioning, was it really necessary for Mrs. K. to receive two dozen of them? Why were five Chem-8s ordered in a single day? Would 10 x-rays and three Chem-8s have done as well? How about five x-rays and two Chem-8s? How did Mrs. K.'s doctors decide on the appropriate number? Was the financial cost of Mrs. K.'s hospital stay considered by her doctors in their treatment strategy? Should it have been? What about the cost in pain and suffering? If Mrs. K. would have preferred a quiet death, should the doctors have ceased their efforts? Is there any way to measure the relative costs and benefits of medical interventions?

3. *The role of experience.* Would physicians of different levels of experience have handled Mrs. K.'s case differently? How? Assuming the components of expertise can be isolated, can novices be taught to think like experts?

4. *Training in medical decision making.* Would training in medical decision making have changed the way Mrs. K.'s doctors handled her case?

5. *Automated clinics versus automated clinicians.* Would automated decision making by computers or computer-aided clinicians have made any difference in how Mrs. K. was treated?

6. *Patient preferences and public policy.* Could Mrs. K. and her relatives have been involved in the doctors' decision making? Should they have been? Given that the public (through higher insurance premiums) ultimately pays the bill for Mrs. K.'s treatment, should public opinion be considered in deciding when heroic life-support measures are used and when they are not? If so, how?

Attempts by psychologists, economists, and medical researchers to answer these (and related) questions constitute the subject matter of this book. In the succeeding chapters, we describe their successes and failures. In order to provide the reader with a context within which to organize these discussions, the present chapter is divided into two main sections. The first provides a brief orientation to psychological research into medical decision making. The second section introduces the topics covered in Chapters 2 through 6. The major purpose of the present chapter is not to present an exhaustive treatment of the various topics, but to show how they interrelate. In other words, the present chapter is designed to provide a framework for the more detailed discussions to follow.

Research in Medical Decision Making: Definitions, Theories, and Methods

The history of medicine has always been more interesting to historians than to doctors. There are probably two reasons for this. The first is the abstract nature of historical knowledge. Doctors tend to be practical people and most historical information is of little day-to-day use. Even medical historians such as Lester King admit this. In his own words: "No one would claim that a sound knowledge of Galen . . . would make it easier for a surgeon to remove a gall bladder" (1982, p. 12). The second reason doctors have tended to avoid medical history is because it is so unpleasant. According to physician and essayist Lewis Thomas, "For century after century, all the way into the remote millennia of its origins, medicine got along by sheer guesswork and the crudest sort of empiricism. It is hard to conceive of a less scientific enterprise among human endeavors" (1979, p. 131).

Thomas is no doubt correct—the history of medicine is largely deplorable. It is also true that historical study rarely leads to discoveries applicable in modern medical practice. Nevertheless, there are some important themes that constantly seem to recur throughout medical history. Certain clinical problems (diagnosis, combining the results of several tests, and so on) are present in all eras. They represent constant basic features of medical practice, no matter how dramatically superficial characteristics may change. Taken together, these constant features of medical practice constitute what is known as the "art" (as opposed to the "science") of medicine. This section begins with a brief look at the difference between the art and science of medicine, a distinction with important implications for the psychology of medical thinking.

The Science of Medicine

Despite its critics, modern medicine is generally perceived as quite successful (Illich, 1977). Just compare today's medicine with that practiced 100 years ago.* In the 1880s, surgeons had only the smallest inkling about aseptic techniques and never wore gloves or masks. European cholera epidemics wiped out thousands each year. There were no vaccines to protect us from typhoid, tetanus, measles, diptheria, yellow fever, polio, or mumps. There were no sulfonamides, no drugs for use against tuberculosis, and no antibiotics. There was no insulin or steroids,

* The figures on illness and life expectancy 100 years ago come from Baida (1984).

no psychotherapy or tranquilizers, and no contraception. Open-heart surgery, transplants, and x-rays did not exist. Pneumonia was the most virulent killer disease, followed by tuberculosis. Life expectancy was only 43 years as compared with today's 74 or more. Sixty times more women died in childbirth 100 years ago than today. Clearly, the advances made during the past century are remarkable. Some writers have even argued that medicine only became scientific during the last 100 years (see Thomas, 1979, for example).

It is certainly true that, prior to the 19th century, medicine was pretty much a hit-and-miss affair. Weird theories (tuberculosis is caused by the night air) and even stranger treatments (cupping, bleeding, purgings) were accepted as if they had some basis in fact. Anything that could be dreamed up was given a try; it did not seem to matter that practically all medical treatments were demonstrably worthless, and that some treatments were worse than the diseases they were meant to cure.

One reason that bizarre and useless treatments continued to be used was that doctors felt compelled to do *something*. The common belief was that untreated patients inevitably got worse and died. According to Thomas, some time in the early 1800s, doctors began to observe that untreated patients occasionally recovered all by themselves; this was the breakthrough that opened the way to modern scientific medicine. Rather than treating everyone, physicians turned to diagnosis. They became particularly interested in predicting which patients would improve and which would not. To accomplish this, doctors observed their patients, noting similarities, differences, and outcomes. Before long, they had accumulated a large body of information about the natural courses of many diseases.

By the middle of the 19th century, accurate diagnosis became the primary purpose of medicine. Textbook writers of the time pointed out the similarity between medical diagnosis and the scientific classification methods used in botany and other branches of biology. For example, in a text published in 1864, students were told:

> "The detection of disease is the product of the close observation of symptoms, and of correct deduction from these symptoms. . . . When . . . the symptoms of the malady have been discovered, the next step toward a diagnosis is a proper appreciation of their significance and of their relation toward each other. Knowledge, and above all, the exercise of the reasoning faculties are now indispensable . . ." (Da Costa, 1864, pp. 14–15)

In modern terms, students were being advised to make observations, listen to the patient describe his/her symptoms, and consider these to be signs of some underlying disease. The validity of the postulated disease could then be assessed by further observation, including tests. Such an approach is surely the essence of scientific reasoning.

By the early 1900s, physicians knew what to expect from many different illnesses. Patients could now be told the name of the disease they had contracted and what was likely to happen to them. Surgical procedures, and even vaccines, became available for some illnesses, but for most, "supportive" therapy was all that could be offered. All this changed in the 1930s with the discovery of the sulfonamides and penicillin and the perfection of immunization techniques. Now doctors could do more than label illnesses; they could also cure some and prevent others. The new discoveries added another link to the inferential chain physicians constructed each time they examined a patient. Not only did they observe symptoms and try to associate these with diseases, they could also link many diseases to specific treatments. In this century, for the first time, doctors were able to use the inferential methods proven so successful in the physical and chemical sciences; they could infer underlying causes from observed symptoms and examine the effects of interventions.

Progress has been rapid during the past 50 years. Today, scientific medicine has totally replaced the haphazard empirical approach of the past. Not all puzzles have been solved, of course. We still have the mysteries of cancer, arthritis, schizophrenia, and many other diseases to solve. Yet, there is great optimism among the medical community that these, too, will eventually succumb to the scientific method. After all, technology has provided modern medicine with powerful diagnostic and treatment tools; it is only a matter of time before many of today's killers are understood. Although the success of modern medicine is correctly attributed to its scientific nature, an important part of medicine remains an art. As we discuss in the next section, progress in the art has lagged behind the science.

The Art of Medicine

For some writers (see Komaroff, 1982, for example), the word *art* appears to be an antonym for *science*. From this point of view, the art of medicine is a kind of mysterious clinical intuition, whereas medical science is a body of specified scientific rules. In reality, however, the art and science of medicine are not nearly so easy to separate. Consider, for example, an incident described by King (1982). A general practitioner made a house call to a family whose six children had all come down with signs of stomach distress after a family picnic. The children had cramps, vomiting, and other symptoms that, along with the picnic, suggested food poisoning. The diagnosis seemed obvious. However, after examining the six children, the doctor said, "These five have food poisoning, but *this* one has appendicitis" (King, 1982, p. 301). The child in question went to the hospital, where the physician's diagnosis was confirmed after an operation.

The doctor in this anecdote was certainly practicing scientific medicine. Noting a discrepancy in the symptoms of one of the children, he inferred a different underlying cause. A less careful physician may have jumped to the "obvious" conclusion that all six children were suffering from food poisoning. The difference between the two doctors is what we mean by the art of medicine; not the opposite of scientific medicine, but its thoughtful application. Specifically, the art of medicine is the skilled application of medical science. In this sense, the art of medicine is no different from the art of engineering or architecture or any other applied science in which a large body of knowledge must be applied to everyday problems. Some engineers and architects are better than others; they are better "artists."

Although the art of medicine is not totally divorced from medical science, it is certainly true that some physicians are less "artistic" than others. Some go about their business in an unsystematic manner that not only wastes scarce medical resources but can also threaten the well-being of their patients. Clearly, it does little good for medical science and technology to make dramatic advances if these advances are going to be applied inefficiently or incorrectly. Traditionally, the bulk of biomedical research efforts have been devoted to medical science while the art of medicine (the application of medical science) has been neglected. The last 30 years, however, have seen an increasing research interest in medical judgment and reasoning. Indeed, judgment and decision making have become important areas of scientific study in their own right, particularly among psychologists. Psychological research into clinical judgment had its beginnings in 1954 when Paul Meehl began what has come to be known as the "clinical versus statistical prediction" debate.

Clinical versus Statistical Prediction

Under one name or another, the clinical versus statistical prediction debate has been going on for centuries. To take but one example, Hammond, McClelland, and Mumpower (1980) noted that Raphael's Renaissance portrait of the celebrated Athenian philosophers arranges them from right to left according to whether they adopted a quantitative (statistical) scientific approach or an intuitive (clinical) approach to understanding human thinking. Meehl (1954) organized psychological research along similar lines. That is, he characterized judgments as based either on clinical or statistical reasoning. Meehl went on to claim that clinical judgments (Is this patient schizophrenic? Does that patient have brain damage?) made by following formal statistical rules are at least as accurate, and sometimes more accurate, than judgments arrived at clinically or intuitively. (The statistical approach is sometimes known as "actuarial" because, just as an insurance company predicts life expectancy from population longevity figures, statistical decision makers create their formulas by examining the statistical likelihood of various outcomes.)

Meehl's claim that statistical judgments are superior to or at least no worse than those reached by intuitive methods was hotly contested by many clinicians, and the debate raged on in the psychology literature for many years (see Elstein, 1976, and Kleinmuntz, 1984, for reviews).

Despite the intense nature of the clinical versus statistical prediction debate, it is important to note that the two approaches do not differ in the data they use, but in the way data are combined and evaluated (Gough, 1962). Consider, for example, the university admissions officer about to interview a prospective medical student. The interviewer might begin by noting the applicant's neat appearance, alert posture, fluent speech, and well-organized fund of scientific knowledge. The admissions officer may also know that the applicant's father is a famous surgeon on the medical school's staff. The interviewer's observations lead to the conclusion that the applicant's intellectual capacity, perseverance and self-discipline, and background are exactly those required for a good doctor. The admissions officer predicts success in medical school and recommends admission.

The medical school admissions officer is using what Meehl termed "clinical" reasoning. The alternative, statistical, procedure requires setting up a decision rule before any applicants are actually interviewed. Based on previous experience, those attributes correlated with success in medical school (including having a father on staff if this predicts success) are identified and weighted according to how well they predict performance. Every applicant is then evaluated on each attribute and those with the best overall profile are admitted.

In the actual clinical situation, the clinical reasoning method involves making largely intuitive judgments on the basis of a patient's history, presenting symptoms, and laboratory tests. The statistical approach requires that judgments be reached through the application of formal quantitative techniques and statistical formulas. Writers on both sides of the debate agree that clinical judgments are rife with uncertainty. Both admit that the relationships between diagnostic signs and diseases as well as between treatment interventions and outcomes is never perfect. Where they differ is on what, if anything, needs to be done about this. Those in the clinical camp believe that clinical intuition applied individually on a case-by-case basis will lead to the most sensitive decision making. Those favoring the statistical approach argue that case-by-case decision making is too easily biased. They prefer to set up *a priori* "decision rules" that can then be applied in all similar cases. An example of such a decision rule is: Always order a throat culture when a patient presents with sore throat and swollen glands.

Although many (but not all) psychologists agree that decisions reached statistically are more accurate and fairer than clinical ones, clinicians have been slow to give up the clinical approach. Elstein (1976) was somewhat bemused that, although medicine is well known to embrace new technology and scientific discoveries from the biomedical sciences, strategies for drawing clinical inferences or reaching clinical decisions remain fundamentally unchanged despite the psychological research of the past 30 years. Even as recently as 1982, Pauker still found it necessary to list the pros and cons of statistical judgments (specifically those based on prescriptive theories) as opposed to clinical decision making.

The tenacity of the clinical approach despite the evidence favoring the superiority of statistical reasoning is largely due to the feeling that the research has not been entirely fair. Holt (1958, 1978), for example, has argued that studies designed to highlight clinical fallibility accomplish their goal by emphasizing tasks that place the clinician at a great disadvantage. Holt agreed that diagnoses may be judged better by statistical formulas when an entire population is concerned, but he believed that clinicians may still do better with an individual case. Moreover, statistical decision rules can only cope with a small part of what the clinician does and are often difficult to apply. Holt's views are shared by many doctors and, as we shall see in later discussions, not without good reason.

Another reason for the continued popularity of the clinical approach is that the outcome of a statistical decision may not coincide with the physician's personal experience. When this happens, some doctors perceive the statistical judgment as risky (Kozielecki, 1981). These same physicians perceive clinical judgment as conservative and prudent. This is just the opposite of the research evidence. We shall return to this discrepancy between research evidence and clinical practice later in this book. For now, we turn to a discussion of several theoretical and methodological approaches to clinical judgment. We begin with several important definitions.

A Few Definitions

All theories in the field of medical judgment and decision making are ultimately directed at the same question: How do people go about making judgments and decisions with only partial information? In philosophy, the word *decision* is taken to mean "a resolution to do something" or, more commonly, "a resolution to behave in a certain way" (Szanawkski, 1980, p. 328). So long as *behavior* is interpreted broadly to include internal thoughts as well as external actions and so long as it also includes resolving to do nothing at all ("let's wait and see what happens"), this definition seems appropriate to the medical situation. In the present book, the term "medical decision making" is used to refer to all patient management decisions made by physicians—even when such decisions mean abstaining from any action.

Making decisions implies that one has a choice between at least two options. Sometimes the choice can be between beginning or withholding treatment (prescribing antibiotics for a sore throat or waiting for the result of a throat culture); sometimes the choice may be from among several treatments. In any case, there must always be some sort of choice.

Although it is sometimes useful to distinguish between judgment and decision making (judgments are inferences from data—"this test indicates a 50% chance of pneumonia," for example, whereas decisions involve a commitment to a course of action), we find that the terms are often used interchangeably. In this book, we try to reserve the word *judgment* for data evaluations (the patient has a fever, for example) and use the word *decision* to describe a choice between two or more actions. However, we recognize that the distinction is somewhat arbitrary and that placing a patient in the category "fever" or "not fever" can be considered a type of decision.

All of the theories of decision making discussed in this book assume that the choices confronting decision makers are clearly distinct. In some medical situations, however, this may not be true. The data upon which medical decisions are made can be decidedly "fuzzy" and open to more than one interpretation. Komaroff (1979), after reviewing the literature on the accuracy of medical data, concluded that medical histories, physical examinations, and laboratory tests yield relatively unreliable information. Some researchers have even reported having difficulty getting doctors to agree on what they mean when they say a patient is suffering from a particular disease.

Indeed, it seems fair to say that uncertainty is the hallmark of medical decision making. If the physician knew exactly what would happen as the result of any particular patient management decision, then medical decision making would consist solely of looking up the "correct" decision for each clinical situation. Uncertainty, however, means that the best choice is not always obvious. It also means that the result of a particular decision is a matter of *probability*. Probability is measured on a scale that goes from 0 to 1. Certainties (the sun will set in the west) are assigned probabilities of 1.00 and impossibilities (the sun will set in the east) have probabilities of 0. Everything else has a probability somewhere between these two extremes. In medicine, probabilities are almost never equal to 1.00. A physician may be fairly sure that a particular antibiotic will clear up a patient's infection, but a cure cannot be guaranteed. At best, the doctor can be very sure—say, a probability equal to .99.

In classical statistics, a probability is simply a long-run frequency. Calculating such probabilities requires taking a large number of samples (rolling a pair of dice 1000 times, for instance) and noting how often various numbers occur. There is another type of probability, however. This is the *subjective probability* used by the weather bureau when they forecast a 50% chance of rain or by the engineer who estimates the chance of a nuclear power accident is 1 in 10 million. This latter type of probability is not directly based on frequency, but rather represents someone's subjective belief in the likelihood of an event. This subjective belief can, of course, be derived from frequency information, but it is not, itself, a frequency. The important difference between the two types of probability is not in their method of estimation but in what they stand for—objective frequency counts or subjective belief.

In medicine, subjective probabilities are used more often than frequency-based probabilities. It's easy to see why. From a frequency point of view, the probability that a particular patient has pneumonia is not meaningful—a single patient obviously has no frequency. So, when a doctor says that the probability of *a particular* patient having pneumonia is .50, the physician is really saying that his/her subjective belief that the patient has pneumonia is about the same as the probability that a tossed coin will come up heads.

In addition to probabilities, medical decisions also involve the patient's preference for each outcome. These preferences are known as *utilities*. The term "utility" comes from economics, where it is often necessary to differentiate objective monetary value from subjective value. For example, when a rich person and a poor person both bet on the same winning horse at the racetrack, the monetary value of their $10 win is identical, but the subjective utility of this win for the poor person—for whom $10 is a lot of money—is much greater than for the rich person, to whom an extra $10 means little. In medicine, utilities include more than just cost. They also include intangibles such as pain and the quality of life. An important assumption underlying the concept of utility is that values attached to all types of outcomes can be expressed using a common scale. To see how utilities affect medical judgment, it is necessary to consider theories of decision making.

Prescriptive Theories

To make a medical decision, doctors should consider (at least implicitly) both probabilities and utilities. According to one popular theory of decision making, *expected utility theory* (EU), probabilities and utilities are combined through multiplication.* In other words, the probability of each outcome is multiplied by the appropriate utility. When the probabilities involved are subjective the theory is usually called *subjective expected utility theory* (SEU).

According to SEU theory, the choice with the highest expected utility (subjective probability × utility) is best. An example appears in Figure 1-1, which is a *decision tree* representation of the process of deciding whether a person should be diagnosed as having pneumonia (adapted from Christensen-Szalanski & Bushyhead, 1979).

In decision trees, the problem-solving sequence goes from left to right, matching the order in which choices are believed to occur. Typi-

---

* When objective values rather than subject utilities are used, this approach is known as expected value rather than expected utility.

Decision Tree

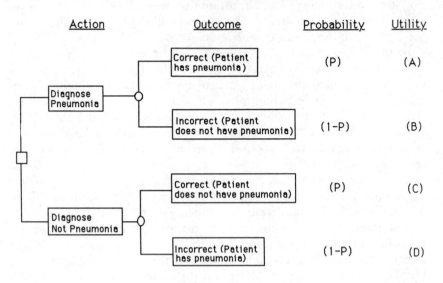

Action	Outcome	Probability	Utility

Correct (Patient has pneumonia)   (P)   (A)

Diagnose Pneumonia

Incorrect (Patient does not have pneumonia)   (1-P)   (B)

Correct (Patient does not have pneumonia)   (P)   (C)

Diagnose Not Pneumonia

Incorrect (Patient has pneumonia)   (1-P)   (D)

Expected Utilities

(1) EU of Diagnosing Pneumonia = $(P)A+(1-P)B$

(2) EU of Diagnosing Not Pneumonia = $(P)C+(1-P)D$

Decision Rule

If 1>2 then diagnose Pneumonia

If 2>1 then diagnose Not Pneumonia

Figure 1-1   A decision tree representation of a diagnostic problem. The initial square represents an action; the circles represent possible outcomes of the action. The utilities for the final outcomes are expressed arbitrarily as A, B, C, or D. Adapted from Christensen-Szalanski and Bushyhead (1979) and reprinted with the permission of the authors.

cally, a square represents a specific choice while a circle indicates that two or more outcomes can take place. In Figure 1-1 each choice can result in two possible outcomes: the patient has pneumonia or the patient does not have pneumonia. The probability that the patient has pneumonia is represented by the letter P. Because the only alternative to the patient having pneumonia is that the patient does not have pneumonia (and since the alternative probabilities must sum to 1.00), the probability that the patient does not have pneumonia is $1 - P$.

The strategy of choosing the alternative with the highest subjective utility is one of many possible *decision rules*; the decision maker must, according to SEU theory, always choose the alternative that serves to maximize utilities. It is worth noting that this decision rule does not necessarily lead doctors to always choose the most likely alternative. Depending on the utilities assigned to each outcome, even an unlikely outcome can wind up maximizing the physician's utilities. This can be seen by examining the final column, labeled "Utility," in Figure 1-1. Each outcome has been assigned a utility represented by the values A, B, C, and D. Although no numbers have been assigned to these utilities, it is safe to assume that, for most physicians, assigning a mistaken pneumonia diagnosis is probably less serious than assigning the nonpneumonia diagnosis to someone who actually has the disease. In the first instance the patient undergoes a usually harmless course of antibiotics, whereas in the second the patient may actually die. The utilities for both these outcomes, of course, are lower than those for correctly diagnosing pneumonia (or for correctly identifying those who do not have pneumonia).

In the decision-making literature, SEU theory is known as a *normative* or *prescriptive* theory. Normative theories represent a subset of the statistical approaches to clinical judgment already mentioned. They provide a set of rules for combining beliefs (probabilities) and preferences (utilities) to make a decision. The terms "normative" and "prescriptive" as used here mean that such theories specify how decisions *should* be made. If you accept the axioms upon which they are based, then the only rational choice is the one specified by the theory. Put another way, normative models are models of an "ideal world." Provided their axioms are met, they will lead to optimal decision making.

Some writers have argued that simply explaining the rationale behind normative theories should encourage decision makers to conform to their demands (Estes, 1980). However, conformity to the axioms underlying normative models of decision making is more wishful thinking than fact. Psychological research has established that people do not always behave as normative theories such as SEU claim they should (Edwards, 1955; Lichtenstein & Slovic, 1971). In one study (Lichtenstein, Slovic, & Zinc, 1969), subjects ignored expected value in making their decisions even after the experimenters had carefully explained the concept to them (see also Kahneman, Slovic, & Tversky, 1982).

Critics have also claimed that the assumptions underlying many normative theories are unrealistic and that the theories are often applied inappropriately (Pitz & Sachs, 1984). These criticisms are discussed in greater detail in Chapters 3 and 4. For now, we wish to note that perhaps the major unresolved question facing theories of decision making is deciding just what is meant by the "best" decision. How to define "the best decision" is an old question in philosophy, one that has never been completely answered. Psychologists have also been interested (see Edwards, Kiss, Majone, & Toda, 1984, for example). Socrates asserted that it is enough to know what is good in order for people to act accordingly. In practice, however, knowing what is good has proved to be far from simple.

Most normative decision rules are based on some version of *utilitarianism* (see Wulff, 1981). This rule simply states that decision makers should choose the action that produces the best consequences for everyone concerned ("the greatest good for the greatest number"). In normal practice, this rule might mean not prescribing antibiotics for patients without clear evidence of bacterial infection because of the possible harm this might do to others if drug-resistant strains develop.

Utilitarianism is not, however, the only decision rule under which doctors operate. There are times when many act to maximize their patients' utilities. According to this latter, usually implicit, rule, the "best" decisions are those with the best consequences for the patient regardless of their effect on society. Determining which consequences are best for the patient can be done by the clinician alone or by the clinician working with the patient. In either case, the decisions reached may be quite different from those reached by the utilitarianism rule. For example, a physician working for a public hospital or health service with (as is usual today) a tight budget who decides to discharge a pneumonia patient before his/her chest films are completely clear is maximizing society's utilities by keeping costs down and waiting lists short. If the doctor decided instead to keep the patient in the hospital until all signs of infection are gone, the patient's utilities are being maximized, not society's. (Mrs. K.'s hospital bill was ultimately paid by society as a whole through increased insurance premiums.)

To make things even more complicated, these two approaches to determining what decision to make do not exhaust all possible decision rules (see Dawes, 1977; Wulff, 1981). The "best decision" often depends on the social context and the individual concerned (see Edwards et al., 1984). Because values (and utilities) vary across people and societies, the "best" decision may turn out to be different depending on the individual case and the society in which the doctor and patient live. Different social contexts may require different decision rules (see Hardin, 1972, for a discussion of how ethical rules relate to social settings). We return to the question "What is meant by the best decision?" later in this book.

Since people do not always behave as SEU and other normative theories say they should, and since there is more than one definition of the "best decision," it is not surprising that the judgments reached using normative theories and informal judgments do not always agree. This is precisely what the "clinical versus statistical prediction" debate is all about. In fact, one of the most important consequences of that controversy was the awakening of interest among psychologists in understanding how clinicians actually make decisions in the real world. This research field has come to be known as the "descriptive" approach to studying decision making.

Descriptive Theories

In Chapter 3, we review several examples in which clinicians have been found inferior to statistical formulas. Often, the fault lies in how they go about making judgments. If these faults can be isolated, then presumably doctors can be taught to correct them. This has been the practical goal underlying much recent psychological research. The result has been the development of decision-making theories quite unlike the normative theories previously discussed. Instead of specifying what physicians *should* do, these theories attempt to describe how clinicians actually behave in clinical situations. Models developed in this way are called *descriptive* rather than prescriptive, and this field of research, as a whole, is known as *behavioral decision theory*. Although there is a fair amount of overlap between these two approaches (formal prescriptive theories may form the basis for descriptive models), it is best to keep the approaches separate because they serve different purposes. Formal models specify in advance how beliefs and preferences should be combined and how optimal decisions should be chosen. Descriptive models derive these "combination roles" from individual decision makers.

Psychological research into decision making traces its origins to Egon Brunswick's book *The Conceptual Framework of Psychology* (1952). In his book, Brunswick showed the importance of studying not only a person's cognitions but also the context in which judgments are made. Brunswick summarized his ideas in his "lens" model, which uses the analogy of a convex lens to show how a subject's perception of the environment compares with the actual state of the environment. Figure 1-2 contains the lens model as it applies to the typical medical environment.

The important sources of information available to the doctor (laboratory tests, examination results, and so on) appear in the center of the figure. Each of these sources of information has a probabilistic relationship to the true state of the world (the patient's actual state of health) on the left and the clinician's judgment on the right. The small rs indicate the correlations between each information source on the one hand and either the true state of health or the clinician's judgment on the other. Since laboratory tests and other sources of information are probabilistically related to both the patient's actual state of health and the doctor's judgment, medical decisions will always be less than perfect. The overall relationship between the patient's true state of health and the doctor's judgment is labeled "validity" in Figure 1-2. This overall validity is, in turn, a function of the r *ENVs* (how well the true environmental state is predicted from the information sources) and r *subjs* (the doctor's ability

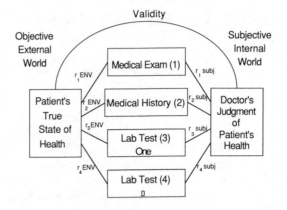

Figure 1-2   The lens model applied to medical decision making. The doctor's subjective perception of the patient's true state of health is mediated by a set of cues (laboratory tests, physical signs, and so on). Each *r ENV* represents the relationship between a cue and a patient's true state. Each *r subj* represents the relationship between a cue and the doctor's subjective impression. The overall relationship between the physician's subjective impression and the true state of the patient is called "validity" and is measured using multiple regression techniques in which the various cues serve as predictors.

to make use of the information available to produce a subjective judgment).

The lens model is probably the most carefully spelled out descriptive model of decision making. Its most important contribution is its emphasis on the importance of the context. Numerous psychological studies have shown that how judgments are presented, the number of alternatives, and even the availability of irrelevant information can affect a decision outcome (see Payne, 1982, for a review). Not only do such findings severely limit the applicability of normative theories (which usually assume that decisions are reached the same way across contexts), they also suggest that there are different decision-making strategies for different situations.

A great deal of psychological research has been directed at clarifying these judgment strategies. This research has led to the identification of certain judgment rules known as *heuristics* (see Kahneman et al., 1982). Heuristics are guides to inference, such as "patients with symptoms similar to those known to have disease *X* probably suffer from the same disease" or *primum non nocere* ("first do no harm"). Descriptive research has also led to the development of several theories about how people reach decisions under uncertainty (Coombs, 1975; Shanteau, 1975). However, there is not yet any widely accepted model of the cognitive mechanisms involved. Further discussion of the information-processing strategies and judgment heuristics underlying medical decision making may be found in Chapter 3. For now, it is sufficient to note that a complete understanding of medical judgment requires both normative and descriptive theories; it also requires more information about the cognitive strategies involved in processing clinical information. In this book, we try to integrate, wherever possible, various theoretical orientations and research methodologies.

Organization of this Book

If we are ever to develop a general theory of medical decision making, we must first have a clear idea of the questions such a theory must be able to answer. Chapters 2 through 6 of this book contain reviews of research designed to help answer the important questions about medical decision making posed earlier in this chapter. In this section, the topics to be discussed in these chapters are introduced. The order and organization of the various topics has been adapted from Einhorn and Hogarth's (1981a) review of the judgment and decision-making research.

Acquisition of Medical Data

In the past, diagnostic and treatment difficulties were generally blamed on the inadequacy of the information available to the doctor. It is easy to see why. Before the advent of modern diagnostic equipment, doctors were required to make their patient management decisions on the basis of very limited data. Prior to the development of the stethoscope, for example, the state of a patient's lungs had to be inferred from overt behavior and appearance. Not surprisingly, inferences based on such data were often wrong. Auscultation, and the stethoscope, changed all that. The new technique and equipment provided more information; the result was that inferences about the lungs became more accurate. Even greater accuracy was achieved with the development of the x-ray. The history of modern medicine contains many similar instances of new technology providing increasingly more accurate data.

Because more information has historically led to better judgment, it is not surprising that a great deal of medicine's research effort has been directed at providing more information. The laboratory tests given to Mrs. K. and the many others available are testimony to the success of this effort. However, the sheer mass of information available to modern doctors has brought its own problems. Foremost among these is the problem of interpreting and integrating information from many different tests. Physicians faced with a bewildering array of data often have no systematic way of using it; they must rely on intuition and *ad hoc* decision rules. The result is less-than-optimal decision making. Some psychologists have gone so far as to suggest that, like computers, there are inherent limitations to the amount of information human beings are capable of handling and, perhaps, even limits to rationality itself (Newell & Simon, 1972).

The traditional philosophical view of human beings emphasizes our rationality ("noble in reason . . . infinite in faculty" was how Shakespeare put it). However, this view has been severely challenged by the findings of psychologists. Beginning with Miller's (1956) demonstration that people are severely limited in their ability to attend to and process sensory information (most people have great difficulty keeping more than six chunks of information in memory simultaneously), many additional studies have confirmed that human information-processing capacity is severely limited. Taken together, these research findings support Simon's (1957) theory of "bounded rationality." Simon's theory asserts that, because of our cognitive limitations, we construct simplified "models" of the world. According to Simon, judgments and decisions are based on these simplified models rather than on the total information available in any judgment situation. The decision maker:

> behaves rationally with respect to this [simplified] model, and such behavior is not even approximately optimal with respect to the real world. To predict this behavior, we must understand the way in which this simplified model is constructed, and its construction will certainly be related to his psychological properties as a perceiving, thinking, and learning animal. (Simon, 1957, p. 198)

The bounded rationality theory has particular relevance for medical decision making because physicians have always been taught to gather as much information about the patient as possible, providing, of course, that gathering the information produces no harm. This exhaustive strategy is sometimes referred to as the "Baconian ideal," after the philosopher who believed that, given enough information, problems can always be solved. The problem with the exhaustive approach (in addition to the expense) is amply illustrated by what happened to Mrs. K. The sheer volume of information becomes so great that it is difficult to make any sense of it.

Recent research has shown that the Baconian ideal may not be so ideal after all. For example, several studies have shown that a carefully selected subset of information is often as useful as the voluminous data obtained by the exhaustive approach (Jennett, 1975; Keighly, Hoare, & Horrocks, 1976). Some studies have even found that providing clinicians with too much data can lead to lower diagnostic accuracy than providing them with what appears to be too little data (Sisson, Schoomaker, & Ross, 1976). A particularly striking example of the debilitating effect of excessive information comes not from the clinical situation but from a study of horserace handicappers (cited in Slovic, 1982). Eight expert handicappers were presented with either 5, 10, 20, or 40 items of information taken from past performance records; their job was to predict where horses would finish in a sample of 45 actual races. Not only did accuracy fail to improve with increased information, in many cases predictive accuracy decreased as the amount of relevant information increased. Such findings suggest that exhaustively gathering information prior to making a judgment may not always be the best strategy. Some clinicians may intuitively realize this. This would explain why they sometimes ignore laboratory test results even though they, themselves, ordered them (Dixon & Lazlo, 1974).

In summary, one of the major questions facing researchers in medical decision making is how doctors gather and use clinical information. Deciding on a test's value, however, is not always easy because, as we shall show, test results cannot be considered independently of diagnoses.

Evaluating Medical Information

Diagnosis is an important—perhaps the most important—job of a clinician. If the diagnosis is correct, and a treatment is available, proper care will generally follow. Even when no specific treatment is available, accurate diagnosis is necessary because: (1) it provides the basis for prognosis, and (2) researchers require homogeneous experimental groups. (An effective treatment may appear ineffective when tried out on a heterogeneous group of patients because some improve while others remain the same.) Ideally, medical diagnoses should be made according to the hypotheticodeductive method, in which a number of alternative hypotheses concerning the patient's problem are generated by the clinician's initial observations. Data are then sequentially and logically gathered until one of these hypotheses emerges as the most likely.

Although the hypotheticodeductive approach is logical, it is not without its problems. The most serious of these is judging whether clinical data support one or another hypothesis. Politser (1981) described several difficulties physicians have in applying the hypotheticodeductive method. For example, doctors may overlook or forget important information, or they may be biased toward a favorite hypothesis. Perhaps the most serious difficulty, however, is the problems doctors face in interpreting evidence in the light of hypotheses. Medical data have been described by Komaroff (1979) as inherently "soft." Few tests or physical examinations can claim 100% accuracy, and therefore the data doctors use are always uncertain. This means that there is no one-to-one relationship between a test result and an underlying disease; a hypothesis can never be 100% confirmed. In other words, the relationship between data obtained in the clinic, or the laboratory, and underlying diseases is probabilistic (see Bursztajn & Hamm, 1979, for a more complete discussion on the probabilistic nature of medical evidence).

There is substantial evidence that many physicians have difficulty thinking probabilistically. Actually, not only physicians have this trouble,

physicists have it too. Einstein always objected to quantum theory because of its insistence that nature was inherently probabilistic: "God" he
said "does not play dice games with the world." The difficulty physicians
have with probability is particularly apparent when conditional probabilities (the relationship between two events) are concerned. Eddy (1982),
for example, found evidence of misunderstanding of conditional probabilities even in medical journals. He reported that one physician equated
the probability that a woman with breast cancer will have a negative
mammogram with the probability that a woman with a negative mammogram will have cancer. In reality, these two probabilities are completely different. Saying they are the same is like claiming that the probability of a woman being pregnant given she has had intercourse is the
same as the probability she has had intercourse given she is pregnant.
The latter probability is, of course, 1.00 (ignoring in vitro fertilization);
the former probability is (fortunately) much lower. Several writers have
remarked that integrating information and using this information to
evaluate hypotheses (a procedure that requires understanding conditional probabilities) is a particularly difficult aspect of clinical judgment
(see Elstein, Shulman, & Sprafka, 1978, for a review). The problems
physicians face in generating hypotheses and collecting, combining, and
interpreting data are reviewed in detail in Chapters 2 and 3, respectively.

Choosing Actions

More often than not, medical treatment involves some degree of risk. In
many cases, the risks are minor, but sometimes they are considerable. In
either case, the ultimate decision about whether the risks are worth
taking will rely on the patient's perceptions. These perceptions, in turn,
depend on the type of information provided to the patient and *the manner* in which this information is presented. For example, Eraker and
Politser (1982) described a study that found that patients who received
more information about a drug's side effects than its benefits perceived
it as more risky than those given more information about benefits than
risks.

There also appear to be large individual differences among patients in
risk perception. For example, one study found that some subjects prefer
radiation treatment for cancer of the larynx to the more certain cure
offered by surgery because they prefer to keep their voice even if it
means an increased risk of death (McNeil, Weichselbaum, & Pauker,
1981).

Psychological studies are beginning to clarify the perceptual and cognitive mechanisms underlying perceived risk (see Slovic, Fischhoff, &
Lichtenstein, 1982a, for example). One aspect of this research is the
development of methods for estimating the costs (both economic and

personal) and benefits of medical decisions. Indeed, in these days of rising prices and patient awareness, costs and benefits are increasingly difficult to ignore. Over the past 20 years, a new technology—cost-benefit analysis—has developed to help decision makers incorporate information about costs and benefits into the judgment process. The technology of cost–benefit analysis can be broken down into six steps (Fischhoff, 1977):

1. Enumerate all the adverse consequences of a particular course of action.
2. Estimate the probability that each consequence will occur.
3. Estimate the cost (loss) should each occur.
4. Calculate the expected loss from each consequence by multiplying the amount of loss by its probability of occurring.
5. Compute the expected loss for the course of action by summing the losses associated with the various consequences.
6. Repeat the procedure for benefits.

It should be readily apparent that cost–benefit analysis is closely related to the EU and SEU approaches to decision making presented earlier. Probabilities and outcome utilities (losses and benefits, in this case) are estimated, multiplied, and summed. As in any decision analysis, once the basic data are collected, there are several decision rules that may be applied. Although it is generally assumed that doctors will choose the course of action that maximizes benefits, there may be times when they will wish to minimize negative outcomes instead (when the information gained from invasive tests, for instance, has only a small influence on patient management).

Performing a cost–benefit analysis involves several rather strong assumptions. It assumes, for example, that all important consequences of an action can be enumerated in advance, that the probability of their occurrence can be reliably estimated, and that different kinds of costs (financial versus pain and suffering) can be compared. All of these assumptions can and have been questioned. But surely the most controversial aspect of cost–benefit analysis is the need to compare disparate costs. Take Mrs. K.'s case as an example. It is easy to see how to measure the cost of her treatment in dollars and cents, but are such costs relevant? After all, most of us believe that good medical care should not be a function of a person's ability to pay. However, society pays in the end, and society as a whole is entitled to have a say about how its resources are used.

Even more controversial is the matter of placing a value on a patient's suffering or on his/her life (Card & Mooney, 1977). One approach to valuing life that has been used in several cost–benefit analyses is to calculate the "net benefit to society" of keeping a particular person alive. The technique involves subtracting the dollar value of a person's lifetime consumption from that of their lifetime earnings. However, as Bishop and Cicchetti (1973) noted, "Under this approach extending the lives of the non-working poor, welfare recipients, and retirees is counted as a cost not a benefit of a health program" (p. 112). For this reason, recent cost–benefit analyses have replaced the "human capital" approach with one based on society's "willingness to pay" for its member's health.

Clearly, no one expects doctors to engage in a cost–benefit analysis for every treatment decision. Such analyses would have to be done in large-scale studies. The important question is whether the results of such analyses are even relevant to clinical practice. Had the results of a cost–benefit analysis been available, would Mrs. K.'s doctors have behaved differently? Various attempts to estimate risks and to examine the value of cost–benefit analysis in medical care are discussed in Chapter 4.

Learning, Feedback, and Decision Aids

Even without definitive information about how experts think, many medical educators already believe that clinical decision making can be improved by courses in "Medical Decision Making." In fact, a recent survey found that about one-fourth of canvassed training institutions in the United States, Canada, and Mexico offer formal courses in medical decision making. Although the content of these courses differs, most involve some combination of instruction on probability, formal decision making, cost–benefit analysis, and risk analysis. The content of the syllabus, as a whole, is commonly referred to as "Decision Analysis."

Decision analysis is a general-purpose technology for making decisions under uncertainty. Beginning with the seminal work of Ledley and Lusted (1959), the past 25 years have seen decision analysis applied in many different areas of medicine (Pliskin & Pliskin, 1980; Weinstein & Fineberg, 1980). Decision analysis consists of four main steps:

1. Specify the decision problem (identify the choices).
2. Specify the sequences in which choices can be made.
3. Specify the information upon which the decision must be made.
4. Make the decision.

Specialized techniques have been developed to help the clinician complete each step. The rationale for courses in decision analysis is that they improve clinical judgment. From this viewpoint, decision analysis, cost–benefit analysis, risk assessment, and the other techniques taught in these courses are considered to be ways of aiding people to make good decisions. Unfortunately, there is little evidence to indicate that physicians who enroll in such courses actually use decision analyses in their clinical work. However, they may be trained to use the *results* of decision analyses in the form of clinical *algorithms*.

"Algorithm" is computer jargon for a plan or strategy for solving a problem. Algorithms are developed by collecting data on the outcome of clinical decisions and devising a rule that maximizes the relevant utilities. (Deciding whose utilities are relevant is, as we shall show, a decision problem in itself.) By capitalizing on the results of follow-up studies, decision analyses can eventually give rise to precise algorithms that can be used in clinical work.

Before physicians became interested in decision analysis, clinical algorithms were rare. Today, there are algorithms for the care of patients with minor illnesses, for medical emergencies, for surgical problems, and even for evaluating disease at the work site (Komaroff, 1982). Algorithms not only improve diagnostic accuracy (Rhodes, McCue, Komaroff, & Pass, 1976), they also make the delivery of medical care more efficient by permitting primary care physicians, nurses, and physician's assistants to apply them without the need for the specialist to always be present (Sox, Sox, & Tompkins, 1973). Algorithms can also be an effective teaching device, a fact that is beginning to be appreciated by textbook authors (see Runyan, 1975, for instance).

Perhaps one of the most important advantages of algorithms is that they are easily computerized. This advantage is likely to become increasingly important as computers take on a greater role in health care. In the future, instead of being examined and receiving advice simply from a doctor, patients will likely find themselves confronting a computer as well. The machine will not simply be there to help the doctor send out bills; it will also be there to help in diagnosing patients and recommending treatments.

The development of computers that operate like medical experts is well on its way. The basic research that has made such machines possible comes from the field of artificial intelligence, the discipline concerned with designing computers that perform intelligent tasks (Michie, 1982). A number of artificial intelligence programs already exist; several more are presently being developed. These programs have come to be known as "Expert Systems."

Psychologists are also interested in expertise. Psychological research on chess experts (de Groot, 1965), physicists (Simon & Simon, 1978), and other experts has repeatedly confirmed that the ability to generate a limited number of likely hypotheses is one of the most important characteristics distinguishing experts from novices. Since experts have more experience than novices, most authors believe that experts' ability to generate likely hypotheses is a function of the information stored in their memories. How this information is organized and how it may be taught to others is the subject of a great deal of interest among psychological researchers. The nature of the medical expertise, training programs, algorithms, computer programs, and decision aids are all discussed further in Chapter 5.

Making Good Decisions

Patients generally want to be involved in decisions that affect them (Al-fidi, 1971); physicians generally agree (Eraker & Politser, 1982). The problem comes in deciding where patient input can and should take place. Many medical decisions are based on technical information not available to patients. For example, we can hardly expect the average neurological patient to be able to choose between tomography and arte-riography as the best test to perform at some point in the diagnostic process. The appropriate place for patient involvement is not in making technical decisions but in expressing their values and preferences for various outcomes. In decision analysis terms, patients can help specify utilities while doctors, who are the technical experts, can provide the subjective probabilities. A formal approach to decision making, there-fore, permits patient involvement in the decision making process even though they are not medical experts (see Eraker & Politser, 1982, for more on how formal decision analysis allows patients to become involved in medical decision making).

Although medical decisions are made by patients and their doctors, indirectly the public is involved as well. A physician who decides to keep a patient in the hospital until he/she is fully recovered may force some-one else onto a waiting list. If borderline patients are placed in intensive care, others may be left out or intensive care wards may have to be made much larger to accommodate the crowds. Insurance companies and state health schemes are funded by all of their members, and ultimately all must pay for decisions taken. As the demands on health services con-tinue to increase, physicians will be forced to balance their responsibility to the patient against their responsibility to society at large. Possible problems in meeting these responsibilities are reviewd in Chapter 6.

Summary

Doctors are constantly making decisions that affect the lives and well-being of others. Although many medical decisions are routine, virtually all are characterized by uncertainty—the available information is never 100% reliable, and the outcomes of particular courses of action are rarely perfectly predictable. Making decisions under uncertainty has been an important area of psychological research for the past 30 years. During this time, both prescriptive theories dealing with how decisions ought to be reached and descriptive theories that portray how decisions actually are reached have been developed. These theories and their relevance to medicine were introduced in this chapter.

Although the application of prescriptive theories (decision analysis) has become widely accepted among medical educators and researchers, such applications are not without problems. Measuring subjective probability, determining utilities, and formulating decision rules are three important problems, but there are others. Some researchers have approached the problems of medical decision making by examining how experts go about solving problems. The idea behind their work is to isolate the cognitive components of expertise and teach these to trainee doctors; formal patient management strategies known as algorithms can also be used for this purpose. No matter how decisions are reached, however, certain ethical and moral problems will always remain. Doctors are used to considering the patient's needs as paramount, but economic and political forces are demanding that society's needs be considered as well. The result is an ethical dilemma.

The remainder of this book is devoted to examining research on the various topics introduced in this chapter. Chapters 2 and 3 are concerned with acquiring and evaluating medical data. Chapter 4 focuses on choosing specific actions. Decision aids, training, and the role of expertise are addressed in Chapter 5. The final chapter examines the ethical and social aspects of medical decision making and attempts to make some predictions about where medical decision-making research and theory may be heading in the future.

2

The Acquisition of Medical Data

*Chance is a word void of
sense; nothing can exist without cause.*

Voltaire

*But in this world nothing can
be said to be certain, except
death and taxes.*

Benjamin Franklin

There was a time in the history of medicine when diagnosis was second-
ary because practically everybody received the same treatment (bleeding, cupping, purging, and so on), but things have changed. Today,
making a diagnosis is one of a doctor's central activities. Indeed, much of
medical education is given over to answering the question: How does
one go about making a diagnosis? As noted in Chapter 1, accurate diagnoses are indispensable because they not only suggest proper courses of
management, they also aid researchers in discovering new treatments.

Diagnosis, as an intellectual activity, is a variant of the more general
skill of classification—assigning entities to different classes or categories.
In medical diagnosis, these categories are usually diseases, but they do
not have to be. In emergencies, the diagnostic process called triage involves placing patients in categories not on the basis of their disease or
injury but on their treatment priority. As the name suggests, there are
only three categories to triage: patients without hope, those requiring
immediate attention, and those who can safely wait for treatment. No
matter how many categories are involved, however, the diagnostic process is essentially unchanged—the doctor must make a choice from
among a number of alternatives. Therefore, according to the definition
given in Chapter 1, diagnosis is certainly a form of decision making.

According to a popular textbook on the subject, diagnosis should proceed along "scientific" lines. Specifically, diagnosis requires "marshalling all the facts . . . an unprejudiced analysis . . . and a logical conclusion" (Harvey, Bordley, & Barondess, 1979, p. 3). From a psychological viewpoint, this description of diagnosis actually involves two different sets of cognitive processes: those involved in gathering data ("marshalling all the facts") and those underlying evaluation and logical inference. The two types of processes each have their special problems.

Gathering data is more complicated than simply conducting a physical examination and ordering some laboratory tests. The physician must know what to look for in the first place. As we have seen in the case of Mrs. K., modern technology has made a large number of tests available to the clinician; "marshalling all the facts" can produce a mountain of data leading to confusion rather than clarity. To avoid unnecessary testing, data selection should be based on some criterion of expected value. That is, the facts "marshalled" by the clinician should be those most likely to yield a diagnosis.

Gathering information, while important, is only the first step in diagnosis; the information must also be interpreted. This is where the second set of cognitive processes—those underlying evaluation and inference—come in. First, the data gathered by the doctor must be combined, a process that involves differentially weighting each item according to its diagnosticity and reliability. Next, the various diagnostic alternatives must be evaluated in the light of the combined data. Finally, a treatment must be selected. This chapter is concerned with the cognitive processes involved in acquiring diagnostic data. Combining and evaluating medical information is discussed in Chapter 3 and treatment selection is addressed in Chapter 4.

Even when the unreliable nature of medical data is appreciated and steps are taken to compensate for the inability to consider all possible data sources simultaneously, there remains one further difficulty in learning to make diagnoses. Physicians must be able to use the data they collect to make classification. That is, they must know what conclusions may be drawn from their findings. Learning to make diagnostic judgments on the basis of probabilistic data is a problem that has been extensively studied by psychologists. Chapter 5 reviews and summarizes this research.

Diagnostic procedures are not completely reliable. Even the so-called objective data gathered in physical examinations or by sophisticated medical tests can often be inaccurate. The effects of unreliable data and unreliable observers on the diagnostic process are reviewed in the first two parts of this chapter. The remaining sections are concerned with how one theory—the theory of signal detection—may be used to understand and evaluate the data-acquisition process.

The Quality of the Data Produced by
Diagnostic Procedures

The Diagnostic System

Although it appears to involve just the doctor and the patient, diagnosis actually requires a system consisting of three separable parts: data-collection devices, an observer to record the data collected by these devices, and a decision maker to decide what the data mean (Swets & Pickett, 1982).

The data collection devices may be laboratory tests (x-rays, blood assays) or they can be part of the normal office routine (history taking, physical examination). In both cases, the resulting data are imperfect. In engineering terminology, the observer's job is to detect "signals" produced by the data-collection devices and to differentiate these signals from the "noise" always present in the background. The decision maker must then classify these signals into normal and abnormal categories, and from this classification, make a diagnosis. Ordinarily, the observer and the decision maker are combined into one person—the doctor. However, as is discussed in Chapter 5, it is sometimes possible for computers to take over one or both of these roles.

For the remainder of this chapter, unless a specific device is indicated, we refer to all data-collection devices (laboratory tests, histories, physical examinations) as "diagnostic procedures." We use the term, "physician–observer" to refer to the part of the diagnostic system that records (or acquires) the diagnostic data; the part of the system that decides what the data mean is called the "decision maker." Together, diagnostic procedures, the physician–observer, and the decision maker constitute the complete diagnostic system.

Textbook writers, like the ones quoted earlier, quite reasonably believe that diagnosis begins with the "marshalling" of all the facts. Clearly, diagnosis could not proceed without facts, but knowing which ones to collect and being able to record them accurately are hardly trivial matters. How well data are gathered depends on the quality of the initial hypothesis generated by the decision maker as well as on the efficiency and reliability of the diagnostic system's data-collection devices. As we shall show, some diagnostic procedures are neither as efficient nor as reliable as many doctors believe them to be.

For the purposes of the present discussion, the problems involved in gathering diagnostic data have been divided into three categories: those involved in generating hypotheses, those inherent in the diagnostic procedures themselves, and those located in the physician–observer. Each of these is discussed separately, although, in reality, they usually interact. For example, an unlikely hypothesis can lead to the collection of irrelevant data or an unreliable observer can misperceive the output of even highly accurate diagnostic procedures. We begin our discussion with hypothesis generation.

Problems in Hypothesis Generation

Before the diagnostic system can begin to do any useful work, there must be some hypothesis for it to test. Without a hypothesis (or several hypotheses) to evaluate, physicians would merely be stockpiling facts haphazardly. Like the baseball statistician, they would have a great number of facts available to them but no way of determining what, if anything, they mean.

Studies of expert diagnosticians (Balla, 1980; Elstein et al., 1978) have found that they tend to generate a small set of hypotheses early in the diagnostic process. These hypotheses are usually based on very limited data. The patient's chief complaint is usually enough. Data are then gathered that support or refute these hypotheses. In this way, the diagnostician gradually narrows down general questions (What is this patient's problem?) to one or more specific ones (Does this patient have an inflamed appendix?) (Elstein & Bordage, 1979).

Elstein et al. (1978) found that physicians generate their initial hypotheses by correlating various clinical signs with their knowledge of patients and diseases, usually without a specific scientific rationale. Instead, the incidence of various diseases is the most important determinant of which hypotheses are considered. Once hypotheses are formulated, they may suggest others. Rarely are more than six or seven hypotheses considered at one time.

Experienced diagnosticians are never without any hypothesis at all; if necessary, even vague notions can guide data collection. Thus, the absence of a hypothesis is rarely a serious diagnostic problem, but untestable hypotheses are another matter (Fischhoff & Beyth-Marom, 1982). Hypotheses are untestable when they are too ambiguous to evaluate meaningfully. For example, some obsolete diagnoses (ague, grip) fell out of favor because their manifestations were too nebulous for anyone to be entirely certain they were present (or absent). Hypotheses may also be untestable because they are too complicated to assess or because the appropriate evidence to confirm or disconfirm them is not available. Examples of both problems are particularly common in psychiatry, where diagnostic hypotheses often concern intrapsychic conflicts that cannot be directly observed.

Uncertainties Arising from Diagnostic Procedures

Medical data are decidedly fuzzy. They are collected with a degree of uncertainty and sometimes inaccuracy. In this section, we describe several sources of uncertainty commonly found in diagnostic procedures.

Patient reports

The diagnostic system depends on patients presenting themselves for evaluation. Patients who, for whatever reason, do not seek medical advice for a problem will remain undiagnosed. Komaroff (1979), in a review of the literature on sources of inaccuracy in medical data, described several studies demonstrating considerable variability in how people perceive their symptoms. For example, Komaroff noted reports claiming that members of different ethnic groups seek help for different types of problems. According to these reports, Italians seek care for symptoms that interfere with social or personal relations, whereas Anglo-Saxons are more likely to visit their doctors when a symptom interferes with work.

There are also individual differences in how people decide when a symptom is serious enough to warrant professional advice. As every doctor knows, some patients seek help when there is little or nothing wrong with them while others let even life-threatening illnesses go on for a long time before visiting a doctor. In one United States study (Elinson & Trussell, 1957), members of an adult sample were interviewed in their homes about their current state of health. These interviews were followed by complete medical examinations. The researchers found that only one-fourth of the diseases turned up by the examination were reported during the interviews. Such underreporting of illness is particularly troubling because in many cases early medical advice can make the difference between living or dying.

Medical histories and interviews

At least some of the variability in how people perceive their current state of health is the result of different value systems; some patients simply do not consider their symptoms very important while others bring even the most trivial problems to the attention of their doctors. However, value systems cannot account for all instances of inaccuracy. There is also patient ignorance to consider. A striking example was provided by Lilienfeld and Graham (1958), who reported that 35% of their sample of 192 men gave an inaccurate answer to the question, "Are you circumsized?"

Patients' perceptions influence more than just their responses to verbal questions; they can also affect their responses to procedures that are part of most physical examinations. When a doctor presses part of the patient's body and asks if it feels painful, it is the patient's definition of pain—a definition that varies greatly among individuals—that will determine whether the answer is yes or no.

It is fair to say, then, that patients' perceptions are an important source of uncertainty (and inaccuracy) in medical data. How a patient interprets a doctor's questions, the patient's background and education, and the patient's attitude toward symptoms and disease can all affect the quality of the data the physician receives. This does not mean, however, that all uncertainty in medical diagnosis derives from patients' perceptions. Physical examinations and laboratory tests can also produce ambiguous data.

Laboratory tests

Each year, millions of laboratory tests are performed at clinics around the world at a cost of billions of dollars. Tests are ordered because they help monitor a treatment or because they are useful in formulating a diagnosis. However, there are some tests that seem to be ordered simply because they are available. The number of tests falling in this latter category may be quite large. A recent survey of the laboratory tests ordered by 111 California doctors (Wertman, Sostrin, Pavlova, & Lundberg, 1980) found that 32% of the tests ordered produced no change in diagnosis, prognosis, therapy, or understanding of the patient's condition. While 2 or 3% of these valueless tests were ordered by physicians seeking to protect themselves from potential lawsuits or for educational reasons (to learn more about the tests rather than the particular patient), the remainder appear to be attempts at "marshalling all the facts" even when these facts are of no particular use. Moreover, when the data provided by the tests are potentially relevant, their use may not always be justified because most tests are neither perfectly reliable nor valid.

Test reliability and validity

Laboratory tests and other diagnostic instruments rarely yield perfectly accurate data. Typically, some proportion of normal patients produce positive results (false-positives) and some proportion of symptomatic patients produce negative results (false-negatives). Sometimes the number of patients misclassified by a diagnostic technique can be quite large. For example, in one study of a formerly used hemoccult test (a screening test for cancer of the colon), 36% of normal patients were classified as "positive" for cancer (Greegor, 1969). Of course, the number of false-positives can often be reduced by raising the test's cutoff point (the level at which a finding is considered "positive"—a temperature above 37°C, for example). Unfortunately, raising the cutoff point will also result in a reduction in the number of true-positives—not always an acceptable outcome, particularly for serious diseases.

The ability of a test to identify correctly those with a particular symptom is known as a test's *validity*. It is taken for granted that tests with high true-positive rates are valid indicators of the target symptom. However, the validity of a test is highly dependent on another test property, its reliability.

The *reliability* of a test is a measure of its consistency. The common fever thermometer, for example, is a highly reliable indicator of a patient's temperature. If the patient's temperature is taken twice in succession, chances are the thermometer will produce precisely the same result. The correlation between the two temperature readings is a mathematical measure of the thermometer's reliability. If this correlation equals 1.00, the thermometer is perfectly reliable.

Reliability is a necessary prerequisite for validity. This is because a test's validity is measured by how well it correlates with some other index of the symptom. For instance, the validity of the skin test for tuberculosis depends on how well it identifies patients with the disease as verified by x-ray and pathology tests. Since a test will always correlate higher with itself than with some other measure, reliability sets a ceiling for validity.

Studies of the reliability of diagnostic procedures sometimes produce rather troubling results. For example, Durbridge, Edwards, Edwards, and Atkinson (1976) studied hospitalized patients who received laboratory tests more than once. Their sample was very large (more than 2000 test repeats). They found that many abnormal findings failed to be confirmed on a second test administration. In the case of one test, serum bilirubin, 47% of abnormal findings disappeared when the test was repeated.

Of course, test results are expected to change as a patient's condition improves or deteriorates, but the failure to produce similar results when tests are repeated in close succession means that those tests are not reliable. Unreliable information makes the physician–observer's task difficult. If a test is administered once, the doctor cannot be sure the result is a true picture of the patient's state of health. This is the reason that tests are often repeated. However, there is no guarantee that simply repeating a test will yield useful information. If the test is reliable then repeating it will confirm the original result but may not tell the doctor anything new (see Neuhauser & Lewicki, 1975, for example). If, on the other hand, the test is not reliable, it may produce different results on each administration and the doctor will not know which to accept. Redundant information is really only useful when it is provided by several different tests each with a different pattern of reliability and validity. A possible exception is the situation in which tests are being used to monitor change. Mrs. K., the woman whose case was described in Chapter 1, had repeated chest x-rays because her doctors were using them to monitor heart–lung function.

In a discussion of the value of repeating a test, Politser (1982) pointed out that physicians generally use one of two informal decision rules to deal with repeated tests. They either "believe the positive" and consider a patient to require further study if just one test result is positive or they "believe the negative" and stop testing patients who produce a negative result. The two rules obviously have different consequences, but neither one is clearly better. Indeed, the same doctor may use both rules (for example, when it comes to blood cultures, believe the positive; for respiratory function, believe the negative).

The relative efficacy of the two rules depends on test reliability. As Politser shows, a test can have high reliability for normal patients but low reliability for truly ill patients (the opposite pattern is also possible). These reliability patterns can interact with decision rules. For example, repeating a test that is perfectly reliable for normal patients but has a low reliability for actual patients (those with the disease) will only produce discrepant results for true patients. For such patients, two different results (a negative followed by a positive or vice versa) indicates a true patient. Physicians will optimize their use of such a test by adopting the "believe the positive" rule. Tests with the opposite pattern of reliabilities require the "believe the negative" rule. Of course, when the reliability patterns for both true patients and normal subjects are the same, then which rule is best to use depends on prior probabilities and the consequences of positive and negative results.

Prevalence and uncertainty

Another source of variability in test data is indirect—the prevalence of a symptom or sign in the population. The importance of prevalence to the meaning of a test may be illustrated by an example from Applegate (1981).

The test in question is a hypothetical hemoccult screening test for colon cancer based on a stool assay. The test is first tried out on a sample of 500 patients, half with known cancer and half of whom are normal. The experimenter calculates the probability of a positive test given that the patient actually has cancer. This is called the test's *sensitivity*. Also calculated is the probability of a negative result given that the patient does not have cancer (the test's *specificity*). Let us say these both turn out to be .90. The test clearly has potential, but now we must try it out in the real world. There are many differences between the laboratory and the clinic, but one of the most important is prevalence. The original sample was constructed to have a prevalence of 50%, but colon cancer actually has a prevalence of less than 1%. The experimenter decides to evaluate the test on 1000 patients who visit a general practitioner's office complaining of abdominal pain. The results appear in Table 2-1.

Since the prevalence of colon cancer is 1%, 10 cases are expected in a sample of 1000. As can be seen, the test identifies 9 of these cases and misses 1, which it misclassifies as normal. The test also identifies 99 normal patients as ill, a fairly high number of false-positives. The percentage of true-positives out of the total number of positives on this test is 8.3% (9/108). This means that *even after a positive test result*, the odds are still 10 to 1 against this patient having colon cancer. [The number of true-positives divided by the total number of positives is known as a test's *predictive value* (Kundel, 1982).]

Table 2-1. Outcome of an Evaluation of a Hypothetical Colon
Cancer Screening Test on 1000 General Practice Patients[a]

Test Results	Patient's Actual State of Health		
	Cancer Present	Cancer Absent	Total
Positive	9	99	108
Negative	1	891	892
Total	10	990	1000

[a] Prevalence = 1%. Adapted from Applegate (1981). Reprinted with the permission of the author and The Southern Medical Association.

Now consider what happens if, instead of a population of general practice patients, the hypothetical test is administered to a population more likely to have colon cancer—say, patients referred to a gastroenterologist with rectal bleeding. Let us assume that the prevalence in this population is 25%. Table 2-2 illustrates the expected results.

Since the prevalence in this population is 25%, we would expect 250 colon cancer cases out of the 1000 people tested. As can be seen, the test correctly identifies 225 of these and misses 25, who are misclassified as normal. The percentage of true-positives out of all positives in this case is 75% (225/300), a great improvement over that obtained in the population with a lower prevalence. In this high-risk population, three out of every four patients who have a positive test result actually have the disease. Clearly, prevalence is an important source of variability in test results.

It should be apparent from the discussion thus far that the data gathered by the medical diagnostic system are far from perfect. Patients do not always seek care for their problems, and when they do they may not report their condition accurately. Physical examinations and laboratory tests, while superficially objective, yield ambiguous data because of their less-than-perfect reliability and because the meaning of a test result changes with the prevalence of a symptom or disease in the population

Table 2-2. Outcome of an Evaluation of a Hypothetical Colon
Cancer Screening Test on 1000 Gastroenterology Patients[a]

Test Results	Patient's Actual State of Health		
	Cancer Present	Cancer Absent	Total
Positive	225	75	300
Negative	25	675	700
Total	250	750	1000

[a] Prevalence = 25%. Adapted from Applegate (1981). Reprinted with the permission of the author and The Southern Medical Association.

being tested. All of these factors create uncertainty about the meaning of diagnostic data.

However, laboratory tests, patient histories, and so on are not the only sources of inaccuracy and ambiguity in the diagnostic system. Some ambiguities arise from within the physician–observers themselves. These are discussed next.

The Quality of the Data Recorded by Physician–Observers

Perceptual Expectancies

In a psychological experiment conducted by Warren (1970), subjects were asked to listen to recorded speech and report what they heard. Some of the words they listened to had sounds removed and replaced by coughs, breaths, or other nonspeech sounds. For example, the sound belonging to the letter "s" in "hesitate" may have been replaced with a cough. Despite this alteration, subjects reported hearing the "s" sound. In fact, they were so convinced that the sound was present that even telling them about the substitution and asking them to listen again did not change their minds. In this experiment, it seemed that subjects' expectancies were causing them to have "hallucinatory" experiences that they could not distinguish from "real" ones. Such experiences are by no means rare. Psychologists have repeatedly shown that common (highly probable) events are much easier to perceive then rare ones (see Broadbent, 1971).

In a recent discussion, Kahneman and Tversky (1982c) labeled these perceptual expectations "passive expectancies" because they are long-term, relatively permanent behavioral dispositions as opposed to the short-term, active expectations created by specific circumstances. An example of the latter type of expectancy is the casino gambler who has been counting cards during the blackjack game and "expects" a face card to turn up in the next few cards.

In general, passive expectances are more important determiners of perception than active ones. This is why subjects in Warren's experiment continued to "hear" the missing sound even when they were told it was omitted (that is, even when they were given an active expectancy opposite to their passive one). Subjects asked to look at visual illusions exhibit similar behavior; they continue to perceive the illusion even when they have been told exactly how it works. According to Kahneman and Tversky, the strength of passive expectancies serves a biological survival function. Rather than admit to ourselves the uncertain nature of our momentary perceptions, we appear to suppress uncertainty and to believe what our passive expectancies tell us we are hearing and seeing.

Laboratory tests, physical examination signs, and other data may also

sometimes be misperceived because of the operation of passive expectancies. This need not only be the result of fatigue, distractions, or other
outside influences. Expectancies can take their toll even when physicians
are completely alert and undistracted. When expectancies are combined
with the uncertainty inherent in many diagnostic procedures, the result
is physician–observer variability.

Perhaps the most dramatic demonstration of physician–observer variability comes from studies that compared several doctors all of whom
examined the same set of patients. In one such study, three physicians
took the peripheral pulse of 192 patients. Their readings agreed only
69% of the time (Meade, Gardner, & Cannon, 1968). Variability also
occurs when physicians are called upon to interpret laboratory tests.
Doctors have been found to disagree about the interpretation of chest x-
rays (Herman & Hessel, 1975), electrocardiograms (Segall, 1966), and
electroencephalograms (Woody, 1968). Not only have doctors been
found to disagree with one another, they sometimes will disagree with
their own previous judgments. A study that required pathologists to
examine the same tissue sample on two different occasions found that
their conclusions (malignant or benign) differed 28% of the time (Coppleson, Factor, Strum, Graff, & Rapaport, 1970).

At least some of these disagreements result from the already noted
uncertain nature of diagnostic data. For example, Waddell, Main, and
Morris (1982) found that several signs commonly relied upon to assess
back pain during a physical examination (spasm, guarding, tenderness)
cannot be reliably assessed, even after extensive practice. Different physician–observers attempting to use these signs to diagnose back pain
must, of necessity, produce varying diagnoses.

The Interpretation of Numbers and Words

Although many diagnostic procedures yield numerical data, it is customary for physicians to communicate with one another using verbal labels
rather than numbers. Terms such as "probably" or "likely" are common
in medical reports and patient histories ("this test indicates a high likelihood of malignancy," for example). In an investigation of how doctors
view the relationship between numbers and verbal labels, Bryant and
Norman (1980) asked a sample of hospital-based physicians to indicate
on a scale that went from 0 to 100% the meaning of 30 commonly used
probability labels. They found little agreement. To take but one example, "sometimes" meant a 5% chance to one physician and a 75% chance
to another. The range of estimates exceeded 50% for more than half the
terms surveyed. Similar results have been reported by others (Haynes,
Sackett, & Tugwell, 1983; Kenney, 1981; Robertson, 1983; Toogood,
1980). Table 2-3 contains a list of 22 frequently used verbal probability
terms and the range of probabilities associated with each by a sample of

Table 2.3 Range of Probabilities Associated with Verbal
Modifiers by Physicians and Nonphysicians[a]

Verbal Modifiers	Range of Probability Estimates	
	Physician	Nonphysician
Not infrequently	45	60
May be associated	40	50
Often	40	59
Majority	39	39
Common	38	40
Frequent	35	45
Not unusual	30	35
Occasionally	30	33
Reported to occur	30	65
Typical	30	30
Sometimes	27	35
Extremely common	25	28
Infrequent	25	29
Most	25	35
Usual	25	30
Characteristic	20	37
Invariably	20	60
Atypical	18	23
Unusual	15	22
Vast majority	15	23
Rare	9	9
Very unusual	7	9

[a] Adapted from Nakao and Axelrod (1983, p. 1063) and reprinted
with the permission of Yorke Medical Books and the authors.

physicians and laymen (adapted from Nakao & Axelrod, 1983). Although the ranges are somewhat smaller for physicians, it seems clear
that numerical adjectives mean different things to different people.
Their use is an important source of communication errors in the diagnostic system.

Nakao and Axelrod (1983), and most other writers on the subject,
recommend that doctors replace frequency adjectives with actual numbers (50%, 30%, and so on). They believe this will lead to greater agreement among doctors. However, indications are that their faith may be
misplaced. Berwick, Fineberg, and Weinstein (1981) surveyed 281 physicians and medical students using a questionnaire designed to assess their
understanding of common numerical terms used in medicine. They
found little consensus among their respondents on the meaning and
interpretation of false-positive rates and probability values. It appears

that numerical estimates of probability do not always lead to greater consistency and better communication than verbal labels.

Illusory Correlations

Imagine the following simple psychological experiment. You are seated in a comfortable chair looking at a projection screen where pairs of words (*Boat–tiger*) appear for 2 seconds each. The left-hand member of each pair is always one of four words: *bacon, lion, blossoms,* or *boat.* The word on the right is always one of three: *eggs, tiger,* or *notebook.* All word pairs are equally likely to appear. You are asked to study the word pairs and, later, the experimenter asks you to reproduce the pairs together with their respective frequencies of occurrence. How do you think you would do? If you are like most people, you will not report that each pair appeared an equal number of times even though they did. Instead, you will claim that when *bacon* was the word on the left, *eggs* most frequently appeared on the right. Similarly, most people report that *lion* was most often paired with *tiger.* In other words, subjects report that word pairs with strong verbal associations occur more often than unrelated pairs. This tendency to perceive associated items as occurring more frequently than they really do is called "illusory correlation" (Chapman & Chapman, 1969).

Chapman and Chapman explored the effect of illusory correlations in a clinical judgment task. Clinical psychologists were given information concerning several hypothetical psychiatric patients. The data for each patient consisted of a clinical diagnosis and a drawing of a person supposedly made by the patient. After studying these, the judges were asked to estimate how frequently a particular diagnosis (paranoia, for instance) was associated with particular features in the drawings (peculiar eyes, for example). Judges were found to greatly overestimate the frequency with which features and diagnoses cooccurred. This was particularly true for those features and diagnoses they naturally associated together (peculiar eyes and paranoia was one of these). These illusory correlations were so strong that they persisted even when the relationships between picture features and diagnoses were arranged by the experimenters to be negative (when paranoia was associated with normal eyes, for example).

In both the word-pair experiment and the one pairing diagnoses and drawings, judges appear to base their frequency estimates on preconceived relationships that they believe ought to exist rather than on true empirical covariation. A similar phenomenon may take place in the clinic, where symptoms and diagnoses (and treatment and outcomes) may appear to covary even when they are unrelated (Arkes, 1981). Indeed, illusory correlations have probably been responsible for the persistence of many unwarranted medical beliefs (tuberculosis is caused by night air, bleeding cures infections). Most important for our present purposes, illusory correlations introduce "noise" into the diagnostic system, thereby reducing the quality of the data used by the decision maker.

Illusory correlations are not the only problem physicians must worry about. Low correlations can also sometimes mask important causal relationships. Einhorn and Hogarth (1982) provided the following example. Suppose some prehistoric cave dwellers have somehow generated the hypothesis that intercourse causes pregnancy. To test this hypothesis, they design an experiment in which 100 females are randomly assigned to an intercourse condition and another 100 are kept celibate. With the passage of time, 20 of the women in the intercourse condition became pregnant and 80 did not. In the nonintercourse condition, 5 females became pregnant and 95 did not. (The 5 represent measurement error—faulty memory, lying, and so on.) In this experiment, the statistical correlation between intercourse and pregnancy is only .34 and the cave dwellers would be justified in believing that the two are practically unrelated. Indeed, with a smaller sample size, the correlation would not be statistically significant. Turning the usual adage on its head, Einhorn and Hogarth correctly state that causation does not necessarily imply correlation.

Information Overload

Thus far, we have considered how patients' beliefs, unreliable data-gathering procedures, and inconsistent physician—observers all combine to make the data available to the diagnostic system rather fuzzy. One factor that has only been mentioned in passing is the effect of the sheer amount of information available to the modern diagnostician. Recent years have seen an exponential growth in the number and complexity of diagnostic procedures. Laboratory tests alone yield over 20,000 individual items of information for every practicing physician each year (Fineberg, 1979). Although doctors were once taught to believe that more information is better than less ("marshalling all the facts"), there are limits to the amount of data anyone can handle. We have already noted in Chapter 1 that some studies have shown diagnostic accuracy to be just as good with a subset of clinical data as with a full set, and at least one study (Sisson et al., 1976) has shown that too many data can actually impair the diagnostic process. As Herbert Simon, whose concept of bounded rationality has already been introduced, put it: "We cannot afford to attend to information simply because it is there" (Simon, 1978, p. 13). Instead, the effective physician—observer must learn to attend to those sources most likely to produce relevant information. The effective physician will not necessarily be the one who refrains from testing, but the one who orders the most relevant tests.

We shall have more to say about information overload in the next chapter. For the present we should note that the complexity of the modern diagnostic process can also lead to another sort of cognitive overload known as "operational failure' (Palmer, Strain, Rothrock, & Hsu, 1983). Operational failures occur when, for one reason or another, important steps in the diagnostic process are omitted, or data are lost or not acted upon. In one study, Palmer et al. found operational failures to be fairly common. They evaluated 858 cases in which positive urine cultures were obtained in children. They found many of these positive results were omitted from medical records. Not surprisingly, they also found a failure to follow up and treat many of these patients. They also found incorrectly treated patients, and so on. In all, 52% of the cases studied showed evidence of one or more operational failures. Although the reasons for these operational failures are complicated, it is fair to say that they become more common as the volume of data increases.

If doctors cannot use all the information they collect then why do they bother collecting it? The answer is that tests are ordered for a variety of reasons, including protection from lawsuits, tradition ("marshalling all the facts"), and sometimes simply to have them "on the record" (see Wertman et al., 1980). What is more, test-ordering behavior varies among doctors depending on their training (Manu & Schwartz, 1983), whether they were trained in a public or private medical school (Eisenberg & Nicklin, 1981), and on test cost in dollars and cents (Hoey, Eisenberg, Spitzer, & Thomas, 1982). Some tests are ordered by consultants who believe that this is what referring doctors expect them to do (Holmes et al., 1982).

The Value of Diagnostic Data

Assuming the risks of various diagnostic procedures are equal, the most valuable diagnostic data are those expected to produce the most useful information. Although some physicians believe that only positive information is useful (Christensen-Szalanski & Bushyhead, 1983), negative findings are also valuable if they allow some hypotheses to be ruled out. Deciding which data to collect requires a "value of information" analysis that considers the rewards and costs of data collection, the consequences of the possible decisions, and the probability of receiving various answers (Brown, Kahr, & Peterson, 1974; Doubilet, 1983; Eddy, 1983).

We shall discuss how the value of information is measured in the next chapter. For now, we simply reiterate that the medical diagnostic system must make do with less-than-perfect data. Patient and physician expectancies, unreliable (and irrelevant) laboratory tests, information overload, illusory correlations, operational failures, and the other factors discussed so far all make it difficult for the decision maker to determine whether the data collected and recorded by the diagnostic system are evidence for a signal (a true symptom) or noise (which can sometimes mimic a signal). Nevertheless, diagnoses get made, most of the time correctly. It would appear that decision makers have learned ways of compensating for the inadequacies of the data. Understanding how unreliable data may still be used to produce accurate diagnoses is one of the goals of signal detection theory—the topic of the next section.

The Development of Signal Detection Theory

When diagnosis is viewed as a problem in detecting "signals" and classifying them as either "true symptoms" or "noise" (normal variants that mimic signals), *signal detection theory* (SDT) can supply a rationale for testing and understanding diagnostic systems. Signal detection theory allows investigators to separate a diagnostic system's ability to discriminate true signals from noise from the factors that determine how perceived signals are translated into diagnostic decisions. In other words, it permits us to separate the processes involved in data collection from those underlying inference and classification.

The present discussion begins with a brief review of the background of SDT and the reasons for its development. This is followed by an introduction to the theory itself, and an illustration of how it may be applied to medical diagnosis.

Psychophysics and Perception

When the first experimental psychologists began studying behavior scientifically, they modeled their efforts on the activities of physicists. Physicists, after all, were the most respected of all scientists and much of their work was of obvious relevance to the new science of psychology. Newton, for example, had analyzed light into its perceived spectrum of colors, and other physicists had conducted research on the detection of sounds. Because much of 19th-century physics was given over to measuring things (the speed of light, the pull of gravity), it is not surprising that the early experimental psychologists also devoted most of their efforts to developing measures—mental measures. Soon, a psychological subspecialty devoted to mental measurement developed; it was called *psychophysics*. Its goal was the measurement of psychological sensations.

Measuring the physical stimuli that give rise to sensations (light intensity, loudness) provided the physicists with little difficulty; there were balance scales, thermometers, and yardsticks suitable for measuring them. Measuring mental sensations was another matter entirely. What was required was a measurement device similar to a thermometer or yardstick but divided into mental rather than physical units. The unit the psychophysicists finally settled on was the *just noticeable difference,* or JND. A JND is the increase or decrease in stimulus intensity required before a subject can report a "just noticeable difference."

Just noticeable differences turned out to be directly related to stimulus intensity; as the intensity of a stimulus increases (as it gets brighter, heavier, louder, or whatever), the JND increases as well. For example, a 102-gram weight can be discriminated from a 100-gram weight, but a 202-gram weight cannot be discriminated from a 200-gram weight. Instead, it takes 204 grams to produce a JND when the comparison weight is 200 grams.

Since all physical measures have some sort of zero point (0 centimeters, 0 kilograms, and so on), the psychophysicists gave their JND scale a zero point too. This was defined as the *absolute threshold*. The absolute threshold of any sensory system is the lowest level of stimulus intensity necessary for a subject to detect its presence 50% of the time. The absolute threshold for loudness, for instance, is the softest sound a subject can reliably detect on one-half the occasions it is presented. The early psychophysicists devised several methods to measure both absolute thresholds and JNDs. These "psychophysical methods" were designed to cope with the tendency of most human subjects to be inconsistent. That is, subjects would not always produce exactly the same JNDs and absolute thresholds. Instead, their responses tended to fluctuate depending on how they were tested and, perhaps, on their interest in the task. The psychophysicists assumed that by taking the mean of many tests administered in several different ways, they could eliminate these fluctuations and be left with true physiological thresholds and JNDs.

Absolute Thresholds versus a Continuum of Sensation

Almost from its inception, psychophysics was controversial. The most important criticism concerned the zero point of the mental sensation scale—the absolute threshold. The problem, said the critics, was that the absolute threshold was defined not as zero physical energy but as the level of stimulus energy required to arouse a response 50% of the time. Since the absolute threshold is defined arbitrarily in statistical terms, some other definition (say the level of energy that produces a response 25% of the time) could also be adopted. In either case, the notion of a physiological "absolute threshold" is hard to defend if stimuli below this threshold are also sometimes perceived.

Over the years, psychologists found it increasingly difficult to maintain the idea of an absolute threshold. Instead of a physiological cutoff point below which sensations are negative and above which sensations are positive, psychologists have come to think of sensations as varying along a continuum. Rather than an abrupt change from no sensation to a sensation as the threshold notion implies, psychologists came to believe that the point at which a sensation is detected varies with a person's interest, attitude, fatigue, and motivation.

From the recognition that sensations vary along a continuum, it was only a short step to the realization that human perception can be thought of entirely in "probabilistic" terms. The probabilistic approach began with observations of radar operators during World War II (see Swets, 1973, for a more detailed description of the origins of SDT). The job of the radar operator is to detect a specific signal against electromechanical background "noise." Usually, the operator can discriminate signals from noise, but not always. Sometimes, operators claim to have perceived signals when none were present; at other times, they fail to register a signal that was actually transmitted. Clearly, this pattern of behavior is not consistent with the notion of an absolute threshold. The performance of radar operators in various detection situations is described graphically in Figure 2-1.

The abscissa of the graph in Figure 2-1 represents the strength of the sensation experienced by the radar operator. These sensations get stronger as we go from the left side of the graph to the right. The bell-shaped curves represent the probability of a sensation of any particular strength occurring. The higher the point on the curve, the greater the probability of a particular sensory effect. The bell-shaped curve on the left is produced by the noise always present in the detection system (by radio activity in the atmosphere as well as neural activity within the observer). The bell-shaped curve on the right is produced by a combination of signal-plus-noise.

If the two bell-shaped curves do not overlap (as in Panel A of Figure 2-1), the signal and the signal-plus-noise distributions are perfectly distinguishable. Put another way, nonoverlapping curves mean that the sensations produced by the signal are so strong they are never confused with noise.

If the two curves are completely superimposed (as in Panel B of Figure 2-1), signal and noise are indistinguishable; they produce the same sensations and, therefore, cannot be told apart. When the two distributions partly overlap, behavior is more complicated. As depicted in Panel C of Figure 2-1, a partial overlap will produce many correct responses, but some responses will be incorrect. Incorrect responses occur when signals fall in the shaded area. Some of these will be true signals mistaken for noise while others will be noise mistaken for signals. Panel C represents the situation in which most radar operators found themselves.

Decision Criteria in Perception

Although the two overlapping curves of Panel C of Figure 2-1 illustrate one of the reasons why radar operators made errors, it turns out to be only a partial explanation. Operators trained to be very conservative—to only report a signal when they were absolutely sure one was present—made very few false reports. They sometimes missed signals because

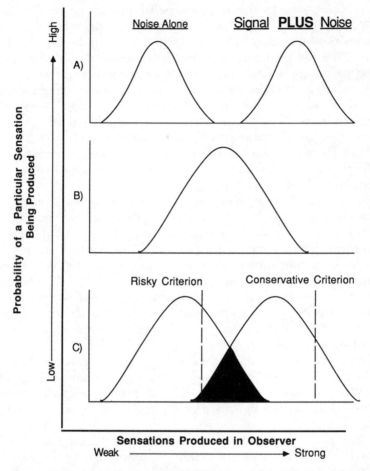

Figure 2-1   Three possible "signal" and "signal-plus-noise" distributions. *Panel A* illustrates completely separate distributions in which signal and signal-plus-noise are perfectly separable. In *Panel B*, the two distributions are identical; signal-plus-noise cannot be discriminated. *Panel C* illustrates the most common situation; partial overlap of the two distributions creates both false-positives and false-negatives. The number of each depends on the decision criterion, which can be risky (many false-positives) or conservative (few false-positives).

when they were unsure their conservative training taught them not to respond, but they made no "false alarms." In contrast, operators trained to report anything they believe might be a signal no matter how unsure they were produced many false alarms but missed few signals. The demonstration of the ability to shift one's criterion for reporting a signal was the final blow to the notion of fixed absolute thresholds. It seems that the threshold for reporting a signal changes in response to training and task demands. Thus, instead of a threshold, the newly developed theory of signal detection postulated a variable "decision criterion" that can be altered depending on the decision context.

The dotted vertical lines in Panel C of Figure 2-1 represent two different decision criteria. The one on the left is a risky criterion; all sensations to the right of it are reported as signals. Anyone adopting this criterion will miss very few signals but is likely to produce many false alarms because sensations falling in the shaded area will be reported to be signals. The decision criterion on the right is a conservative one. Since sensations to the right are reported to be signals, only true signals will be detected. However, some signals (those falling to the left of the criterion) will be classified as noise.

According to SDT, then, there is no such thing as an absolute threshold or a standard JND. Instead, the probability of a signal being detected depends on two factors: the overlap of the noise and signal-plus-noise distributions and the decision criterion. If a new radar process is developed that greatly reduces background noise, the two distributions are moved further apart and signal and noise are less likely to be confused. If radar technology remains unchanged but the decision criterion is made more lenient, fewer signals will be missed. In both cases, the probability that a signal will be detected changes, but not for the same reason. Noise reduction affects the quality of the data gathered by the detection system, whereas changes in decision criteria affect how the observer assigns data to classifications. In most cases, these two influences on detection are independent.

Readers familiar with hypothesis-testing statistical procedures will have already noticed similarities between SDT and the rationale underlying many common statistical tests. In testing hypotheses, the results of an experiment are classified as produced either by chance or by a "real" experimental effect. Chance can be thought of as similar to noise and a true experimental result as signal-plus-noise. The decision criterion is the test's critical value, the value at which a result is considered real and not due to chance. The similarity between statistical hypothesis testing and signal detection will be returned to later in this book.

Summarizing to this point, psychophysics was originally developed to determine the relationship between properties of physical stimuli and sensory experience. The concept of an absolute physiological threshold for the perception of signals left out any role for nonsensory determinants of detection (Swets, 1979). Observations of radar operators whose detections varied depending on the decision criterion they adopted led to the development of SDT—a theory that views detection as determined both by the probability of a signal being observed and by the decision criterion adopted by the observer.

Although SDT has its origins in the study of radar operators, it soon

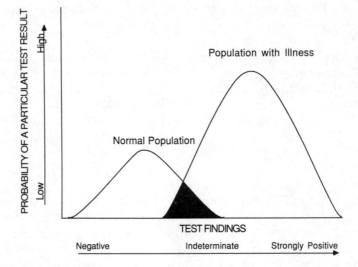

Figure 2-2   Test results can be viewed as signals in a noisy background. The probability of a positive test result is higher among those with the illness, but some overlap with the normal population (false-positives) may still occur.

found application in other areas, including medicine (see Lusted, 1984, for a brief history). Its medical applications, particularly in diagnosis, are the subject of the next section.

Medical Applications of Signal Detection Theory

To see the relevance of SDT for medicine, it is first necessary to examine the diagnostic process in more detail. It is especially important to understand the probabilistic nature of most medical data.

As we have already noted, few diagnostic procedures yield results that can be assigned to a unique diagnostic category. A particular diagnostic procedure may indicate that a patient is abnormal or normal or that a tumor is benign or malignant, but the result always carries some degree of doubt. In fact, the distribution of a test's results for actually positive and negative cases may overlap like the noise and signal-plus-noise distributions illustrated in Panel C of Figure 2-1. The physician must decide whether any particular test result is positive or negative by setting a decision criterion above which results will be classified positive and below which they will be considered negative. In medical diagnosis, however, the distributions are not typically equal. Instead, they look like those depicted in Figure 2-2.

Diagnosis, like signal detection, depends on two factors: the capacity to discriminate among alternatives (malignant versus benign, for instance) and the decision criterion used to select one alternative over another. The first factor, the ability to discriminate, is influenced by the sensitivity of the tests themselves. As diagnostic procedures improve, discriminating capacity improves as well. For example, early radiographs were unclear and abnormalities were difficult to detect. As x-ray machines improved, however, the overlap between "signal" and "noise" decreased and abnormal films were less often confused with normal ones.

Improved tests (and more highly trained observers) mean fewer misclassifications, but since the distributions of normal and abnormal continue to overlap to some degree, cognitive "decision" factors still influence the diagnostic process. These factors determine where the decision criterion will be placed. Normally, physician-decision makers set their decision criterion so as to make more correct than incorrect judgments. ("Correct" in this context means judging cases as positive when they actually are positive and negative when they actually are negative.) There are instances, however, when the diagnostician does not necessarily want to maximize the number of correct judgments. In the pneumonia example discussed in Chapter 1 (see Figure 1-1), the physician may be resigned to diagnosing at least some normal patients as ill if this means that no sick patients are misclassified. Most medical situations are similar; it is the total expected value of a diagnostic decision that is important. Thus, where the decision criterion is set depends not only on the likelihood that a particular positive result is "correct" but also on the costs and benefits associated with correct and incorrect decisions. Put another way, where the decision criterion is set depends on the consequences of the possible diagnostic outcomes.

Diagnostic Outcomes

There are at least four possible outcomes to any diagnostic procedure. A true-positive result occurs when an abnormality is present and the test indicates that it is present. A true-negative is exactly the opposite—no abnormality is present and that is what the test indicates. The two remaining outcomes are incorrect. A false-positive occurs when a normal patient is classified as abnormal and a false-negative result indicates that a patient is normal when an abnormality is actually present. Although it is customary to refer to test results as true and false positives and negatives, these terms are really shorthand abbreviations for a set of conditional probabilities. Conditional probabilities have already been introduced, but since they appear throughout the book, they will be expanded upon here.

A *conditional probability* is the probability of an event occurring given that another has already taken place. Conditional probabilities should be distinguished from *joint probabilities*, which refer to the probability of two events occurring together. To see the difference, imagine you are tossing coins. Assuming that the coins are fair, the conditional probability of one coin coming up heads given that you have just tossed a head is 1/2, because the earlier toss has no effect on the later one. The joint probability of tossing two heads in a row, however, is 1/4 (1/2 × 1/2).

In the clinic, we are interested in the output of the diagnostic system given certain inputs. That is, we want to know the conditional probability of normal and abnormal diagnoses given certain test results. For example, a true-positive result is really the conditional probability of an "abnormal" diagnosis when the patient actually is abnormal. In mathematical notation, this probability is written as:

$$P(\text{Diagnosis Abnormal/Patient Abnormal})$$

where the P stands for probability. The expression is read as the probability that a patient is diagnosed abnormal *given* that he/she really is abnormal. For convenience, we follow Swets and Pickett (1982) and abbreviate our terminology. For the remainder of this book, A will stand for abnormal and N for normal. If the letter appears in upper case, it refers to the output of the diagnostic system (the final normal or abnormal decision as made by the system). In lower case, the letters refer to the data received by the collection device; that is, the "true state" of the patient. We can now translate the earlier terminology into conditional probabilities:

True-positive = $P(A/a)$
True-negative = $P(N/n)$
False-positive = $P(A/n)$
False-negative = $P(N/a)$

Although there are four possible outcomes, only two are independent. This is because $P(A/a) + P(N/a) = P(A/n) + P(N/n) = 1.00$. This means that if one knows $P(A/a)$ and $P(A/n)$ then the remaining probabilities can be calculated by simple algebra.

At first glance, there seems little need for calculating even two probabilities. Why not simply judge the usefulness of a diagnostic procedure by calculating the proportion of cases for which it produces a "correct" result? (Provided, of course, that we have some independent means of determining whether the test is correct.) The problem with this approach to measuring test accuracy is that it can produce misleading data, particularly for rare conditions. If a symptom is present in only 3% of patients, a diagnostician can be correct 97% of the time simply by classifying every patient as normal. Relying just on the number of patients correctly classified also ignores the costs and benefits associated with particular decisions. We have already seen that there are times when physicians may prefer classifying some normal patients as ill so as to be certain not to miss any who are potentially sick. In other cases, where the treatments themselves may be dangerous, the diagnostician may prefer to err on the side of missing a few ill patients to ensure that normal ones are not subjected to the treatment. An index of diagnostic usefulness based solely on the number of patients correctly classified ignores these important considerations.

Realizing that test usefulness is a relative matter, medical researchers have generally evaluated diagnostic techniques by concentrating on $P(A/a)$ and $P(N/n)$, which are generally referred to as sensitivity and specificity, respectively (Galen & Gambino, 1975; Krieg, Gambino, & Galen, 1975). Diagnostic procedures are considered useful if both probabilities are high. While this approach represents an improvement over concentrating solely on true-positives, it is still inadequate because it does not tell us how the diagnostic decision responds to changes in the decision maker's response criterion (Swets & Pickett, 1982). Does a small change in specificity lead to a large change in sensitivity or is sensitivity largely unaffected by changes in specificity? Answering this question requires more information than that available from these two probabilities. To know how $P(A/a)$ responds to changes in the decision criterion requires that $P(A/a)$ be compared with $P(A/n)$ across the entire range of decision criteria. Signal detection theory accomplished this using a method based on the *receiver operating characteristic* (ROC).

Receiver Operating Characteristic

The ROC received its name from the early studies of radar operators, but its use has become routine in many areas of psychology and medicine. Basically, a ROC curve consists of a graph plotting $P(A/a)$ against the $P(A/n)$ under different decision criteria. An example of a ROC curve appears in Figure 2-3.

The abscissa of the ROC curve is the $P(A/n)$ or the false-positive rate; the ordinate is the $P(A/a)$ or the true-positive rate. The points on the curve represent the relationship between these two probabilities for different decision criteria. Figure 2-3 indicates three possibilities. The conservative criterion produces very few false-positives but at the cost of a low true-positive rate. The risky criterion identifies most true-positives but at the cost of a relatively high false-positive rate. The intermediate threshold produces results midway between these two extremes.

Although only three criteria are marked on the graph, each point actually represents a separate criterion. The beginning and end points of the graph are fixed at 0 and 1 because all tests can be labeled negative or positive, but the remaining points depend on the characteristics of the test. The better the test is at separating true- from false-positives, the steeper the ROC curve will be. Figure 2-4 illustrates a family of ROC

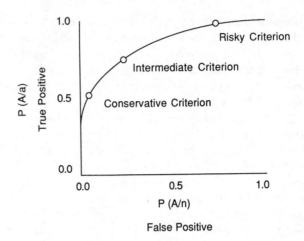

Figure 2-3   A hypothetical ROC curve. Each point represents performance under a different decision criterion.

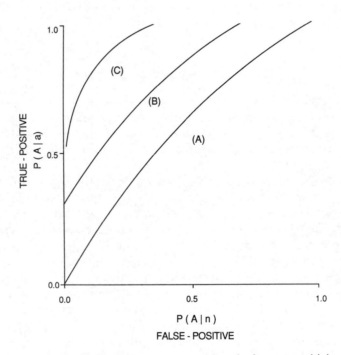

Figure 2-4   A family of ROC curves. *Curve A* has the lowest sensitivity, *curve C* the highest.

curves, each representing a different level of discrimination between true- and false-positives.

Curve A in Figure 2-4 illustrates a test whose discriminative ability is only slightly better than chance. Increases in true-positives are always accompanied (for this test) by increases in false-positives of almost the same magnitude. Such a test would correspond to the situation depicted in Panel B of Figure 2-1, in which the signal and the signal-plus-noise distributions almost completely overlap. Curve B in Figure 2-4 depicts a test with a higher level of discriminative ability, and Curve C shows a test with a very high ability to discriminate between true- and false-positives.

Figures 2-3 and 2-4 together illustrate the two types of information available from ROC curves: the ability of a test to separate true- from false-positives and the changes that occur when the decision criterion is altered. Rather than refer to whole ROC curves, investigators have found it handy to derive mathematical indices from the curves that represent these two types of information. Over the years, many different indices have been developed (see McNeil & Hanley, 1984, for a review), but two are most common. The *discriminating ability* of a test (its ability to separate signal from noise, normal from abnormal, and so on) is indexed by d', the difference between the means of the signal and signal-plus-noise distributions in units of the standard deviation. Typically, d' is known as a test's "sensitivity," but this should not be confused with the earlier definition of sensitivity, the $P(A/a)$. The usual index of the decision criterion is the slope of the ROC curve at any particular point. This is usually known by the Greek letter β.

There are two ways to generate a ROC curve. The direct way is to simply arrange to have the probabilities of true- and false-positives vary from one testing session to the next and record an observer's responses (normal or abnormal). Asking observers to change their decision criteria across sessions (only respond "abnormal" if you are absolutely certain) will also produce ROC curves. However, these procedures are tedious. A more common way to produce ROC curves is to require observers to produce confidence ratings (in five or six categories) giving their degree of belief that a result is normal or abnormal. Typically, the rating method involves assigning verbal labels to the various confidence levels (definitely abnormal, probably abnormal, possibly abnormal, and so on) and asking the observer to indicate which label best describes each of his/her observations. The data are analyzed by treating each label as a category. First, only the probability of a "definitely abnormal" response is calculated. This is followed by the probability of the top two categories combined ("definitely abnormal" and "probably abnormal"), then the top three combined, and so on until all categories are exhausted. Since each response category is considered to be a separate decision criterion, the rating scale technique requires the observer to hold several decision

criteria in mind simultaneously, thereby permitting researchers to determine several points on the ROC curve in a single session.

To date, the most common use of ROC analysis has been in the evaluation and comparison of diagnostic data. Using ROC curves, researchers
have been able to determine which of several alternative data-collection
procedures is the most valuable (see Swets & Pickett, 1982, for some
examples). Receiver operating characteristic analysis has also been used
to measure whether new tests add any useful data to those derived from
already existing tests.

An example of how ROC analysis can be used to evaluate a diagnostic
procedure is provided by Turner, Ramachandran, and Ali (1976; see
also Turner, 1978). These researchers wished to compare two brain-
imaging procedures, computerized tomography and a brain scintillation
camera, as alternative methods of scintigraphy.

First, patients with and without focal brain lesions were assessed using
both techniques. Three judges evaluated the results, making judgments
in one of five categories ranging from definitely abnormal to definitely
normal. Since there were five categories used in the rating scale, the
researchers were able to calculate four points on the ROC curve for each
technique. (The fifth rating category is not independent of the others
because the total of each rating scale must equal 1.) The resulting ROC
curve for one of the judges appears in Figure 2-5. Note that the observer
performed better with tomographic scans than with scintigrams produced by the camera. The ROC curve for tomography shows greater
discriminating ability at every decision criterion than the camera technique. Additional details and further examples of ROC analysis in medicine may be found in Metz (1978) and Swets (1979).

Signal detection theory, ROC analysis, and their derivatives have been
used extensively in medicine to evaluate diagnostic procedures (Goin,
Preston, Gallagher, & Wegst, 1983; Goodenough, Rossman, & Lusted,
1972; Swets, 1979; Swets & Pickett, 1982) and patient care decisions
(Greenfield, Cretin, Worthman, & Dorey, 1982). In recent years, the
ROC approach has generalized to include more than two judgments.
Instead of simply normal and abnormal, these approaches permit a
"can't say" category as well (Swets & Pickett, 1982). However, our
present interest is not mainly in diagnostic procedures, but in decision
making. Receiver operating characteristic analysis has proven useful for
understanding this as well. For example, Starr, Metz, Lusted, and
Goodenough (1975) showed how radiologists' ability to localize lesions
may be measured using a modified ROC procedure, and Goodenough
(1975) showed how ROC curves may be used to test doctors' ability to
diagnose pneumoconiosis from chest radiographs.

The main value of ROC analysis in understanding diagnostic performance is its ability to separate detection from decision making. According to SDT, the probability that a symptom or sign will be detected

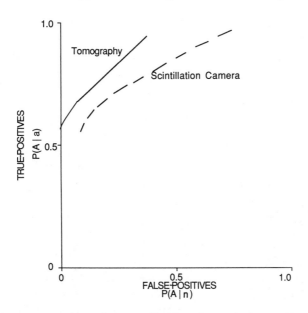

Figure 2-5   A comparison of two medical imaging techniques using ROC analysis (see text for details). Adapted from Turner et al. (1976) and reprinted here with the permission of the author and the Radiological Society of North America.

accurately is determined by the discriminating ability of the diagnostic procedure and the observer. The likelihood of a particular diagnosis, however, depends on decision factors—on how the signal is interpreted and where the decision criterion is set. Doctors with a stringent decision criterion will be biased against "positive" responses; those with a lenient criterion will be biased toward "positive" responses.

The term "bias" is not used here in a pejorative sense. Instead, it refers to the amount of evidence a doctor requires to make a diagnosis. A strong bias means a tendency to respond in a particular way. The degree of bias is determined by the probability of the various diagnostic alternatives (rare illnesses usually require stringent decision criteria, common illnesses require lenient ones), as well as the costs and benefits associated with various diagnostic decisions. (The clinician who suspects a serious illness may prefer a false-positive to a false-negative in order to be certain that no "sick" patients are misclassified as normal.)

A study that used ROC analysis to investigate how diagnostic skill changes with experience was reported by Berwick and Thibodeau (1983). Their technique required physicians working in the emergency room of a large hospital to predict the outcome of the chest x-rays and throat cultures they ordered for patients in the course of their normal working day. Attached to every x-ray request form was a question of the following form: Out of 100 patients with a history and physical examination just like this patient's, how many would you expect to have pulmonary density on their chest x-ray consistent with pneumonia? The question attached to the bacteriology request form asked: Out of 100 patients with a history and physical examination just like this patient's, in how many would you expect the bacteriology laboratory to report the presence of Group A β-hemolytic streptococcus on throat culture? Respondents were grouped according to years of experience.

Berwick and Thibodeau obtained the actual outcome of each test from the radiology department or the pathology laboratory and classified each test as positive or negative. Although they performed several analyses of these data, those of primary interest were their comparisons of the physicians' probability estimates with the actual test outcomes. For each experience group, the experimenters ranked the probability estimates from least to most probable. This was done by grouping probabilities into 100 intervals (each with a width of .01). They also computed the proportion of positive and negative results falling into each of these 100 intervals. Receiver operating characteristic–type curves were generated from these data by plotting the cumulative proportion of positive results in each interval (correct detection) as compared with the proportion of negative results. Figure 2.4 displayed some potential outcomes of their approach.

Curve C represents perfect performance. A physician behaving this way assigns a greater probability of positive to all tests with a positive result than to any test with a negative result. Curve A illustrates zero ability to discriminate between negative and positive results. A physician who produces this pattern is as likely to make a correct response as a false-positive. Curve B represents intermediate performance. A physician behaving this way produces many false-positives in order to detect the same number of true-positives as the physician whose behavior resembles curve C.

Berwick and Thibodeau found that their experienced group showed greater ability to discriminate positive from negative cases than the less-experienced group (their ROC curves are closer to curve A than curve C), but the difference between groups was greater for x-rays than for throat cultures. It would seem that the signs of streptococcal throat infection are more difficult to pick up in a physical examination (even by experienced diagnosticians) than are signs of pneumonia.

If the signs relied upon by experienced physicians can be distilled and taught to the less-experienced ones, the ROC analysis could serve as a test of learning. As their skill increases, the trainees' ROC curves should resemble those of the experienced doctors. The ROC curve can also be used to establish probability cutoff points for test ordering. For example, the experienced physicians correctly predicted 80% of the positive x-rays when negative x-rays made up 40% of the total. To increase the proportion of true-positives to 90%, the physician must order x-rays for 80% of the negative cases. Perhaps the cost of an x-ray is so small that a large increase in false-positives is tolerable. For more costly or danger-ous procedures, however, we may wish to set the cutoff at the point at which 80% of the positives are detected in order to avoid large numbers of false-positives. However, cutoffs are also dependent on experience. For the inexperienced group to achieve a true-positive rate of 80%, they will have to order x-rays for almost everyone.

Since ROC analysis provides separate indices of sensitivity and bias, experiments using this technique have been able to isolate the factors influencing each. Several factors affecting the quality of information gathered by the medical diagnostic system were described in this chap-ter. All exert their effect on the system's sensitivity. Chapter 3 is con-cerned with how the data gathered by the diagnostic system are evalu-ated and interpreted. Chapter 4 examines how decision criteria are set and how diagnostic and treatment decisions are made.

Summary

Diagnosis is the doctor's main activity; virtually all of modern medicine's formidable treatment apparatus depends on first obtaining an accurate diagnosis. Although diagnoses are performed by individual physicians, usually working alone, diagnosis is best viewed as a system consisting of data-collection devices, a physician–observer who records information from these devices, and a physician–decision maker who evaluates the data and decides what they mean. In many ways, diagnosis is similar to signal detection, in which operators must distinguish true signals from noisy backgrounds. Signal detection theory, originally derived from studies of radar operators, provides a way of separating the data-collec-tion aspect of diagnosis from decision making.

Factors affecting the quality of data collected were reviewed in this chapter. Some of these factors are inherent in the data-collection devices themselves. These include patient perceptions and test unreliability. Physician–observer factors can also affect the quality of diagnostic data. Among these variables are perceptual expectancies, the interpretation of what numbers mean, illusory correlations, and information overload. All these variables have the effect of reducing test sensitivity, thereby mak-ing signals more difficult to distinguish from noise. In the next chapter, we look at how data collected by the diagnostic system are evaluated.

3

Evaluating Medical Information

*The art of being wise is the art
of knowing what to overlook.*

William James

Modern doctors have access to a large variety of clinical data. These data, whether gathered from patient histories, physical examinations, or laboratory tests, are rarely able to discriminate perfectly between truly symptomatic and "normal" patients. Yet doctors have no choice; they must somehow learn to use probabilistic data to make patient management decisions.

Most people (doctors included), have great difficulty thinking probabilistically. The mathematical complexity of probability calculations, and the amount of information that must be evaluated, have led to the development of judgment heuristics—rules of thumb—that help us to cope with uncertainty. Although usually helpful, these judgment heuristics may, under certain conditions, introduce bias (distortion) into the decision-making process.

The present chapter is concerned with how data obtained by the diagnostic system are evaluated and integrated. The chapter begins with a discussion of probability revision; how new data may be used to alter judgments about the likelihood of particular diagnoses and treatment outcomes. In the first section, we present and discuss a normative approach to probability analyses—the Bayesian method. Although Bayesian mathematics represents the optimum (mathematically correct) method for revising judgments based on probabilistic data, research has revealed that most of us do not behave as Bayes' formula suggests we should. Instead, we appear to rely on the simplifying heuristics described in the second section of this chapter. The chapter's final section contains a discussion of the problems involved in integrating information from various sources to reach a diagnostic or treatment decision.

Probability Revision and Bounded Rationality

The following clinical problem is adapted from one discussed by Diamond and Forrester (1983):

> A patient is suspected to be suffering from coronary artery disease; he is asymptomatic and middle-aged. The prevalence of this disease, in the middle-aged, male population, is 5 per cent. An electrocardiographic stress test reveals a pattern which is manifested by 13 per cent of patients with coronary artery disease. However, one per cent of disease-free patients manifest the same test pattern. What is the probability that this particular patient has coronary artery disease?

One way to answer this question is to employ the formula developed by the 18th-century mathematician–philosopher, the Reverend Thomas Bayes.

The Bayesian Method

As discussed in Chapter 2, the diagnostic process begins with the formulation of hypotheses about the cause of a patient's condition. Evidence can then be gathered to support or refute these hypotheses. Indeed, from a Bayesian viewpoint, logical reasoning is a matter of evaluating hypotheses. If a diagnostic procedure does not yield information suitable for this purpose, then it is valueless at least so far as Bayesians are concerned (Eddy, 1982). Unfortunately, as we have already seen, many diagnostic procedures fall into the "valueless" category.*

In its simplest form, Bayes' formula states that:

$$P(H/Proc.+) = \frac{P(H) \times P(Proc.+/H)}{P(H) \times P(Proc.+/H) + P(Alt.\ H) \times P(Proc.+/Alt.\ H)} \quad (1)$$

where H is the hypothesis being evaluated, *Proc.+* is the probability of a positive diagnostic procedure, and *Alt. H* is the probability of an alternative hypothesis. This last probability is included because Bayesian thinking always involves contrasting a hypothesis with one or more alternative hypotheses. These alternative hypotheses can be either another diagnosis or simply "no disease."

Equation 1, which embodies what is known as Bayes' theorem, states that the conditional probability (see Chapter 2 for a definition of conditional probability) that a patient is suffering from a hypothesized illness given a positive diagnostic procedure (known in Bayesian terminology as the "posterior probability") is a function of $P(H)$, the prevalence of the hypothesized disease (known to Bayesians as its "prior probability"), the

---

* It should be kept in mind that this discussion is concerned with tests as aids in diagnosis. But tests are done for other reasons as well (monitoring, prognosis, prevention, and so on). Their value for one purpose may not be the same as for another purpose.

conditional probability of a positive procedure given that the patient actually has the hypothesized disease, $P(\text{Proc.}+/\text{H})$, and the prevalence and conditional probabilities associated with the alternative hypothesis, $P(\text{Alt.H})$ and $P(\text{Proc.}+/\text{Alt.H})$ From a Bayesian perspective, the probabilities inserted into Equation 1 can be either genuine frequencies (gathered from epidemiological or other studies) or subjective probabilities. (See Chapter 1 for the differences between these two types of probability.) It is also possible to use Bayes' formula with "noninformative" prior probabilities (equal priors for all hypotheses, for example).

Equation 1 can be used to solve the coronary artery disease problem, as illustrated in Equation 2. The probability that the patient who produced a positive stress test has coronary artery disease is a function of the prior probability of this disease in similar patients (.05) multiplied by the conditional probability of a positive test given that the patient is suffering from coronary artery disease (.13) divided by these probabilities plus the appropriate probabilities for the alternative hypothesis (the patient is not suffering from coronary artery disease.) As can be seen, a positive test result produces a posterior probability of .41. Thus, even after a positive test, the probability that this patient actually suffers from the hypothesized disease remains less than 50%.

$$P(\text{Coronary Art. Disease/Test}+) = \frac{.05 \times .13}{(.05 \times .13) + (.95 \times .01)} \quad (2)$$

A simple example illustrating the practical use of Bayes' formula (and also one of the earliest attempts to employ Bayes's formula in a medical situation) can be found in Steinhaus' work on establishing paternity (cited by Kozielecki, 1981). Paternity cases are fairly common legal proceedings. Typically, a mother sues a man claiming that he is the father of her child. The grounds for the suit are that the couple had sexual intercourse approximately 9 months prior to the child's birth. Naturally, the man denies he is the father or there would be no need for a lawsuit. Depending on who the court believes, the putative father may or may not be required to pay for the child's support.

Thirty years ago, when Steinhaus' research was conducted, the only objective evidence available to the court was serological; that is, the blood type and group of all concerned individuals. Sometimes this evidence was definitive. For example, a man with group B blood cannot be the father of a group A child if the mother is group O. Unfortunately, definitive tests occurred in only 10% of cases. In the remaining 90% the serological data were only suggestive.

Steinhaus began by searching the legal literature for an estimate of the relevant prior probability—the probability that an accused man is later determined to be the true father. He found that 71% of men sued for paternity were ultimately found to be true fathers, so he adopted .71 as his prior probability. Now, it is clear that this is only an estimate.

Whether putative fathers are found to be true fathers depends on cultural, legal, and social factors; for this reason, the prior probability may well be expected to vary from time to time and from place to place. Steinhaus also reviewed the relevant literature noting how frequently particular blood characteristics are shared by children and their real fathers and by children and men who turn out not to be their real fathers. These various items of information were incorporated into Bayes' formula as follows:

$$P(F/C) = \frac{P(F) \times P(C/F)}{P(F) \times P(C/F) + P(\text{Not } F) \times P(C/\text{Not } F)} \qquad (3)$$

In Equation 3, F stands for real father, *Not F* for an innocent accused, and C for some blood characteristic shared between the accused man and the child. As might be expected, Steinhaus found that the posterior probability depended on exactly what blood characteristic was measured. In many cases, he was able to say whether an accused was the real father with a probability exceeding .995.

Bayes' Formula and ROC Analysis

It should be obvious that the probabilities in Bayes' formula are similar to those used in ROC analysis as described in Chapter 2. Both make use of true- and false-positive rates; to these, Bayes' formula adds the prior probabilities of hypotheses and combines the lot to produce a posterior probability. Bayes' formula makes clear the importance of a disease's prevalence to the meaning of the findings of a diagnostic procedure. If everything else remains unchanged, increasing prevalence results in an increased posterior probability. If, subsequently, a second diagnostic procedure is performed, use of the formula can be repeated. This is why Bayes' theorem is said to provide a method for revising prior probabilities.

The relationship between Bayes' theorem and ROC analysis also makes it possible to assess the value of an additional diagnostic procedure on the posterior probability. Looking at Bayes' formula (Equation 1), it is easy to see how increasing a test's sensitivity [in this case, the true positive rate, $P(\text{Proc.}+/H)$] while maintaining a low false-positive rate [$P(\text{Proc.}+/\text{Alt. } H)$] increases the posterior probability. Indeed, if the false-positive rate is reduced to 0, the posterior probability will equal 1.00 and we will be 100% certain that the patient is suffering from the hypothesized illness. Since they both affect posterior probabilities, both positive and negative test findings are important, as Bayes' formula shows us.

The importance of negative as well as positive diagnostic procedures is not always understood by diagnosticians (Christensen-Szalanski & Bushyhead, 1983; Gorry, Pauker, & Schwartz, 1978). Diagnostic proce-

Table 3-1.   Probability of Positive and Negative
Mammograms for Benign and Malignant Growths[a]

Test	Patient's Actual State of Health	
Results	Malignant Growth	Benign Growth
Positive	.792	.096
Negative	.208	.904

[a] Numbers taken from Snyder (1966).

dures that exert a great effect on posterior probabilities are said to have high "diagnosticity." Since a procedure's influence on the posterior probability is a function of its sensitivity (given a specific decision criterion), it is possible to determine the diagnosticity of a test before it is actually administered by calculating the degree to which every possible test outcome can influence the posterior probability (Gregg, Rao, & Friedell, 1976; Metz, Starr, & Lusted, 1976b).

Although Bayes' formula represents the accepted normative method for revising probabilities, psychological research has shown that most people are not intuitive Bayesians. In other words, when left to our own devices, most of us do not revise probabilities as Bayes' formula says we should (Kahneman & Tversky, 1972; Phillips and Edwards, 1966; see also Slovic, Fischhoff, & Lichtenstein, 1977). One reason appears to be confusion about the meaning of probabilities.

Doctors' Understanding of Probabilities

Confusion about probabilities has been explored by Eddy (1982), whose research focused on doctors' interpretations of mammography test results. Eddy used a hypothetical, but common, situation as his experimental task. A female patient with a breast mass is examined by a doctor. Based on prior experience with similar patients, the doctor is 99% certain that the mass is benign. Put another way, the doctor's prior probability for the hypothesis that the patient has cancer is .01. The doctor orders a mammogram and receives a positive (cancer present) report. Clearly, the physician must take this new information into account, but how? One possibility is to turn to the relevant clinical literature. A study of mammography by Snyder (1966) produced the data contained in Table 3-1. As may be seen, mammography has fairly high true-positive and true-negative rates, but it also has a substantial false-negative rate as well.

The doctor now has all the information necessary to apply Bayes' formula: a subjective prior probability of .01 and the objective true- and false-positive rates in Table 3-1. The result is contained in Equation 4:

$$P(\text{Cancer/Pos. Mamm}) = \frac{.792 \times .01}{.792 \times .01 + .096 \times .99} = .077 \qquad (4)$$

The probability that the patient's breast mass is cancerous is about .08. However, when Eddy presented this hypothetical problem to a sample of 100 physicians, 95 estimated the probability that the patient has cancer to be about .75. This estimate appears to be based solely on the test's true-positive rate, ignoring both prior probabilities and false-positives. Similar findings have been reported by Schwartz, Gorry, Kassirer, and Essig (1973).

If Eddy's physicians ignored prior probabilities and false-positives, then they were violating a fundamental axiom of Bayesian statistics that asserts that the impact of any observation can only be interpreted by comparing two hypotheses. A high true-positive rate, by itself, cannot tell us whether a particular hypothesis is very likely unless it is accompanied by a low false-positive rate. Physicians and others who interpret their observations solely in the light of a single hypothesis have been described by Beyth-Marom and Fischhoff (1983) as succumbing to "pseudodiagnosticity." They believe that a high true-positive rate is diagnostic by itself without reference to false-positives.

Pseudodiagnosticity has been reported in medical situations. Kern and Doherty (1982), for example, showed that student diagnosticians preferred information on many symptoms applicable to a single disease (redundant information) to data that would have helped them rule out competing hypotheses. Pseudodiagnosticity resulted because, although the students gathered a large number of positive results pointing toward one diagnosis, the same results could not completely rule out alternative diagnoses. Wolf, Gruppen, and Billi (1984) found first-year residents to behave the same way as the students.

Clearly, physicians do not always revise probabilities in line with the requirements of Bayes' formula. In one sense this is not too surprising. After all, few doctors are even familiar with the formula and fewer still would combine probabilities in the way the formula requires purely by intuition. For this reason, some experimenters have tried to improve probability estimates by calling attention to the need to consider both true- and false-positives (Beyth-Marom & Fischhoff, 1983). Although this appears to help, there is still a discrepancy between the average doctor's judgment and the one reached by Bayes' formula. Part of the reason is a misunderstanding about the nature of conditional probabilities. Eddy (1982) cited many instances in which articles on mammography published in medical journals confuse posterior probabilities with the likelihood of various test results. That is, they confuse P(Cancer/Test+) with the P(Test+/Cancer).

The P(Test+/Cancer) is the probability of obtaining a positive diagnostic test result given that the patient actually has the disease. If the probability is high, the implication is that the disease may be responsible for the test result. The P(Cancer/Test+), on the other hand, is the probability of the disease being present given a positive test. If the probability is high, the test is considered "diagnostic." There is little doubt that what physicians would most like to know is the P(Cancer/Test+). Unfortunately, the information typically available to doctors is P(Test+/Cancer). These are almost never the same. As illustrated in Chapter 1, in our example of the relationship between sexual intercourse and pregnancy, there is no direct relationship between these two conditional probabilities. Einhorn and Hogarth (1982, 1983) provided several additional examples of how diagnostic and causal influences can easily become confused by those unfamiliar with the mathematics of probability.

Although a contributor, confusion about conditional probabilities is not the entire explanation for why an individual's probability estimates do not behave in accord with those dictated by Bayes' theorem. Even those well versed in probability theory and considered experts in statistics do not always conform to Bayesian prescriptions (Tversky & Kahneman, 1973). In recent years, psychologists have come to believe that we fail to conform to Bayes' theorem because we simply lack the cognitive capacity to combine the required information in a systematic manner. This is the explanation for non-normative behavior offered by the principle of "bounded rationality."

Bounded Rationality

The principal of bounded rationality states that:

> The capacity of the human mind for formulating and solving complex problems is very small compared with the size of the problems whose solution is required for objectively rational behavior in the real world—or even for a reasonable approximation to such objective rationality. (Simon, 1957, p. 18)

The claim that rationality is bounded is really another way of saying that there are limits to the human capacity to process information. Our ability to keep data in memory, to retrieve them when needed, and to manipulate them as required is not limitless. Many complex judgment tasks make cognitive demands that are beyond our information-processing capacity. When this happens, we create simplified "problem representations" (subjective models of the real world) that permit us to handle the task with the available cognitive resources (see Newell & Simon, 1972).

In addition to simplified problem representations, cognitive load can be reduced by using a number of stereotyped decision-making strategies. These simplifying cognitive procedures, or rules of thumb, are known in the literature as *judgment heuristics*. Although judgment heuristics usually lead to good decisions, this is not guaranteed. In the past 15 years or so, psychologists Amos Tversky and Daniel Kahneman (as well as many others) have described a number of general judgment heuristics (see Fischhoff, 1975, 1982b; Fischhoff & Beyth, 1975; Fischhoff, Slovic, & Lichtenstein, 1977; Kahneman, Slovic, & Tversky, 1982). They have also shown the circumstances under which these heuristics lead to errors in probabilistic reasoning. Because many of these errors result from an attempt to apply the normally useful heuristics to situations in which they are inappropriate, errors are often referred to as cognitive "biases." Several of these biases are sufficiently predictable and orderly to have been given names. The main types are discussed in the next section.

Judgment Heuristics and Biases

We begin this section by permitting the principal authors in the field to provide a rationale for their approach:

> There are three related reasons for the focus on systematic errors and inferential biases in the study of reasoning. First, they expose some of our intellectual limitations and suggest ways of improving the quality of our thinking. Second, errors and biases often reveal the psychological processes and the heuristic procedures that govern judgment and inference. Third, mistakes and fallacies help the mapping of human intuitions by indicating which principles of statistics or logic are non-intuitive or counter-intuitive. (Kahneman & Tversky, 1982b, p. 124)

Although this rationale appears compelling, it contains an implicit assumption worth noting. The conclusion that people make errors in reasoning can only be reached if we first have a clear idea of what constitutes correct probabilistic reasoning. For Kahneman, Tversky, and the others who have conducted research on judgment heuristics, correct probabilistic reasoning is defined by Bayesian axioms. However, alternatives to Bayesian probability revision do exist (see Cohen, 1981, for example). It is entirely possible that behavior that appears biased when judged according to one set of rules will not appear biased in the light of another set (see Einhorn & Hogarth, 1981b, for more discussion on this subject). In reading the discussions that follow, the reader should keep in mind that biases and errors are always defined as deviations from some normative (usually Bayesian) theory and may not be considered errors in another context.

Availability

Physicians are often called upon to estimate prior probabilities subjectively. In the mammography example discussed earlier, the prior probability that the patient had cancer was estimated to be .01. This estimate was assumed to have been based on the physician's experience with similar patients. Indeed, unless the doctor conducts an epidemiological survey, there is nowhere else the estimate could have come from.

From a Bayesian viewpoint, there is nothing inherently worrying about doctors making subjective estimates of prior probabilities, but it is possible that doctors with different backgrounds (general practitioners versus oncologists, for example) may make different probability estimates. Studies of the effect of experience on probability judgments by Tversky and Kahneman (1973) produced evidence for what has come to be called the "availability" heuristic.

Tversky and Kahneman found that subjective probability estimates are at least partly determined by the ease with which events similar to those being estimated can be retrieved from memory. To take a simple example, people asked to estimate the probability that a marriage will end in divorce do so by trying to recall all the cases of divorce with which they have firsthand experience (as well as those they have read about). Those who are acquainted with many cases of divorce estimate a higher probability that marriage will end in divorce than those who have rarely encountered divorce (Kozielecki, 1981). In other words, subjective probability estimates for an event or outcome depend on how "available" other instances of the event are to the estimators.

Ordinarily, events that are easier to recall (more available) are also more likely, so the availability heuristic leads to accurate probability estimates. However, this is not always the case. There are times when availability is not related to probability. Tversky and Kahneman (1973) created such a situation using an artificial laboratory task. They asked their subjects if the letter 'k' appeared more often as the first or third letter of a word. The correct answer is third letter, but the investigators expected their subjects to say the first letter because it is easier to think of examples of 'k' beginning a word than of 'k' as the third letter. Their results conformed to their expectations. As many as 68% of their subjects judged that 'k' was more frequent as the first letter even though a typical text contains twice as many instances of 'k' in the third-letter position. Tversky and Kahneman concluded that the true probabilities were ignored because the availability heuristic suggested a different conclusion.

One factor that can exert a strong effect on availability (and therefore on estimates of subjective probability) is media coverage (Combs & Slovic, 1979; Slovic, Fischhoff, & Lichtenstein, 1979). For example, when asked to estimate the risk of dying from several different causes, the participants in these studies systematically overestimated the death risk posed by "sensational" events such as homicide and storms and underestimated the risk associated with such mundane killers as emphysema, asthma, and diabetes, which receive much less media attention.

Slovic explained his findings as resulting directly from the availability heuristic. Since sensational deaths are given greater media coverage than everyday causes of death such as diabetes, instances of death by storms, homicide, and so on are easier to retrieve from memory (they are more available). Because they are easier to retrieve from memory, sensational causes are judged to have a higher probability than more common, but less available, killers. Indeed, Slovic and his colleagues were able to demonstrate a significant relationship between the newspaper column space devoted to a cause of death and subjects' subjective estimates of its likelihood.

Medical journal coverage appears to exert a similar effect on physicians. Christensen-Szalanski, Beck, Christensen-Szalanski and Koepsell (1983) asked doctors to estimate the mortality rates of 42 different diseases. They found a tendency to overestimate the lethality of diseases that receive a great deal of journal coverage.* In accord with the earlier research by Slovic and his colleagues, Christensen-Szalanski et al. found the number of journal articles devoted to a disease, regardless of their actual content, a good predictor of physician mortality estimates. They concluded that journal coverage affects availability, which, in turn, determines judged frequency. The same authors also noted that the availability heuristic may influence medical testing. For instance, if the doctor believes, on the basis of journal coverage, that a disease is more lethal than it actually is, screening tests may be ordered unnecessarily.

Another investigation of the availability heuristic by Detmer, Fryback, and Gassner (1978) required surgeons to estimate mortality rates for various types of hospitalized patients. The researchers found that judgments of overall hospital death rates were lower for surgeons in low-mortality specialties (plastics, orthopedics, and urology) than were judgments of surgeons in high-mortality specialties (cardiovascular, neurosurgery, and general surgery). Interestingly, 60% of the surgeons in this study estimated the overall mortality rate to be higher than their own. Their reasoning seemed to imply that "it didn't happen because of me."

Still another example of the availability heuristic at work in the clinic comes from a study by Schiffman, Cohen, Nowick, and Selinger (1978), who reported that, when doctors viewed a list of differential diagnoses, they usually judged the first disease on the list as more probable than the last. The researchers explained this finding as the result of the longer amount of time the first diagnosis resided in memory as compared with later ones. They assumed that longer residence in memory made these earlier diagnoses more available. A possible problem with this finding is that differential diagnoses are often written with the most probable coming first. It is possible that the doctors in this experiment merely assumed that the differential diagnosis had been written in the usual way.

It should be obvious that, when forming an opinion about the implications of a set of diagnostic data, each item should be evaluated on its

* An even better predictor of physician estimates was the number of patients with a specific diagnosis previously encountered.

merits regardless of whether it is gathered first or last. Unfortunately, a physician's initial hypothesis may influence the way in which evidence is evaluated. For example, inconsistent findings that come late in the diagnostic workup may be downplayed (see Slovic, Fischhoff, & Lichtenstein, 1977; Slovic & Lichtenstein, 1971); sometimes new data may even be ignored if they contradict a hypothesis generated earlier (Elstein et al., 1978).

The domination of later items of information by earlier ones (known as the "primacy" effect) has been demonstrated by Wallsten (1981), who asked medical students and graduate physicians to "workup" 27 hypothetical patients. They were permitted to do as thorough a history, as complete a physical examination, and as extensive an array of laboratory tests as they considered necessary. Wallsten reported that both groups subjectively distorted evidence in the latter part of the workup to support opinions formed earlier in the diagnostic process.

These distortions can take several forms. One possibility, suggested by Elstein et al. (1978), is that neutral data may be taken as positive (confirmatory). For instance, Smedslund (1963) gave nurses hypothetical case material in which the relationship between a particular symptom and a particular disease was presented in each of four different ways: (1) when the symptom was present, the disease was also present; (2) when the symptom was present, the disease was not present; (3) when the symptom was absent; the disease was also absent; and (4) when the symptom was absent the disease was present. Since all four possibilities occurred equally often in the case histories, there was effectively no relationship between the symptom and the disease (the correlation was 0). Nevertheless, the nurses maintained that the relationship was positive, and they pointed to the many instances when this was true, ignoring the large number of cases for which the relationship did not hold. The nurses appeared to give more weight to data that supported their initial hypothesis than to data that refuted it.

Clearly, the availability heuristic can bias medical judgments by giving easily imagined events more importance than their objective frequency warrants. When the events being estimated are likely to be rare (side effects in drug studies, for example), the availability heuristic can seriously bias judgment. The importance of the availability heuristic in drug studies is summarized by Hogarth (1980), who wrote, "To the extent that judgment by availability is a common strategy, it suggests that physicians need to think very carefully about the specific instances they recall when making assessments of possible adverse reactions" (p. 449).

In addition to explaining how estimates of subjective probability can be influenced by factors other than objective frequency, the availability heuristic can also provide an explanation for the illusory correlations discussed in Chapter 2. If subjects in Chapman and Chapman's (1969) paired-word experiment were using the availability heuristic then we would expect them to say that semantically related pairs were more frequently associated than they really were simply because meaningfully related word pairs are easier to retrieve from memory than unrelated pairs. The same explanation holds for experiments in which psychiatric symptoms such as suspiciousness were associated with features of drawings (such as peculiar eyes). Because the associations between these words (or between symptoms and signs) are very strong, they appear to occur more frequently (with greater probability) than do unrelated pairs. Thus, the availability heuristic leads people to perceive correlations where none exist.

Research on the availability heuristic demonstrates the importance of memory in making judgments. Usually, ease of recall is a valid cue for estimating probability, but, as we have shown, there are instances when the availability heuristic leads to biased judgments. The same is true of the next heuristic to be discussed, representativeness.

Representativeness

The representativeness heuristic, in its simplest form, states that the probability of an event or outcome can be estimated by the degree to which it resembles general population characteristics. To illustrate the representativeness heuristic in operation, Kahneman and Tversky (1972) posed students the following problem:

> All families of six children in a city were surveyed. In 72 families the exact order of births of boys and girls was GBGBBG. What is your estimate of the number of families surveyed in which the exact order of births was BGB-BBB? (p. 432)

Although, mathematically, these two sequences are equally likely (as are all other sequences), more than 80% of their subjects believed the first birth order to be more than twice as probable as the second. Kahneman and Tversky explained this finding as the result of relying on the representativeness heuristic to estimate probability. Their subjects knew that the ratio of boys to girls in the general population is close to 1. The first sequence maintained this ratio and was, to the subjects, more "representative" of the general population than the 5-to-1 ratio of boys to girls in the second sequence. Since the first sequence appears more "representative" it is judged more likely.

Tversky and Kahneman (1974) identified six potential cognitive errors associated with relying on the representativeness heuristic: insensitivity to prior probabilities, insensitivity to sample size, misconceptions about randomness, insensitivity to predictability, the illusion of validity, and misconceptions about statistical regression. Each of these errors contravenes some aspect of normative statistical theory (Bayesian statistics) and each leads the decision maker to produce judgments on the basis of typicality. We discuss the various cognitive errors in turn.

Insensitivity to prior probabilities

Bayes' formula requires that specific test information (true- and false-positive rates) be combined with prior probabilities (prevalence rates) to make accurate judgments of posterior probabilities. We have seen in the mammography example that prior probabilities may sometimes be ignored in favor of specific information—on how "representative" the case is. The result can be a biased judgment.

A well-known example of how ignoring prior probabilities can lead to biased judgments was reported by Kahneman and Tversky (1973). Their experiment employed three groups of subjects. The first group was asked to estimate the number of students enrolled in each of nine academic fields. The second estimated how similar a mythical student called Tom W. was to the typical student in each of these fields. The data upon which their typicality judgments were based consisted of brief personality sketches such as the following one:

> Tom W. is of high intelligence although lacking in true creativity. He has a need for order and clarity, and for neat, tidy systems in which every detail finds its appropriate place. His writing is rather dull and mechanical, occasionally enlivened by somewhat corny puns and by flashes of imagination of the sci-fi type. He has a strong drive for competence. He seems to have little feel and little sympathy for other people and does not enjoy interacting with others. Self-centered, he nonetheless has a deep moral sense. (p. 238)

A third group of subjects was also given the personality sketches and told that they were compiled on the basis of projective personality tests (ink-blots and so on). This group was asked to rate the likelihood that Tom W. was enrolled in each of the nine academic fields.

If we take the first group's estimates as the prior probability of a student being in each academic field and the likelihoods produced by subjects in the second group as indicating the probability that a student in each of the fields would be described in the same way as Tom W. (that is, the typicality ratings indicated the perceived "diagnosticity" of the personality sketch), then Bayes' formula can be used to calculate the posterior probability that Tom is a student in each of the academic fields. The output of Bayes' formula (the normative response) can then be compared with the probabilities produced by subjects in Group 3. Any deviations from the probabilities produced by Bayes' formula represent non-normative responding.

When Kahneman and Tversky compared the normative probabilities with those produced by subjects in Group 3, they found major discrepancies. Instead of producing estimates based on both the prior probabilities and the typicality ratings, subjects based their estimates solely on the latter. In fact, the probability estimates of the third group were almost perfectly correlated with the typicality ratings of the second group. Fields of study were judged likely for Tom precisely to the extent that his personality profile represented the common stereotype of what students in that discipline are like. Awareness that the fields differed markedly in the size of their memberships (as shown by the estimates of the first group) had virtually no impact on Group 3's probability ratings. For example, 95% of the students in Group 3 rated computer science as a more likely field for Tom than humanities or education, even though the members of the first group estimated computer science to have only one-third as many students as the other two fields.

This reliance on the specific case while overlooking prior probabilities might have been reasonable if the subjects in Group 3 firmly believed that the personality sketches purportedly made on the basis of projective personality tests were highly diagnostic. Highly diagnostic tests would produce such a strong likelihood that Tom belonged in the field indicated that any differences in prior probability would have been overwhelmed. However, Kahneman and Tversky's subjects (graduate psychology students) actually held projective tests in low esteem and did not believe that they are a helpful guide to career choice. Thus, the subjects in Group 3 relied on specific diagnostic information that they believed was not very diagnostic at all while ignoring prior probabilities that, according to the normative Bayesian theory, provide an important source of information about posterior probabilities.

In a more stringent test of the power of the representativeness heuristic to bias judgments, Kahneman and Tversky (1973) again provided subjects with thumbnail personality sketches, this time supposedly of engineers and lawyers. Subjects were asked to rate the probability that each sketch described a member of one profession or the other. Half the subjects were told the population from which the sketches were drawn consisted of 30 engineers and 70 lawyers; the other half were told that there were 70 engineers and 30 lawyers. The results were an impressive demonstration of the representativeness heuristic in operation. The prior probabilities (the number of engineers and lawyers) were essentially ignored. Instead, subjects assigned probabilities by judging how similar each sketch was to their stereotype of an engineer ("he likes building things") or a lawyer ("he is a good debater").

Prior probabilities, in the form of prevalence rates, are often important in medical decision making. Elstein and Bordage (1979) have described what could happen if doctors rely on representativeness and ignore prior probabilities:

> Suppose the clinical picture of a particular case resembles but does not exactly match the typical picture of two alternative conditions, one more common than the other. Because the observed findings of the case fit both larger classes equally well, many clinicians would judge both alternatives

equally probable. In so doing, they have ignored the different prior probabilities of the two alternatives and have employed the representativeness
principle. (p. 353)

Elstein and Bordage's point is illustrated by studies conducted by Bennett (1980) using a medical equivalent of Kahneman and Tversky's "lawyers and engineers" problem. Bennett's subjects were nurses who were
told that a panel of doctors and nurses had examined cases of postoperative hemorrhage and peritonitis following abdominal surgery. The
nurses were given five case histories supposedly drawn at random from
100 such cases. Their task was to estimate the probability that the patients described were hemorrhage patients. As in the Kahneman and
Tversky study, the prior probabilities were systematically altered so that
sometimes there were 30 cases of hemorrhage and 70 cases of peritonitis and *vice versa*. In addition, extreme prior probabilities (90 hemorrhage and 10 peritonitis) were also included. Bennett also manipulated
the degree to which the case histories resembled each condition. Some
cases were highly stereotypical whereas others were ambiguous enough
to suggest either condition.

In line with earlier findings, Bennett reported that nurses tended to
rely on the representativeness heuristic, ignoring prior probabilities in
favor of case-specific information. Although the more extreme prior
probabilities seemed to have exerted a moderating effect (as did altering
the diagnosticity of the descriptions), Bennett concluded that even occu-
pationally relevant medical judgments may be biased when judges rely
on the representativeness heuristic.

Bennett's finding that the diagnosticity of the description can affect
whether the representativeness heuristic is employed was confirmed in a
study reported by Fischhoff and Bar-Hillel (1984a). They found that
prior probabilities were ignored when case descriptions were strongly
stereotypical. When case descriptions were ambiguous, however, prior
probabilities became more important. Even in the latter situation, however, prior probabilities did not exert the influence they should according to normative statistical considerations.

Insensitivity to sample size and misconceptions about randomness

Consider the following problem posed to experimental subjects by
Kahneman and Tversky (1972):

> A certain town is served by two hospitals. In the larger hospital about 45
> babies are born each day, and in the smaller hospital about 15 babies are
> born each day. As you know, about 50 per cent of all babies are boys. The
> exact percentage of baby boys, however, varies from day to day. Sometimes
> it may be higher than 50 per cent, sometimes lower. For a period of one
> year, each hospital recorded the days on which . . . more . . . than 60 per

cent of babies born were boys. Which hospital do you think recorded more such days? (p. 443)

Most subjects believed that the hospitals were equally likely to record days when the percentage of male births exceeded 60 per cent. In other words, they did not perceive the size of the hospital as relevant even though the larger hospital, which records many more births, is more likely to produce data reflecting the population mean (50% boys and 50% girls) than the smaller hospital, which represents a much smaller "sample." Kahneman and Tversky described subjects who ignore sample size when making probability judgments as believing in the "Law of Small Numbers." Instead of the statistically valid law of large numbers, which states that the larger the sample the more accurately it reflects population parameters, the law of small numbers seems to suggest that any sample, no matter how large, is an equally "representative" estimate of population parameters.

Faith in the law of small numbers is not limited to the statistically naive. Tversky and Kahneman (1971) questioned scientists trained in statistics about the statistical decisions they make when designing scientific studies and interpreting their results. They found that, despite their training, these scientists often rely on intuitions about appropriate sample sizes for testing experimental effects and for interpreting any statistically significant effects they obtain. Scientists were found to have unreasonably high expectations about the replicability of results from a single sample and undue confidence in the results obtained from small samples. Often, they gambled their research hypotheses on small samples without being aware of the extremely high odds against detecting the effects they are studying. Perhaps most disturbing was the scientists' reluctance to attribute unexpected results to sampling variability. Instead, they tried to come up with a causal explanation for every observed "effect."

A belief in the law of small numbers may also result in misconceptions about randomness. An illustration is provided by Kahneman and Tversky (1972), who asked people to judge the probability that a coin tossed six times would produce the sequence H-T-H-T-T-H (H=head, T=tail) more often than the sequence H-H-H-T-T-T. This problem is identical to the one about the sequence of boys and girls in large families described earlier and the results were identical as well. Most subjects believed the former sequence to be more likely than the latter even though both sequences are equally probable. It seems that the regular nature of the second sequence does not "represent" what most people think of as a random order. Their belief in the law of small numbers leads them to believe that every sample, no matter how small, will represent their notion of randomness.

Kozielecki (1981) described a related phenomenon discovered in a study conducted by several Polish mathematicians. This study actually resulted in a practical strategy for maximizing gambling winnings by capitalizing on other people's misconceptions about randomness. The game studied by the mathematicians was a version of Lotto in which players must select a small set of numbers from a larger set by marking the numbers on a grid. If the numbers selected match those chosen by a random process, a prize is awarded. The researchers found that players were reluctant to choose regular sequences. For example, they almost never chose the numbers 1, 2, 3, 4, 5, 6 or 30, 31, 32, 33, 34, 35. They also avoided choosing numbers that fell in a single row or column, or mathematical sequences such as 2, 4, 6, 8, 10, 12. It appears that players believed that such regular sequences were less likely than others; to them, such sequences did not seem random. The mathematicians suggested that a player could maximize his/her winnings simply by choosing the regular sequences that most players avoid. They are no more likely to come up than any other sequence, but when they do, there will be fewer players with whom to share the prize.

Misconceptions about randomness, and the law of small numbers, also appear to be responsible for what is commonly known as the "gambler's fallacy." This fallacy occurs when a series of independent events are treated as if they influenced one another. The gambler who has just seen a tossed coin land heads six times in a row and who invokes the mythical "law of averages" to predict that the next toss "has got to be tails" is engaging in the gambler's fallacy. Once again, the problem appears to be a reliance on the representativeness heuristic. Six heads in a row does not represent the gambler's idea of random—it is too regular. The gambler believes that all samples must represent the population mean of an even number of heads and tails; thus the next toss should be tails so that the outcomes will begin to "even out."

There is no reason to believe that doctors are any less susceptible to a belief in the law of small numbers than anyone else. In fact, at least one study has demonstrated that doctors are also susceptible to a version of the gambler's fallacy (Detmer, Fryback, & Gassner, 1977; cited by Hogarth, 1980). In this study, surgeons were given information about the incidence of certain postoperative complications for the past year and for the first 6 months of the current year. Specifically, they were told that the annual rate is 20% and that the rate for the first 6 months of the current year is 14%. They were then asked to predict the rate for the remainder of the year. Few surgeons reasoned that "techniques must be improving and that the complication rate may be down to 10 per cent in the next six months." Instead, roughly half of the 38 participating surgeons predicted a rate of 25–26%. In other words, the surgeons believed that every sample must equal the annual mean (20%) and were predicting a higher rate for the second half of the year to compensate for the lower rate in the first half.

A belief that every sample, regardless of size, must conform to population parameters is also responsible for the results of a study that discovered that apprentice medical laboratory technicians were required by their instructors to produce blood counts that exactly mirrored population characteristics even when the variability in the individual samples made this impossible (Berkson, Magath, & Hurn, 1940; cited by Hogarth, 1980).

Although these examples make it clear that insensitivity to sample size and misperceptions about the meaning of randomness may lead to biases in estimating probabilities, they are not the whole story. A misplaced belief in invalid signs and tests can also result in biased probability estimates. The sources of such misplaced beliefs are discussed next.

Insensitivity to predictability and the illusion of validity

Although it seems obvious that a test that does not predict an event or outcome should not be used to estimate the probability of that event occurring, this is exactly what happened when Tom W. was judged more likely to be a computer science student than a humanities student. The projective personality tests upon which this judgment was based were not considered to be diagnostic of career choice by the very people who were relying on them.

The value of a medical test lies in its ability to affect a physician's judgment. A test result should change a doctor's posterior probabilities or there is no reason for ordering it. Yet doctors, like students, have been found willing to make predictions on the basis of evidence that they later admit has little diagnostic value (see Eddy, 1982, for several examples).

Belief in the validity of nondiagnostic information can be explained as a reliance on the representativeness heuristic: to the extent that a diagnostic procedure yields results that appear representative of the event to be predicted, the actual predictive accuracy of the procedure will be overlooked. Such procedures have the "illusion of validity" (Tversky & Kahneman, 1974). The most likely reason why diagnostic procedures sometimes appear to be valid predictors when they are not is incomplete feedback about the accuracy of decisions to decision makers (Einhorn & Hogarth, 1978). A medical illustration of incomplete feedback is provided by Bushyhead and Christensen-Szalanski's (1981) study of the diagnosis of penumonia.

Pneumonia, they pointed out, is a diagnosis that is ultimately confirmed by examination of chest radiographs, but before these films can be examined they must be ordered. If doctors only order chest x-rays for patients they strongly suspect have pneumonia, they may assume that those not x-rayed do not have the disease. Such an assumption would be justified if the doctors' judgment about who should be x-rayed is 100% correct. In practice, however, some pneumonia patients are not x-rayed.

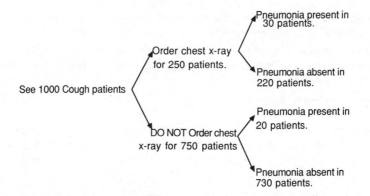

Figure 3-1 Incomplete feedback can lead to distorted estimates of disease prevalence. In the tree diagram, the 20 patients with pneumonia who do not get x-rayed are never diagnosed. The result is that the doctor believes the prevalence of pneumonia to be 30 out of 1000 cough patients when the true prevalence is 50 in 1000. Taken from Bushyhead and Christensen-Szalanski (1981, p. 116) and reprinted here with the permission of the Society for Medical Decision Making.

This results in incomplete feedback to the doctor—patients with pneumonia who are not x-rayed fail to be identified. As illustrated in Figure 3-1, the doctor never learns that 20 patients for whom radiographs were not ordered also have pneumonia. As a consequence, the doctor perceives the prevalence to be 3% when the true prevalence is 5%.

Bushyhead and Christensen-Szalanski also pointed out that incomplete feedback can distort the clinician's perception of the predictive value of a diagnostic procedure. A particular diagnostic sign (the presence of abnormal chest sounds, for example) may be correlated with pneumonia in patients who receive a chest radiograph but *not* among patients who are not x-rayed. Since physicians only receive feedback about the first group, they may believe that a diagnostic sign predicts penumonia when, in fact, it does not (see Kern & Doherty, 1982, for another example of illusory validity and Gray, Begg, & Greenes, 1984, for a ROC analysis of incomplete feedback).

Misconceptions about statistical regression

A source of judgment bias that can result in misuse of the representativeness heuristic is the misunderstanding of statistical regression to the mean. Suppose every child in a school was given an intelligence test. Some children score above, some below, and others right at the mean. If the children are retested with an equivalent test, most of the children who scored above-average on the first test administration will achieve a somewhat lower score and most of those who scored below-average the first time will obtain a somewhat higher score the second time around. The reason their scores behave this way is that random fluctuations can produce deviations from the "true" score that are not likely to be repeated. Instead, scores tend to return (regress) to the population mean. This phenomenon is known as "regression to the mean," and it is quite common in everyday life. As Kahneman and Tversky (1973) stated:

> Regression effects are all around us. In our experience, most outstanding fathers have somewhat disappointing sons, brilliant wives have duller husbands, the ill adjusted tend to adjust and the fortunate are eventually stricken by ill luck. (pp. 249–250)

Failure to appreciate the importance of regression to the mean can lead to serious misjudgments. For example, Tversky and Kahneman (1974) described how flight instructors would praise trainee pilots after very good flights only to find their next performance was not quite so good. Scolding them after a bad flight, however, lead to better performance the next time around. The flight instructors concluded that punishment works better than praise when teaching trainees to fly! It would seem that the flight instructors believed that every test result was truly "representative" of a trainee's flying ability.

In medicine, the practical implications of ignoring regression effects can be quite serious, as in this example given by Hogarth (1980):

> consider that a patient's blood-pressure can be thought to oscillate irregularly around some average level. If blood-pressure is monitored regularly, occasional high or low levels will be observed. What is likely to happen after a patient exhibits exceptionally low (or high) blood-pressure on a particular occasion? Assume that a physician orders the administration of a drug and subsequently observes the level of blood-pressure to be close to the normal average. Is he justified in believing that the drug has brought about the observed change? Not necessarily, for if the fluctuations are indeed random, the next observation is highly likely to be closer to the average anyway (i.e. low blood-pressure will probably increase, and high blood-pressure decrease). (p. 444)

It should be obvious that the representativeness heuristic is frequently employed when individuals are required to estimate the probability of events. Although it can take several forms and can produce a variety of different judgment biases, the representativeness heuristic always involves emphasizing case-specific information while ignoring prior probabilities. Although availability and representativeness are the most commonly studied judgment heuristics, they are not the only judgment strategies relevant to medicine. "Anchoring and adjustment," a common method of estimating probabilities, can also bias outcomes. This strategy is discussed next.

Anchoring and Adjustment

Tversky and Kahneman (1974) demonstrated anchoring and adjustment by asking their subjects factual questions that required estimates of various frequencies (the number of African countries in the United Nations, for example). Before making their judgments, the subjects were given arbitrary starting points between 0 and 100. (Starting points were assigned by spinning a wheel with numbers printed along its circumference and observing which number stopped opposite a pointer.) The subjects were required to indicate whether the starting values were too high, too low, or just right, and they were also asked to give their own estimates of the true frequency. Tversky and Kahneman found that the randomly derived starting values had an impressive effect on frequency estimates. The higher the initial starting value, the higher the estimate. Although the starting points were totally arbitrary, it seemed that people used them to "anchor" their estimates; "adjustments" were made either up or down from the starting point in line with each individual's knowledge of Africa and the United Nations. Typically, these adjustments were crude and imprecise; the crucial point, however, is that the anchor was an important determinant of the final estimate.

Although anchoring and adjustment has not been well documented in the clinic, it is potentially quite relevant. Hogarth (1980), for example, has hypothesized that physicians trying to anticipate the effect of a drug on a particular patient may use the known effect of the drug on other patients as an anchor, and then make adjustments based on the characteristics of the current case. Diagnostic hypotheses may also serve as anchors, with "adjusted" hypotheses entertained as additional information becomes available. If the initial hypothesis is way off base, it may take some time before the adjustments result in the most likely hypothesis (see Schiffman et al., 1978, for an example).

An empirical study of anchoring and adjustment in diagnosis was reported by Friedlander and Stockman (1983), who presented psychiatrists, psychologists, and social workers with case material for two patients, one suffering from anorexia nervosa and one from suicidal depression. The case histories were arranged so that definitive diagnostic information appeared either early or late in the data-acquisition sequence. The experimenters found that early information often served as an anchor for later diagnoses. This finding suggests that the experiments reported earlier, in which the availability heuristic was invoked to explain why data gathered first exert a stronger influence on diagnosis than data gathered later in the diagnostic sequence (the "primacy" effect), may also have been demonstrating the effect of anchoring and adjustment.

Interestingly, a replication of Friedlander and Stockman's study (Friedlander & Phillips, 1984), using undergraduate students and case material more appropriate to this sample, *did not* find a significant anchoring effect. These authors concluded that anchoring may be more prevalent in experienced clinicians because "as more coherent, clearly defined and elaborated clinical prototypes are acquired, the clinician's exclusive attention to the prototype [*may lead to*] disregard of new salient information" (p. 370).

Reliance on judgment heuristics may lead not only to biased judgments but also to the illusion that one's judgments are actually more accurate than they really are. Overconfidence in one's ability to make probability judgments is addressed in the next section.

Overconfidence

As we have seen, physicians sometimes engage in an exhaustive data-gathering strategy in an attempt at "marshalling all the facts." However, as we have also noted, too much information can be misleading. Human information-processing capacity is limited and easily overloaded. When this happens, errors in judgment can occur. Curiously, however, these errors are rarely perceived by decision makers who generally report great confidence in their judgments. In fact, the more information they have available, the more confident they become.

A classic study by Oskamp (1965) serves as an illustration. Oskamp presented his subjects (many of whom were experienced clinical psychologists) with increasing amounts of case material. At various stages in the case presentation, the participant's understanding of the case was tested. Oskamp found that his subjects became more convinced of their understanding of the cases as the amount of information available to them increased—even though objective testing found them to be no better at predicting outcomes than they were with fewer items of information. Several studies have confirmed that a small set of data is often as useful as a large set in reaching accurate diagnoses (Braakman, Gelpke, Habbema, Maas, & Minderhound, 1980; Fryback, 1974b; Gorry & Barnett, 1968; Neutra & Neff, 1975). In these situations, additional information is often redundant. Repeated, nonindependent, tests appear mainly to boost confidence, not accuracy.

Overconfidence may also arise from the data distortions produced by selective attention and memory. For example, Arkes and Harkness (1980) assessed memory for the details of case histories. They found that symptoms that were not presented, but were consistent with the final diagnoses, were falsely remembered as having been presented. The opposite was also true. Symptoms that actually were part of the case materials, but that were not consistent with the final diagnosis, were selectively forgotten. In both cases, the result was a "cleaner" (less ambiguous) case history and greater confidence in the accuracy of the final diagnosis.

Studies of overconfidence focus on how well subjective probability estimates match some objective criterion. In the decision-making literature, the correspondence between subjective estimates and objective criteria is known as "calibration." The closer subjective estimates are to real-world probabilities, the better calibrated the individual is said to be. For example, a weather forecaster whose estimates of the probability of rain conform to the actual data is said to be well calibrated, and this is what has typically been found (Murphy & Winkler, 1974, 1977).

Numerous studies across a wide variety of tasks and subjects have found that people often believe they are better calibrated than they really are. For example, Fischhoff et al. (1977) asked subjects to answer general-knowledge questions and found that subjects were often extremely confident their answers were correct even when they were wrong. Some subjects were so sure they were correct that they were willing to wager at odds of 50 to 1 that their incorrect answers were, in fact, correct. (This may be a good way for researchers to supplement their income but, in this study, all moneys were returned.)

Doctors' calibration was studied by Christensen-Szalanski and Bushyhead (1981). They asked physicians to estimate the probability that patients presenting with coughs had pneumonia. All told, 1531 patients were evaluated. Although performance varied, the doctors' calibration was not very high. For one subgroup of patients, the probability of pneumonia was estimated to be 80% when the true incidence was only 20%. Similar low calibration was reported by De Smet, Fryback, and Thornbury (1979) and by Lusted (1977).

Why are weather forecasters better calibrated than doctors? The reason probably lies in the nature of their respective tasks. Weather forecasters make very repetitive judgments (Will it rain?) and receive prompt feedback (at least for short-term forecasts). In contrast, doctors must weigh a wide variety of possibilities, and feedback may be delayed or unavailable. As is discussed in Chapter 5, useful feedback is necessary for learning to make probability judgments.

Hindsight bias

A particular form of overconfidence studied by Fischhoff (1982b) has been labeled "hindsight bias." According to Fischhoff, hindsight bias occurs when we are told that an event has occurred and this knowledge increases our feeling that the event was inevitable. Despite our inability to predict the event before the fact, learning that it has occurred leads us to believe that we "knew it all along."

Fischhoff (1975) illustrated hindsight bias in an experiment using psychotherapy case histories. One group of subjects, the foresight group, read the histories and then judged the likelihood of four possible therapeutic outcomes. The hindsight group read the histories and were told that one of the four outcomes had actually occurred. Their task was to give the probability they would have assigned to this outcome if they had not known it had occurred. The hindsight group assigned higher probabilities to the actual outcome than the foresight group. In other words, in hindsight, the outcome appeared more likely than it did in foresight.

Hindsight bias in medical diagnosis has been reported by Arkes, Wortmann, Saville, and Harkness (1981). They gave a group of physicians a case history and asked them to assign probabilities to four possible diagnoses (Reiter's syndrome, rheumatic fever, gout, and serum hepatitis in the preicteric phase). The physicians were divided into five groups, one foresight group and four hindsight groups. The foresight group estimated the prior probability of each diagnosis. The hindsight groups were each told which of the four diagnoses was found to be true and then asked how probable they would have believed each diagnosis to be on the basis of the case history. Arkes et al. found that the hindsight groups assigned greater probabilities to the diagnoses they believed to be correct than did the foresight group. The difference between the groups was especially large when the diagnosis was rare. The authors concluded that the doctors in the hindsight group tried to make sense out of what they "knew" happened rather than objectively analyzing the case materials.

This situation facing the hindsight groups in this experiment is similar to the one faced by doctors who are asked to give second opinions or to assume the care of a patient previously managed by someone else. Medical students who have access to the diagnosis made by senior physicians are also liable to succumb to hindsight bias. The result, in each of these situations, may be overconfidence in one's ability to make accurate diagnoses, and a tendency to believe that "I was right all along." In a review of the hindsight research, Arkes (1981) wrote, "There is always enough evidence to nourish all but the most outlandish diagnoses. . . . Given enough data, many diagnoses can appear obvious" (p. 326).

Warning doctors about the perils of hindsight bias and overconfidence may reduce their pernicious effects, but previous attempts to design educational programs to reduce these biases have not been very successful. Overconfidence and hindsight bias have proven very resistant to change (Fischhoff, 1982a,b).

Is Research on Judgment Biases Biased?

The picture of human judgment drawn so far is not very flattering. Decision makers, including doctors, seem to neglect prior probabilities in favor of case-specific information, particularly when the latter is easily called to mind or fits a representative stereotype. We seem to be easily lured into overconfidence in our subjective probability judgments; we are even willing to accept and make use of test results whose validity is illusory. Not surprisingly, some writers have challenged this rather pessi-

mistic portrait (see Jungerman, 1983). Instead of judgment biases resid-
ing in experimental subjects, critics claim that the biases reside in the
researchers and in the tasks and analyses they have designed. Psychologists, they claim, have tested people in artificial situations on largely
unfamiliar tasks; in the real world probability estimates are generally
adequate. The critics have a point. Human beings may not always be
perfectly rational, but they are rarely completely irrational either.

Arguments about rationality, and the extent to which human beings
are "naturally" rational, are hardly a new development. John Locke was
referring to just such a debate when he wrote, "God did not make man
barely two legged and leave it to Aristotle to make him logical." An
extensive review of this debate is beyond the scope of this book. For an
overview of the various positions, the reader is referred to Bar-Hillel
(1983), Berkeley and Humphreys (1982), L. J. Cohen (1979, 1981),
Edwards (1983), Einhorn and Hogarth (1981a), Fischhoff (1983),
Jungerman (1983), Nisbett, Krantz, Jepson, and Kunda (1983), Phillips
(1983), and Wallsten (1983). For our present purpose, we summarize
two major lines of argument against the view that human judgment is
fundamentally flawed. These are: (1) the norms to which judges are
being compared are inappropriate, and (2) the experiments are improp-
erly conducted.

Are normative theories really normative?

Cohen (1981) questioned whether the axiomatic probability theory (as
represented by the Bayesian approach) that underlies research on judgment heuristics and biases actually reflects accepted notions of rationality. He argued that if normative theories are not a criterion for rational
judgment then a failure to behave as they require cannot be used as
evidence for judgment bias, much less for irrationality.

Other critics have also questioned whether a normative statistical theory should be used as a criterion for rational judgments. They argue that
a person's goals may be different from those assumed by normative
theories (see Jungerman, 1983). It is also possible that individuals may
perceive a judgment problem differently from the way experimenters
intended (Phillips, 1983). If idiosyncratic goals and perceptions exist, it
is inappropriate to compare an individual's judgments with normative
theories that assume that all decision makers construe problems similarly
and share the same goals.

Although the question of whether normative theories are really normative is important, it is difficult to see how any amount of purely
philosophical argument will really resolve the issue. It is possible to
devise strong arguments supporting both points of view (see the peer
comments following Cohen, 1981). There is some danger that the critics
of research on judgment bias may overreact, taking the extreme position
that judgment and decisions are never biased, a proposition just as un-

likely as its extreme opposite (see Einhorn & Hogarth, 1981b, for more on this point).

Has psychological research on judgment bias been properly conducted?

Some writers have argued that research on judgment heuristics is too artificial to be generalizable to the "real world" outside the laboratory (Edwards, 1983). It does appear as if psychologists purposely design studies they know will produce biases in statistical reasoning. Indeed, "sometimes considerable ingenuity is required in order to locate the bias" (Berkeley & Humphrey, 1982, p. 243). Furthermore, most judgment errors are identified *post hoc* and cannot be predicted in advance (Wallsten, 1983).

Attempts to examine physicians' behavior in actual clinical settings have found doctors' judgments to be superior to those reported by laboratory studies. For example, Christensen-Szalanski, Diehr, Bushyhead, and Wood (1982) found both experienced physicians and their assistants make probability judgments and behave in a manner generally consistent with what is required by normative theories (see also Thornbury, Fryback, & Edwards, 1975).

Christensen-Szalanski (1985), in a discussion of the practical relevance of psychological research on judgment bias, admits that cognitive biases exist but claims that they have little effect on the *outcome* of actual clinical decisions. He bases this claim on the results of several studies of physicians evaluating patients suspected of having pneumonia (Bushyhead & Christensen-Szalanski, 1981; Christensen-Szalanski & Bushyhead, 1981, 1983). Most of the relevant findings have already been mentioned in this chapter; that is, the doctors were found to be poorly calibrated, they ignored symptoms that supported alternative hypotheses, and they were influenced by incomplete feedback obtained from chest x-rays. Despite these biases, Christensen-Szalanski noted that the outcomes of most of these doctors' diagnostic decisions were close to optimum. He calculated that the elimination of all judgment biases would have helped the average doctor in one of these studies to avoid one mistaken diagnosis per year. In addition, since even misdiagnosed patients usually received the same antibiotic treatment as those who were correctly diagnosed, judgment biases had little practical effect. Christensen-Szalanski concluded that most trivial judgment biases can be safely ignored in the clinic because correcting them may not be worth the effort involved.

While these findings are encouraging because they suggest that clinical judgment is trustworthy, it should be noted that researchers typically observe only the outcome of clinical decisions, not the process by which they were reached. It is possible that doctors were making the "right" decisions but for the "wrong" reasons.

This point is illustrated in a cleverly designed study of the diagnostic process reported by Fox (1980). Fox contrasted a probability-based, normative theory of medical judgment (Bayesian probability revision) with a cognitive, non-probabilistic theory. The latter relied on a set of heuristics and judgment algorithms. Fox found that he could predict final diagnostic decisions by *both* the normative theory and the cognitive model, but the latter gave a better account of the diagnostic process. In other words, even when physicians appear well-calibrated and even when they produce normatively appropriate behavior, they may not be doing so because they actually adhere to the normative theory (see Kleinmuntz & Kleinmuntz, 1981 for a related discussion).

It seems reasonable to conclude this section on judgment heuristics by reiterating that, more often than not, they do not lead to errors. There are occasions, however, when they do. These appear more commonly in the laboratory than the clinic, but examples were given in which real-world clinical judgments have also been affected. All of the factors determining when biases will occur are not yet known, but it seems certain that one important one is the sheer amount of information that must be evaluated. Cognitive overload can easily lead to the adoption of simplifying strategies of information processing and, in some cases, biased judgment. Combining several, potentially conflicting, items of information is a common requirement of clinical work. In the next part of this chapter, we take a closer look at how physicians accomplish this task.

Information Integration

Doctors must integrate information from diverse sources to make diagnostic and treatment decisions. Since most of this information is probabilistic and "noisy," deciding which items are important—and how important—presents serious difficulties.

The signal detection approach to data integration (see Chapter 2) is based on the assumption that data from each diagnostic procedure are given subjective "weight" in accord with their relative importance (diagnosticity). The sum of these weighted items is then evaluated to determine whether it represents a "signal" (true-positive) by comparing it with a decision criterion (Shaw, 1982). Most theories of decision making involve similar assumptions (Pitz & Sachs, 1984). We have already introduced one such theory, subjective expected utility. The decision maker, according to SEU theory, multiplies the subjective probability of various outcomes by their respective utilities and chooses the course that leads to maximal utility. We have designated SEU theory as normative or prescriptive because it dictates how decisions should be made. Such theories may be contrasted with descriptive models that attempt to represent how people actually do make decisions. The research on judgment biases indicates that individuals do not always behave as SEU theory prescribes. In this section, we discuss several important descriptive decision models. We return to SEU theory in Chapter 4.

Linear Models

In Chapter 1, we noted that Meehl's (1954) book comparing "clinical" with "statistical" judgment concluded that clinically relevant judgments are more accurate when made by a statistical formula than by using clinical judgment. The formula he had in mind makes use of what has become known as a "linear model."

A linear judgment model consists of a set of predictor variables on the one hand and some criterion (the outcome to be predicted) on the other. Usually, the predictor variables are weighted in such a way as to maximize the correlation between their weighted sum and the criterion, but linear models can also be used for other purposes (such as to differentiate groups of patients). When linear models are being used to predict judgments, the statistical technique of multiple regression analysis represents a straightforward way to determine the weights to be assigned to the various predictors. In fact, multiple regression analysis was designed specifically to determine the optimum combination of weighted predictors.

To use multiple regression analysis to produce linear models two things are required—numerical measurements of the predictors and the criterion, and some examples of how they covary. For example, a linear model for predicting malignancy from radiographs of a gastric ulcer may be constructed by observing the relationships between a set of pertinent predictors (Is the ulcer extraluminal? Is the contour regular? Is it located on the greater curvature?) and the outcome of pathology reports (the criterion). The evidence provided by each of these predictors can then be weighted according to its diagnosticity and summed. The higher the sum, the greater the likelihood that the ulcer is malignant (Wilson, Templeton, Turner, & Lodwick, 1965). Of course, the accuracy of such a prediction is entirely a function of the diagnosticity of the predictors. The multiple correlation (or, more often, the square of the multiple correlation) provides an index of the strength of the relationship between the predictors and the criterion. The closer the multiple correlation is to 1.00, the better the predictive relationship.

Modeling judgment using multiple regression analysis

Multiple regression has been used to model judgment and decision making by Hammond and his colleagues (see Hammond, Rohrbaugh, Mumpower, & Adelman, 1977, for example). Their preferred approach is to present complex problems to decision makers in the form of computer-generated bar graphs each of which requires a single judgment. After a series of such presentations, multiple regression analysis is used to determine the relative importance of different data sources to the final outcome.

An example of how multiple regression can be used to model medical judgments is an unpublished study of orthopedic surgeons we conducted with our students. We wished to model the decision to perform a total hip replacement. This operation involves removal of a person's hip joint and its replacement with an artificial one. When successful, the operation results in a relatively pain-free, mobile joint and, consequently, increased mobility. As usual, with any operation, there are some risks. There is the always-present risk of a reaction to the anesthesia and there are specific risks as well: infection, breakdown in the artificial joint, and dislocation. Since the risks and benefits vary with the characteristics of the patient, surgeons face a serious judgment problem. Our interest was not to measure the specific risks and benefits of the surgery, but rather to determine how patient characteristics affected the decision to operate.

To determine which patient characteristics are most important, we interviewed an "expert" orthopedic surgeon with many years' experience performing hip replacements. This interview, and a review of his previous cases, resulted in a list of five variables that he believed to be the main factors to consider when deciding whether or not to perform the operation. These were: age of the patient, the patient's general health status, severity of the limb pathology (as indicated by x-rays, etc.), the degree of independence loss, and the amount of pain the patient reports.

To evaluate the relative importance of each of these factors, we presented a sample of five orthopedic surgeons (not including our expert) with a series of bar graphs each representing one hypothetical patient's profile on each of the five variables. An example appears in Figure 3-2. The first bar in the graph represents the hypothetical patient's age, the second indicates the patient's overall health status, the third is an indicator of limb pathology as revealed by radiography, the fourth is a measure of independence loss, and the fifth reflects the amount of reported pain. Using this format, we presented many simulated patients. Each new simulation was produced simply by varying the height of the bars.

After studying each patient's profile, the surgeons were asked to indicate whether they would recommend this patient as suitable for surgery. They were asked to make their judgments on a numerical scale ranging from 1 (definitely not recommend surgery) to 10 (definitely recommend surgery). A rating of 5 indicated that the surgeon was uncertain either way. These ratings then served as the criterion in a multiple regression analysis in which the height of each of the five bars in the graphs served as predictors. The result of this analysis was a set of regression weights indicating how important each variable is in determining overall suitability judgments.

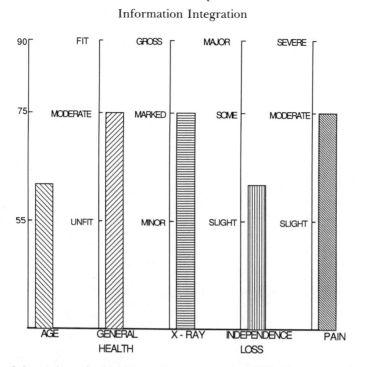

Figure 3-2   A hypothetical hip replacement patient. The doctors received information about the patients in the form of a bar graph such as this one. Each bar represents one important cue dimension.

These weights can also be plotted in the form of a bar graph where the height of each bar indicates its relative importance in determining a surgeon's judgment. An example of one surgeon's weights appears in Figure 3-3. This surgeon was influenced mainly by the patient's age and pain reports. The younger the patient and the greater the amount of reported pain, the more likely the surgeon was to operate. Independence loss and general health were next in importance. Although x-ray reports were hardly considered, this is not surprising. Operations are conducted for functional reasons, not on the basis of pathology as evidenced by x-ray. Actually, the correlation between functional loss and x-ray pathology is not very great. Another way of putting this is that the surgeon took the pathology for granted given the independence loss and pain.

The overall squared multiple correlation for all of our five surgeons was .95. This means that their judgment can be predicted with great accuracy simply from a knowledge of these five variables. A low squared multiple correlation would have meant that their judgments are not predictable either because important predictor variables were omitted from the cases or because they were responding inconsistently. An example of inconsistent responding is a surgeon who sometimes views

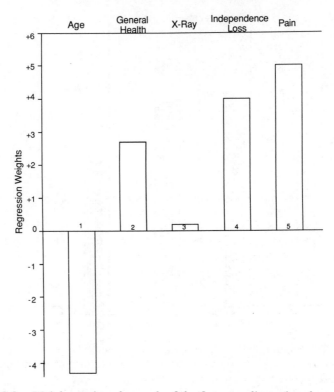

Figure 3-3   Weights assigned to each of the four cue dimensions by one ortho-pedic surgeon as determined by multiple regression. The negative weight for age simply means that, as age increased, the likelihood of this surgeon operating decreased.

increasing age as a reason not to operate while at other times considers it as a reason to operate.

The multiple regression technique can also be used to compare groups of decision makers. For example, after gathering data from the five surgeons, we presented the cases to a group of general practitioners who were asked to make the same judgments as the surgeons. Although the general practitioners' judgments turned out to be even more predict-able than those of the surgeons (their squared multiple correlation was .98), they did not weight the variables in the same way. The general practitioners put most of their emphasis on the x-rays and much less on age or reported pain. In other words, the patients that the general practitioners believed to be the best candidates for hip replacement sur-gery (and, presumably the ones they are most likely to refer to the orthopedic surgeons) are not necessarily the same ones the surgeons would choose.

Another example of how the multiple regression approach may be applied to medical questions comes from a study by Fisch, Hammond, Joyce, and O'Reilly (1981), who used the technique to describe how general practitioners evaluated and prescribed for depression. They asked doctors to judge the severity of the depressive disorder in 80 patients for whom they had been given symptom profiles. Physicians either based their judgments on cues provided by a well-known depression scale or on their own self-defined cues. Agreement among the doctors was found to be low. Doctors were found to be more consistent when using their own cues than when restricted to the depression scale.

The value of the multiple regression technique is not limited to modeling; it may also assist in training. Hammond et al. (1977) demonstrated that, in addition to determining importance weights for the predictor variables, multiple regression analysis can also be used to help improve judgments by providing decision makers with feedback about how well they are performing. We show how feedback can lead to improvement in Chapter 5. For now, we wish to note that the technique may also be applied when the relationship between predictor variables and the criterion is not strictly linear. Using additional mathematical techniques, curvilinear relationships may also be accommodated. For example, in the hip replacement study, the relationship between age and suitability for the operation was found to be linear and negative. This relationship is depicted graphically in Figure 3-4 (Panel A). However, the simulated patients presented to the surgeons fell within a restricted age range. It is possible that, had a greater variety of ages been used, the relationship may have turned out to be curvilinear (as in Figure 3-4, Panel B). That is, doctors may prefer not to operate on either the young or the very old.

An important limitation to the multiple regression approach is the assumption that all relevant predictors are known. The squared multiple correlation can serve as a guide to whether a doctor's judgments are predictable, but it cannot indicate what important variables have been omitted. For this, we must rely on experts and, to a certain extent, trial and error (see Elstein et al., 1983, for more on this point).

When the purpose of an investigation is to distinguish among different diseases, a better technique than multiple regression is discriminant analysis, in which predictor variables are weighted in such a way as to maximize the discrepancy between various groups. Diehr et al. (1981) used this approach to isolate those symptoms that best discriminate between migraine and tension headaches.

Paramorphic models and bootstrapping

It should be apparent that multiple regression analyses are closely related to the linear models introduced in Chapter 1. Linear models are concerned with weighting and summing a set of predictors to predict a criterion. Multiple regression analysis is one way of getting these

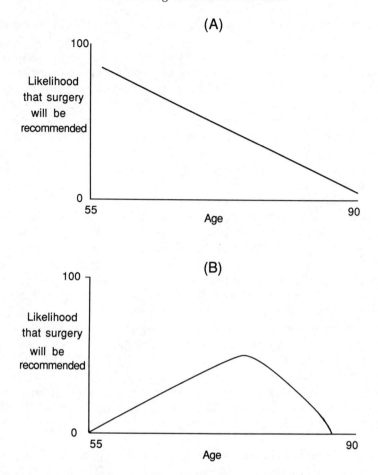

Figure 3-4   *Panel A* illustrates a linear relationship between age and the recommendation to operate. *Panel B* represents a curvilinear relationship. Note that the probability of recommending surgery is lower for the younger and older patients than for those in the middle.

weights. As their name indicates, linear models are concerned only with linear relationships, not curvilinear ones.

Taking into consideration the caveats noted in Chapter 1, research does seem to support the view that statistical linear models are better at predicting clinical outcomes than unaided clinical judgment (see Dawes & Corrigan, 1974, for a review). Their ability to predict, however, does not mean that linear models mimic how decision makers actually think. Just as it is possible for a decision maker to appear well calibrated from a Bayesian perspective while actually employing a set of non-normative judgment rules (as in Fox, 1980), it is also possible to behave as linear models predict without actually weighting and combining data linearly.

For this reason, linear judgment models are generally described as "paramorphic" representations of human judgment (Hoffman, 1960). They are taken to be abstract simulations of human cognition and not concrete theories of how human beings actually process information.

Although the finding that linear models can often predict behavior is important, an even more interesting finding is that a paramorphic model can *outperform* the human decision maker upon whom the model was originally based. That is, a linear model using the predictor variables specified by the decision maker—and the decision maker's own weights—will often do a better job of predicting the criterion than the decision maker (see Dawes & Corrigan, 1974, for examples). This phenomenon, which has been noted repeatedly in the literature, is called "bootstrapping" after the colloquial expression "to pull yourself up by your own bootstraps." According to Goldberg (1970), bootstrapping occurs because:

> the clinician is not a machine. While he possesses his full share of human learning and hypothesis-generating skills, he lacks a machine's reliability. He "has his days." Boredom, fatigue, illness, situational and interpersonal distractions all plague him, with the result that his repeated judgments of the exact same stimulus configurations are not identical. . . . If we could remove some of this human unreliability by eliminating the random error in his judgments, we should thereby increase the value of the resulting predictions. (p. 423)

Goldberg's suggested method for removing human unreliability is to rely on paramorphic models instead. To the extent that boredom, fatigue, distraction, and so on reduce human reliability, paramorphic models will perform better than people. Several of the "decision aids" described in Chapter 5 are based on paramorphic models and owe their success to bootstrapping.

Human unreliability is also responsible for the "robustness" of improper linear models (Dawes, 1976; 1979 and Goldberg, 1968). In contrast to a proper linear model, in which predictors are assigned weights in such a way that their composite predicts a criterion, an improper linear model assigns weights intuitively or sets them all equal. Dawes (1979) showed that even improper linear models can be superior to clinical judgment when predictions must be made from numerical predictors. In other words, even linear models that make no attempt to be paramorphic can outperform human judges. So long as the relationship between predictors and criterion are linear, all we really need to know to make good predictions is "what variables to look at and how to add" (Dawes & Corrigan, 1974, p. 105).

Despite the undeniable ability of linear models to predict clinical judgment, there is strong doubt about whether they are really descriptive. Lichtenstein, Earle, and Slovic (1975) and Birnbaum (1976) both reported that people often prefer to average the information provided by predictors rather than sum across predictors as linear models assume. The importance of averaging data has been emphasized by Norman Anderson, whose approach to information integration is discussed next.

Algebraic Information Integration

Anderson's (1972, 1974) approach to studying information integration, like multiple regression analysis, usually involves presenting judges with hypothetical cases and asking them to make global judgments. Generally, the cases are chosen to represent a completely "crossed" (full-factorial) analysis of variance experimental design. For example, if we wish to examine, algebraically, the way orthopedic surgeons make hip replacement decisions, we must present them with a series of simulated cases in which every level of a predictor is ultimately paired with every other level of a predictor. If each predictor (each bar in the graph shown in Figure 3-2) could take on three values (high, medium, and low) then a full-factorial algebraic design would require surgeons to evaluate 243 different cases (3^5). Clearly, the algebraic approach is best suited to judgment situations with only a small number of predictors.

Anderson uses the statistical technique of analysis of variance to determine how information is integrated. A statistically significant main effect is taken to indicate that a predictor is affecting a judgment, while a statistically significant interaction means that the effect (or meaning) of one predictor depends on the level of another. When statistically significant interactions are present, judgments are said to be *configural*. Configural judgments are not particularly common, but they do occur in clinical practice. To take a simple example, vomiting may be taken as a sign of illness in one situation and as a drug side effect in another. The context, the presence of other variables, determines how vomiting is interpreted. Configural judgments represent a problem for linear models of judgment, which assume that each predictor is evaluated independently.

Anderson and his coworkers have shown that algebraic models of information integration produce good descriptions of judgment in various situations. Typically, he has found that the importance weights assigned to predictors are averaged by decision makers rather than summed as linear models assume.

A medical example of the algebraic approach may be found in Hoffman, Slovic, and Rorer's (1968) study of radiologists (see also Slovic, Rorer, & Hoffman, 1971). In this study, radiologists were asked to rate a set of hypothetical ulcer patients on a 7-point scale ranging from 1 (definitely a benign lesion) to 7 (definitely a malignant lesion). The predictor variables (the data given to radiologists) consisted of seven x-ray signs (for example, the ulcer is extraluminal, or the ulcer contour is regular). Since each sign could be either present or absent, 256 hypothetical cases could be constructed. However, since some combinations of signs were medically implausible, only 192 cases were actually rated.

Their results indicated that radiologists did not all use diagnostic information in the same way. Some doctors differed from others on as many as 40% of the cases. Although there were some statistical interactions among the predictors (indicating configural judgment), these were minor influences compared with their main effects (see also Medin, Alton, Edelson, & Freko, 1982).

Although algebraic models often provide adequate descriptions of judgment, there is no guarantee that these models are more valid indicators of cognitive processes than linear models or any other psychological theory. In fact, it is safe to assume that algebraic models of information integration, like those derived from linear models, are "paramorphic" (Anderson & Shanteau, 1977).

Models of medical judgment have also been developed by comparing expert to novice doctors. Several researchers have shown that novices in a judgment area are more likely to average predictor information, whereas experts tend to sum the weighted predictors (see Wallsten & Budescu, 1981, for instance). Hammond (1980) has suggested that averaging represents an intuitively plausible strategy for combining information in complex, unfamiliar tasks, whereas experts use more complicated decision rules. If Hammond is correct, then medical students may benefit from instruction that concentrates on how experts integrate clinical data. We shall return to this subject in Chapter 5.

For completeness sake, we should note that at least one set of experiments indicates that information may sometimes not be integrated at all prior to making a decision. According to Shaw (1982), decision makers may form a judgment on the basis of each predictor separately and then, somehow, combine these subjudgments into one overall decision. The tendency to behave this way may be particularly strong in clinical situations where data are often gathered sequentially. We have more to say about the sequential (dynamic) nature of medical judgment late in this chapter. First we introduce yet another approach to integrating information, one based on set theory.

Set Theory and Information Integration

One of the first attempts to create a formal mathematical model of how information from various sources is combined to produce an overall clinical judgment was Ledley and Lusted's (1959) set theory approach (see also Lusted, 1968). Ledley and Lusted based their work on symbolic logic in the form of set theory, but also included notions of conditional probability. Their basic building block was the symptom–disease complex (SDC), a list of symptoms and diseases. The clinician must map observed signs (predictors) onto disease categories.

3. Evaluating Medical Information

Table 3-2. Truth Table Representation for Two Symptoms and Two Diseases[a]

Symptom (S) or Disease (D)	Possible Relationships				
S(1)	1111	1	111	0000	0000
S(2)	1111	0	000	1111	0000
D(1)	1100	1	100	1100	1100
D(2)	1010	1	010	1010	1010

[a] Adapted from Kleinmuntz (1984). Used here with the permission of Pergamon Press.

An example of Ledley and Lusted's approach appears in Table 3-2. Two symptoms and two diseases are represented. Each column is an SDC; a 1 in a row indicates that the patient displays that disease or symptom while a 0 means the patient does not show the symptom or the disease. Table 3-2 displays all of the SDCs that can be formed from two symptoms and two diseases. The boxed column represents the SDC for a patient with symptom 1, but no symptom 2, and having diseases 1 and 2.

Although Table 3-2 contains all possible SDCs, a physical examination may indicate that this particular patient has only symptom 2 and not symptom 1. This information allows us to eliminate all SDCs that do not show this pattern. The result is the reduced Table 3-3. We now know that the patient has one of four SDCs. This can be narrowed even further because it is known that some SDCs never occur.

It should be apparent that the values used in an SDC are discrete. A particular symptom or disease is either a member of a particular SDC or it is not, but we already know that the data dealt with in the clinic can be less than perfectly reliable. A test may indicate that a sign is present, but we can rarely be absolutely certain. The unreliability of medical information can be incorporated into the set theory approach by thinking of the

Table 3-3. Reduced Truth Table Representation for Two Symptoms and Two Diseases[a]

Symptom (S) or Disease (D)	Possible Relationships			
S(1)	0	0	0	0
S(2)	1	1	1	1
D(1)	1	1	0	0
D(2)	1	0	1	0

[a] Adapted from Kleinmuntz (1984). Used here with the permission of Pergamon Press.

various SDCs as "fuzzy" sets in which membership is continuous rather than all-or-none.

Fuzzy sets and fuzzy logic (Zadeh, 1973) provide a more realistic picture of medical judgment than traditional set theory, but even fuzzy sets fail to capture much of what is unique about clinical judgment. (The same can be said about linear and algebraic models as well.) For example, doctors often know more about diseases than just their correlated signs. They may also know something about cause and effect. Given a set of predictors, they may be able to infer what other predictors will indicate; they may also be able to make prognoses that can lead to the verification or refutation of certain diagnoses. In other words, clinical decision making is "dynamic." In the clinic, "decisions are made sequentially in time; the task specifications may change over time . . . information available for later decisions may be contingent upon the outcome of earlier ones; and the implications of any decision may reach into the future" (Rapoport & Wallsten, 1972, p. 325). Information integration in dynamic decision making is discussed next.

Dynamic Decision Making

The decision models discussed thus far assume that all necessary information has been collected before judgments are made. However, this is rarely the case in the clinical situation, in which information is gathered sequentially and where new tests are ordered based on the results of earlier ones. Probably because dynamic decision making is more difficult to study than static decision making (see Slovic et al., 1977, for some reasons why), it has not been investigated as fully. Nevertheless, studies have been done. Most of these rely on the analysis of verbal protocols. Decision makers are asked to think aloud and then attempts are made to model their thinking processes, usually in the form of a computer program (see Wortman, 1972, for instance).

In protocol analysis, much attention has been devoted to the sequence in which information is gathered (Payne, 1980). It is usually taken for granted that the decision maker's verbal reports accurately reflect the decision-making sequence. However, verbal protocols may be biased even though they appear to be consistent (Fidler, 1983; Nisbett & Wilson, 1977). An approach to protocol analysis that may eliminate many potential biases was described by Kleinmuntz (1984). This technique requires that a clinician pretend to have a disease while another physician tries to discover what it is. The physician playing the role of diagnostician asks the "patient" questions about the relevant symptoms and signs and their entire interaction is recorded. The interaction is then coded into a kind of decision tree in which each node represents a question and each branch an answer. Trees constructed from the protocols of several different doctors (or the same doctor on several occasions)

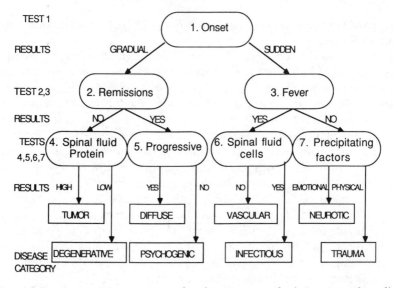

Figure 3-5   A summary statement showing one neurologist's approach to diagnosis. The tree is based on the questions asked by the neurologist during simulated diagnostic sessions. From Kleinmuntz (1984) and reprinted here with the permission of Pergamon Press.

can serve as a generalized model of how information is gathered and integrated. Figure 3-5 illustrates such a model for one expert neurologist. As may be seen, she began by asking whether the problem's onset was sudden or gradual. If the answer is gradual, she pursues a set of questions designed to distinguish tumor from degenerative and psychogenic causes. On the other hand, if the onset was sudden, then traumatic causes as well as infections and vascular causes are explored.

A computer program can be developed based on the flow chart in Figure 3-5. In fact, this is just what Kleinmuntz recommends. The computer program can then be tested to see whether it is as successful as the expert diagnostician. Several computer programs have been developed this way (see Wortman, 1972, for instance) and several have turned out to be good diagnosticians (De Dombal & Gremy, 1976).

Although dynamic models of information integration and decision making are probably more realistic representations of clinical judgment than static ones, they also have their shortcomings. For example, the strict control over the sequence of actions implied by flow charts seems too rigid to be realistic. Not even experts always follow the same information-gathering sequence. There is no objective way to determine which of several sequences is "better." Since it is quite possible to produce a computer program that makes excellent clinical judgments but does not do so in the same way as a human clinician (see Shortliffe, 1976, for example), diagnostic accuracy by itself cannot assure that a program is behaving as a clinician would (see Taylor, Aitchison, & McGirr, 1971).

One way that dynamic decision making may be improved is by incorporating relevant findings from related areas of psychological research. A start has been made in this direction by Fox (1980), whose studies of the diagnostic process have already been mentioned. Fox designed a computerized judgment task in which medical student subjects had to decide whether a patient suffered from tonsillitis, meningitis, laryngitis, hepatitis, or parotitis based on symptoms such as dysphagia, vomiting, headache, earache, and pyrexia. The computer program provided the students with a presenting symptom and then the students were permitted to interrogate the program about any or all of the remaining symptoms. Whenever they felt confident enough, the students could make a diagnosis, at which point the computer program provided feedback on their accuracy. The program defined accuracy as the most likely diagnosis according to Bayes' formula. Over the course of the experiment, the students made many diagnoses and received feedback many times. Thus, the students were learning which symptoms go with which diseases. As a test to see how much the students learned, Fox interspersed the diagnostic trials with memory tests that required them to verify statements such as "Pyrexia goes with meningitis."

Fox found that diagnostic accuracy was very high. By the time the students had gone through 50 diagnostic problems, their diagnoses were the same as the Bayesian ones 85% of the time. As was expected, performance on the memory tests also improved during the course of the experiment. Fox was able to draw a tree diagram depicting his subjects' data-gathering strategy. He wrote two computer programs based on the information in the decision tree. The first program used Bayes' rule to revise probabilities in the light of symptom information. The second program was based on the psychological research on judgment heuristics. Its rules took the following form: "For the first disease that comes to mind, ask about the first symptom associated with it that is already known" or "For the first two diseases that come to mind, ask about the first symptom that is thought of that will discriminate between them" (1980, p. 208). The program based on heuristics actually produced a closer fit to the students' behavior than one based on Bayesian probability revision. Although only a first step, Fox's research shows how computer models may be improved by the incorporation of psychological research on human judgment and decision making. Unfortunately, most psychological theories cannot yet be stated with the precision of mathematical theories, but attempts are being made to make them more formal (Lopes, 1982).

Summary

Faced with an enormous potential data base, modern physicians must somehow learn to choose which information sources to examine, decide what the data mean, and then integrate these data into some overall judgment. Although medical textbooks often view the process of hypothesis formation and evaluation as relatively straightforward, in reality doctors are hampered by the same cognitive limitations that affect all types of human information processing. Rationality appears to have bounds. Cognitive overload, the need to understand probabilistic data, and the usual desire to take *some* action has led to the development of certain rules of thumb. Rather than adhere strictly to normative decision rules, decision makers use heuristics, which most often lead to good judgments but can also result in biases.

The decision heuristics reviewed in this chapter appear more likely to create biases in the psychology laboratory than in the clinic, leading some writers to suggest that their importance has been overstated. However, they do sometimes appear even in the clinic and, more importantly, they do appear to describe how clinicians think (see Fox, 1980).

Decision models developed to describe how information is integrated have taken either a mathematical approach (additive, algebraic) or an information-processing one. The former have the advantage of being stated in clear-cut mathematical terms, but they appear unlikely to describe the cognitive operations underlying how human beings actually go about making judgments. Information-processing models, while more likely to capture the dynamic nature of medical judgments, are more difficult to create and to test. Clearly, the ideal model would capture the best aspects of both. Attempts to produce such models by analyzing the judgments of experts are discussed in Chapter 5.

Chapters 2 and 3 have been concerned with data gathering and evaluation. We have concentrated on the nature of medical data and the ways in which physicians gather and interpret it. In the next chapter, we look at how doctors use their interpretations to choose a course of action.

4

Choosing Actions

The value of life lies not in the length of days but in the use you make of them.

Montaigne

Gathering and interpreting clinical data, the subjects of Chapters 2 and 3, respectively, are only means to an end—choosing an appropriate course of action. The action chosen can be one of several possible treatments or simply a decision to wait and see what happens. The present chapter is concerned with the factors that determine which action is chosen. There are many ways to answer the question: Which action is best? There is one answer that is overwhelmingly favored by decision analysts. For them, the only sensible action is the one specified by subjective expected utility (SEU) theory.

In Chapter 1, we introduced SEU theory as a way of making decisions when outcomes were uncertain. We noted that SEU theory incorporates a normative choice principle that requires the decision maker to estimate the probability and utility of the various possible judgment outcomes and to combine these by multiplication. Subjective expected utility theory also specifies the rule by which actions should be chosen. Typically, this rule states that the "best" action is the one that maximizes utilities. (Exactly whose utilities should be maximized is a matter we leave for later discussion.) Decision analysis, a technique introduced by Raiffa (1968) and Schlaifer (1969), is designed to apply the normative approach embodied in SEU theory to practical decision problems. Recently, decision analysts have devoted considerable effort to showing doctors how to use decision analysis to guide patient management decisions (see Weinstein & Fineberg, 1980, for example).

Although decision analysis provides a powerful technology for making clinical judgments, there are a number of pitfalls awaiting the unwary. Generating appropriate hypotheses, assessing subjective probabilities, interpreting conditional probabilities, knowing which data are relevant, and the ability to integrate information from diverse sources are all skills required for the successful application of decision analysis. As we have seen, these skills are less than perfectly developed in the average clinician. Because no one consistently makes optimum decisions and because behavior sometimes fails to conform to the requirements of normative theories, psychologists have tried to develop descriptive theories as a way of understanding how physicians make patient management decisions (see Elstein, 1982, for several examples). In this chapter, we examine both types of theories. Specifically, the focus is on how doctors use the information they have gathered (and interpreted) to choose actions.

To provide a frame of reference for the discussions that follow, the chapter begins with an outline of the steps involved in making decisions when outcomes are not known with certainty—a situation known as risky decision making. This is followed by an example of medical decision making that follows this outline step by step. The remaining sections of the chapter are concerned with psychological research on risky decision making. Each step in the process is examined in detail. As in earlier chapters, we attempt to show how psychological research can help clarify why decision makers sometimes fail to conform to the dictates of SEU theory and, perhaps, how medical judgment may be improved.

Steps in Risky Decision Making

Although they are not always stated explicitly, there are five broad steps that decision analysts generally agree are involved in making risky decisions:

1. The decision maker first forms an internal cognitive representation of the decision task.
2. The probability of the various outcomes is assessed. These probabilities may be estimated from the relevant literature. When the required data are unavailable or equivocal, subjective probabilities must suffice.
3. The consequences of the various outcomes are assigned a utility.
4. The probabilities assessed in Step 2 are combined with the utilities of Step 3 for all relevant outcomes.
5. The decision maker chooses a course of action according to some decision rule. Usually, this is the action that maximizes expected utility.

These five steps are common to any approach to decision making based on SEU theory. Their validity depends, therefore, on the axioms of that theory and on certain "operational" assumptions (Kozielecki, 1981). The most important of these assumptions are:

1. Probability and utility assessments for the various outcomes are made independently. That is, the probability of an outcome does not affect its subjective value and vice versa.
2. The probability of all possible outcomes totals to 1.00. This means that no relevant outcome has been omitted from consideration.
3. Probabilities and utilities are mutually compensating so that a high value for one can compensate for a low value for the other.

In the discussions that follow, we examine how well these operational assumptions are met in real world clinical decision making. First, however, we show how these steps are supposed to work by describing an example.

A Prescriptive Example

The power of decision analysis as a method of making patient management decisions is brilliantly illustrated by the "Clinical Decision Making Rounds" that appear in the journal *Medical Decision Making*. In this series of articles, Stephen Pauker and his colleagues apply decision analysis to a variety of cases. Taken as a group, the articles provide an exceptionally complete course in how to apply decision analysis to medical problems. The case to be discussed here is adapted from a report by Klein and Pauker (1981). It was chosen because of its interest and its completeness.

The patient, a 25-year-old woman called E.W., was 3 months pregnant when she developed pain and swelling in her left thigh. A venogram revealed a blocked vein leading to the diagnosis of deep venous thrombophlebitis (DVT), a problem she had also suffered from 2 years earlier. E.W. was treated with intravenous heparin (an anticoagulant) and her condition improved. E.W.'s doctors wanted to maintain her on anticoagulants because they feared she might produce a pulmonary embolism—a potentially fatal development. At the same time, there was the possibility that anticoagulants could harm her unborn baby.

Structuring the Problem

Because E.W. wished to continue the pregnancy, there were really two decisions to be made. First, it had to be decided whether or not she would receive anticoagulants. The potential risk to her life from a pulmonary embolism argued for continuing anticoagulant treatment while the risk to her unborn child argued against. The second decision depended upon the first. If drug treatment was to be continued, E.W.'s physicians had to decide which anticoagulant to use. The choice was between warfarin, which is an effective treatment for thrombophlebitis but is known to produce "fetopathy" (fetal abnormalities and possibly death), and heparin, which also increases perinatal mortality but is not associated with fetal abnormality. Unfortunately, heparin's effectiveness against DVT when administered subcutaneously (as it would have been in this case because E.W. was not confined to the hospital) is unclear. Thus, E.W. and her doctors had somehow to choose between an increased risk of fetal abnormality with warfarin and the uncertain efficacy of heparin.

Assessing the Risks

Once the problem has been structured, the next step in a decision analysis involves evaluating the probability of the various outcomes. In the present example, three questions had to be answered:

1. What is the incidence and mortality of pulmonary embolism among patients with DVT?
2. How effective are warfarin and heparin?
3. What is the incidence of fetal complications with each drug?

Klein and Pauker sought an answer to the first question from the medical literature. Across studies, estimates of the incidence of pulmonary embolism among patients with DVT range from 9% to 30%. Estimates of the mortality of pulmonary embolism range from 18% to 30%. In other words, patients with DVT have a substantial probability of producing a pulmonary embolism and many who do so will die. With regard to the efficiency of anticoagulants, Klein and Pauker's examination of the relevant literature indicated that warfarin treatment substantially reduces the likelihood that a pulmonary embolism will be produced. When patients receiving warfarin are compared with untreated patients, studies show that the drug reduces the likelihood of a pulmonary embolism by 52% to 100%. Subcutaneous administration of heparin has also been found to reduce the probability of pulmonary embolisms. When the two drugs have been compared directly, warfarin was found somewhat more likely to reduce the recurrence of DVT, but no real data are available to indicate which drug is better at preventing pulmonary embolisms. The side effects produced by the two drugs are fairly similar; both, for example, can produce serious, even fatal, bleeding. As for fetal complications, warfarin administered to women in the second or third trimester of pregnancy has been associated with a 13% risk of perinatal death while heparin has a 20% risk. In live births, warfarin increased fetal abnormalities by 10% whereas heparin appeared to produce practically no abnormalities at all. (See Klein and Pauker for the relevant literature citations.)

Klein and Pauker present the decision facing E.W. and her doctors in the form of two tree diagrams, which are reproduced in slightly amended form in Figures 4-1 and 4-2. Figure 4-1 depicts the possible outcomes of the decision to administer (or not administer) anticoagu-

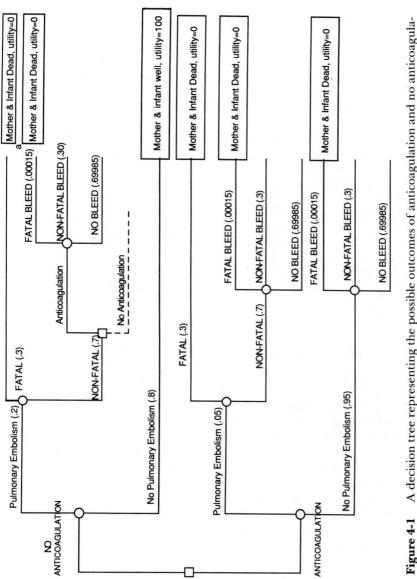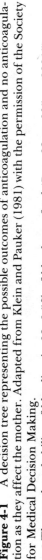

Figure 4-1   A decision tree representing the possible outcomes of anticoagulation and no anticoagulation as they affect the mother. Adapted from Klein and Pauker (1981) with the permission of the Society for Medical Decision Making.

ª The total probability of bleeding is .03; 0.5% of bleeds are fatal ($P = .03 \times .005 = .00015$).

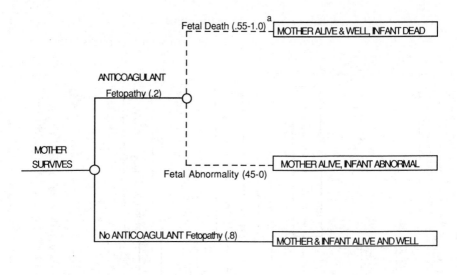

(^{a}.55 for Warfarin, 1.00 for Heparin)

Figure 4-2 A decision tree representing the possible outcomes of the decision to treat with anticoagulants as they affect the unborn child. Adapted from Klein and Pauker (1981) with the permission of the Society for Medical Decision Making.

lants. The problem-solving sequence in this, or any, tree diagram, goes from left to right. The square at the extreme left represents the therapy choice decision. The outcomes of each step in the decision-making sequence, as they affect the mother, are represented by circles. The relevant probabilities gathered from the literature (and a few guesses) appear in parentheses. Thus, it can be seen in Figure 4-1 that, if E.W.'s doctors choose not to administer anticoagulants, the probability that she will develop a pulmonary embolism, as indicated by the literature, is .20. The probability that she will not produce an embolism is .80 (1 − .20). If E.W. does produce an embolism, the probability that it will be fatal is .30; the probability that she would survive such an event is therefore .70. Because a nonfatal embolism may be treated with anticoagulants, the decision tree allows for the possibility of withholding anticoagulants until a nonfatal embolism occurs.

Figure 4-1 does not include fetal abnormalities as possible outcomes of the decision to administer anticoagulants. These are depicted in Figure 4-2. As may be seen, anticoagulants can cause fetal death or fetal abnormalities, but, in the best of all possible outcomes, the drugs may not harm the child at all and both mother and baby will be fine.

Utility Measurement

According to SEU theory, the appropriate course of action is usually the one that maximizes expected utility. Since Klein and Pauker's decision analysis depends on SEU theory for its logic, they measured the utility of the various outcomes. Although all possible outcomes were relevant, Klein and Pauker focused on only four. They ignored nonfatal maternal bleeding because they believed such an outcome would produce only "minor changes in utility" (p. 188). The four outcomes considered were:*

1. Mother and infant both alive and well
2. Mother well but infant born with abnormalities
3. Mother well but infant dead
4. Mother and infant both dead

Since they believed that the first outcome was the most favorable one, it was arbitrarily assigned a utility value of 100. The outcome they considered least favorable (mother and infant both dead) was assigned an arbitrary utility value of 0. These "end-point" utilities appear at the extreme right of Figure 4-1. The two remaining outcomes have utilities somewhere between these two extremes; these utilities must be determined in order to complete the decision analysis. Klein and Pauker described one method for estimating utilities, which is discussed, along with others, later in this chapter. For now, it is important to note that Klein and Pauker did not actually discuss utilities with E.W. Instead, they examined what effect a wide range of utilities would have on the decision to initiate anticoagulant therapy.

Calculating Expected Utilities

Once utilities are specified, the expected utility of the primary decision (should anticoagulants be administered) may be calculated by multiplying the utilities at the end of each branch in the decision tree by the probabilities at each chance node and adding these together.

Klein and Pauker realized that they had made a fair number of assumptions and compromises in their decision analysis, any of which may have influenced the outcome. To see how much influence their various estimates of the parameters had on the final outcome, they undertook what is known as a *sensitivity analysis*. The goal of a sensitivity analysis is to determine what effect alterations in one or more parameters has on the decision outcome. If changes in a parameter (a probability or a utility) lead to a different decision, the decision is said to be "sensitive" to alterations in that parameter.

---

* The utility of negative outcomes (fetal death, for example) often strikes readers as a strange notion. In the present example, it is probably best to think of the negative outcomes as the "least of all evils," second least, and so on.

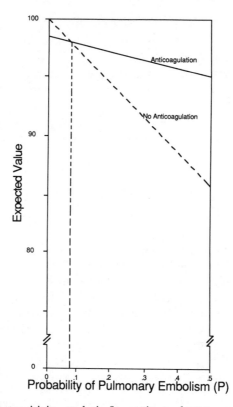

Figure 4-3   A sensitivity analysis for anticoagulant treatment. At a very low probability of embolism (less than .1), no treatment leads to a higher expected value than treatment. However, at probabilities greater than this anticoagulation treatment is preferred. Reprinted from Klein and Pauker (1981) with the permission of the Society for Medical Decision Making.

Figure 4-3 illustrates one of their sensitivity analyses. The figure depicts what happens when the probability of a pulmonary embolism is varied between 0 and .5. (In the original decision analysis, this probability was taken to be .2.) As can be seen, if nothing else changes, anticoagulation therapy is preferred—it has a higher subjective utility than no treatment—so long as the probability of a pulmonary embolism remains above .084. Only when an embolism is extremely unlikely should no treatment be given. Put another way, the decision analysis is not very sensitive to changes in the probability of an embolism; the final decision only changes when this probability is reduced by more than 50%.

Similar sensitivity analyses conducted on the other probabilities and utilities in the decision analysis indicated that the outcome was also relatively insensitive to changes in these parameters (provided all other probabilities remain unchanged). However, since it is possible for two or

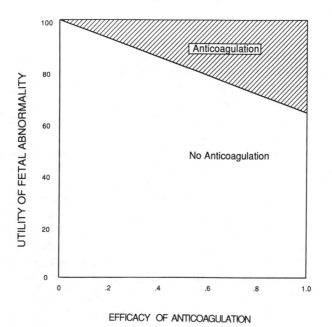

EFFICACY OF ANTICOAGULATION

Figure 4-4   A two-way sensitivity analysis. When the utility for fetopathy is high and the efficacy of anticoagulant treatment is low then it is best not to treat. However, as the probability of successful treatment increases, or as the utility for fetopathy decreases, treatment becomes the preferred option. Reprinted from Klein and Pauker (1981) with the permission of the Society for Medical Decision Making.

more probabilities to vary jointly, Klein and Pauker also considered what happens when several related probabilities change at the same time. An example of a "two-factor" sensitivity analysis appears in Figure 4-4. This figure shows the relationship between the mother's utility for fetopathy and the efficacy of anticoagulation drugs when changes in one of these variables produces a change in the other. For example, if more efficacious drugs were available, therapy could be recommended at lower levels of utility.

Overall, the sensitivity analyses showed that the decision to use anticoagulants was relatively insensitive to changes in the probabilities of pulmonary embolism, anticoagulant-produced fetopathy, and maternal anticoagulant complications. The decision then became a matter of which drug was best. The answer to this question depended on E.W.'s attitude toward fetal death and abnormality and the efficacy of low-dose heparin. If fetal death is easier for her to bear than an abnormal infant, heparin is the drug of choice. However, if an abnormal baby is preferred, then warfarin is the better drug. The point on the utility curve at which warfarin is administered instead of heparin depends on the doctor's estimate of each drug's effectiveness. This relationship is depicted in Figure 4-5. This figure also illustrates that the product of this decision analysis is not a simple yes-or-no answer to the original questions but a rational basis for selecting therapy that can be adapted to the attitudes of any woman facing a similar problem. The analysis can also be adapted to new developments such as the availability of more effective drugs.

In addition to the assumptions already noted, Klein and Pauker's decision analysis is based on several implicit meta-assumptions. For example, they assume that the subjective value of different outcomes (fetal death versus fetal abnormalities) can be measured accurately on a single arbitrary scale. They also assume that the risks and benefits of treatment alternatives can be compared directly and that all significant potential outcomes are known. That is, they assume there are no missing branches to the decision tree. Of course, they also assume that SEU theory provides a normative set of rules for making decisions. The remainder of this chapter examines these, and related, assumptions in greater detail. We begin by looking at how problems are structured.

Structuring the Decision Task

Before a risky choice can be made, the significant elements of the decision, as well as their relationships, must first be identified. This is accomplished in the first step in the decision-making sequence by forming a cognitive model of the decision problem (Kozielecki, 1981). This model is created from the decision maker's stored knowledge about similar decisions made in similar situations, the decision maker's utilities for various outcomes, and specific information gathered about the present problem. Since decision makers vary in experience, values, and their effectiveness in gathering and organizing data, different decision makers may formulate different models of the same decision task.

An illustration of how a task's representation can affect decision making appears in Figure 4-6. The two tree diagrams in this figure represent cognitive models formed by two hospital administrators. The decision they face concerns whether or not to equip their respective hospital laboratories to perform a new blood assay. The assay in question can presently be ordered from private pathologists on a fee-for-service basis, but doing it in the hospital laboratory may be less costly. The assay is a useful adjunct to diagnosis, but the presently available techniques are crude and require expensive equipment that may become obsolete as new techniques become available. Figure 4-6 shows that the two hospital administrators do not emphasize the same aspects of the problem. Their different representations can lead them to different decisions.

Once a problem representation is created, the calculations required for a decision analysis are fairly mechanical. In fact, it may well be said

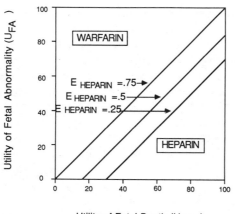

Utility of Fetal Death (U_FD)

Figure 4-5   Choice of drug depends on the utilities for fetal abnormality and for fetal death. Heparin is preferred when the utility for fetal death is relatively high and the utility for fetal abnormality is relatively low. When the opposite is the case, warfarin is preferred. The dividing point between the two depends on the efficacy of the drugs. Thus, the outcome of the decision analysis need not be a rigid choice, but rather a rational guide to appropriate clinical behavior. Reprinted from Klein and Pauker (1981) with the permission of the Society for Medical Decision Making.

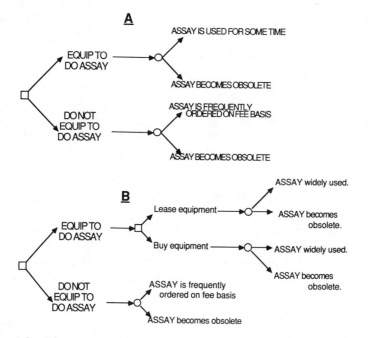

Figure 4-6   The way a decision is represented can exert an important influence on the final outcome. This figure illustrates two different ways of considering whether a hospital should equip to do a new assay.

that the decision analyst's major task is to structure the decision problem. If the problem is conceptualized incorrectly, all subsequent calculations (probabilities, utilities, and so on) will be invalid. Unfortunately, before a decision is made and an outcome observed, it is difficult to know whether a task has been well structured. To make things even more difficult, there is no absolute criterion for deciding exactly what a "well-structured" decision task is. In recent years, psychologists have devoted considerable effort to studying how people create internal cognitive models of decision tasks. One of the findings of this research is that tasks viewed as probabilistic by decision analysts are not always viewed that way by those involved in making decisions. These findings are discussed next.

Probabilistic versus Nonprobabilistic Representations

Decision analyses based on normative theories such as SEU assume that the decision problem is represented adequately and that all relevant outcomes have been identified. They take it for granted that decision makers recognize the probabilistic nature of their risky decisions and are aware of the role of random factors in determining potential outcomes. Peterson and Beach (1967) went as far as to argue that people are "intuitive" statisticians who rarely commit serious errors in interpreting the meaning of probability. As we have shown in Chapter 3, more recent research on judgment heuristics gives us reason to doubt that most people are intuitive statisticians. Psychological research has also provided us with reason to doubt that our mental representations are faithful models of real world decision tasks.

Payne and Braunstein (1971), for example, explored cognitive task representations using a technique called "duplex gambles." Duplex gambles consist of pairs of wagers in which the total probability (across both wagers) of winning or losing is equal but in which the pairs differ in their specific characteristics. An example of a duplex gamble appears in Figure 4-7.

To see how these gambles work, imagine that each of the circular discs is really a revolving wheel with a pointer attached to its center. In Gamble 1, the larger portion of the first wheel occupies 60% of the disc; the smaller, 40%. On the second wheel in Gamble 1, the two portions are equal. Let us now assume that the pointers in Gamble 1 are set in motion simultaneously. Depending on which portion of the wheel the pointer comes to rest in, you will win or lose the amounts indicated. (If the pointer stops in the zero portion of the wheel, there are no consequences.) There are, therefore, four possible outcomes, and the probability of each can be calculated simply by assigning each portion of the wheel a likelihood equivalent to its size. The outcomes and their associated probabilities are:

Gambles

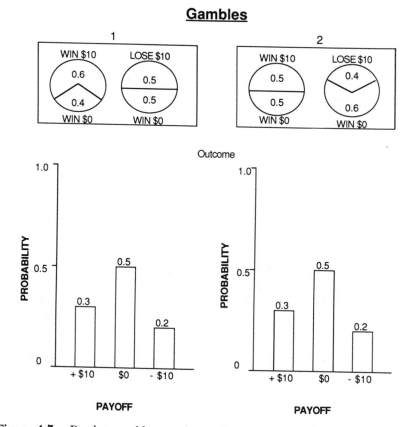

Figure 4-7   Duplex gambles require a choice between two pairs of gambles. The top part of the figure illustrates the gambles in the form of "wheels of fortune." The bar graphs illustrate that the probability distributions are the same and that the two gambles have the same expected value. The overall payout is what should be important, so the two gambles should be equally preferred, but they are not. Adapted from Wright (1984) with the permission of Penguin Books. Copyright © George Wright, 1984.

1. Win $10, Lose $10 = .6 × .5 = .3
2. Win $0, Win $0 = .4 × .5 = .2
3. Win $10, Win $0 = .6 × .5 = .3
4. Win $0, Lose $10 = .4 × .5 = .2

Since outcomes 1 and 2 both lead to identical results (no gain and no loss), their probabilities can be summed, producing the following distribution for the various outcomes:

Win $10 probability = .3
Lose $10 probability = .2
Even probability = .5

If the same procedure is applied to duplex Gamble 2, it will be found to have precisely the same probability distribution for the same three outcomes. Nevertheless, Payne and Braunstein's subjects expressed distinct preferences for one gamble over the other. These preferences appeared to arise from the way the task was structured. Instead of generating mental models of the various probabilities, the subjects in this experiment focused on what they believed to be important attributes of the gambles. Specifically, they examined qualities such as the payoff level and the size of potential losses. Each of these attributes was treated as a separate judgment criterion, and the gamble that "scored" highest on the various criteria, irrespective of their expected utility, was the one they preferred. For example, since the probability of losing $10 is greater in Gamble 1 (.5) than Gamble 2 (.4), many subjects viewed Gamble 2 more positively than Gamble 1. Other subjects focused on the probability of winning $10 and, therefore, preferred Gamble 1, in which this probability was greater.

It seems that Payne and Braunstein's subjects examined the probabilities and payoffs associated with the various gambles but did not use this information in the way that SEU theory dictates. One explanation for their behavior is simple ignorance. It is possible that Payne and Braunstein's subjects were just unfamiliar with the concept of expected value and the necessary computations (Cohen & Hansel, 1956). However, studies by Lichtenstein et al. (1969) and Gawryszewska (cited in Kozielecki, 1981) have found that people do not use expected value (or expected utility) as a guide to choice even when the concept, and calculations, are explained to them. These researchers found their subjects willing to allow their utilities (as reflected by their preferences) to be influenced by the probabilities of the various outcomes—a clear violation of one of the operational assumptions underlying SEU theory.

The duplex gambles studied by Payne and Braunstein are clearly artificial. It is also true that calculating outcome probability distributions may be beyond the knowledge of most of their subjects. Nevertheless, their findings are still relevant to clinical decision making. Recall that E.W.'s doctors had to decide whether to continue anticoagulant therapy and, if so, which drug to administer. In making their decisions, they had to consider drug effectiveness, the probability of fetopathy, and the probability of maternal death. Their decisions can be described in the form of duplex gambles with different probability distributions. For example, E.W. and her doctors had to choose between two probabilities of forming a pulmonary embolism (with and without anticoagulants) and two probability distributions for fetal abnormalities and death (with and without anticoagulants). It seems quite possible that, faced with these "duplex gambles," E.W. and her doctors may behave similarly to Payne and Braunstein's subjects. That is, they may base their preferences not on expected utility but on qualitative aspects of the gambles without regard to expected utility.

One way to conceptualize Payne and Braunstein's findings is in terms of "risk." From this viewpoint, some of their subjects based their preferences for one or another set of gambles on what they perceived to be the greater "risk" of losing $10 in Gamble 1. Others were willing to take a chance on Gamble 1 because, to them, it appeared to lead to greater potential gain. Mathematically, both lines of reasoning are incorrect; the potential gains and losses of the two sets of gambles are identical. Psychologically, however, they appear different. Since risk perceptions seem to affect preferences, predicting behavior requires more than a consideration of SEU alone. It also requires an understanding of how people think about, and perceive, risk.

What is Risk?

The most general definition of a risky decision is one in which the outcome of an action (or actions) cannot be predicted with certainty. For example, when you decide whether to buy a health insurance policy, you do not know whether or not you will become ill. Because you are uncertain about what will happen, choosing one of the two alternatives (buy or not buy) involves some degree of risk. If you do not insure and you require medical care you will have incurred a loss. On the other hand, if you buy insurance and stay healthy, you will have wasted the premium. Clearly, the decision faced by E.W.'s doctors was also a risky one. Prescribing anticoagulants could increase the risk of death or abnormality to the child; foregoing anticoagulants could lead to the death of E.W. herself.

Risk is a fact of life. Many of the decisions we make each day (Should I wear a seatbelt?; Should I have one more drink?) involve some degree of risk. Since it is impossible to avoid risk entirely, we, like E.W.'s doctors, must learn to deal with it. Decision analysis is one method for choosing among risky alternatives, but the validity of decision analysis rests upon an important assumption—that risks can be quantified in a way that makes them amenable to expected utility calculations.

Definitions of Risk and Related Concepts

It is possible to find references to many different types of risk in both the popular and professional literature: social risks, economic risks, safety risks, political risks, and health risks, to name a few. Workers in each field define the term "risk" rather differently (Fischhoff, Watson, & Hope, 1984). In an attempt to provide some standard definitions, Kaplan and Garrick (1981) adopted a generalized quantitative approach. The following definitions are based on their work.

Risk versus uncertainty

Although the concept of risk always involves some degree of uncertainty, the two are not identical. A pregnant woman may be uncertain about whether her child will be a girl or boy, but it can hardly be said that these two outcomes put her at risk. Risks involve both uncertainty and loss or damage. Kaplan and Garrick illustrated this relationship with a symbolic equation: Risk = Uncertainty + Damage (p. 12).

Risks versus hazards

Kaplan and Garrick also distinguished between risks and hazards. Hazards are a source of danger that may or may not pose a risk depending on the specific situation. For example, the ambient radiation produced by radiography constitutes a hazard to technicians who fail to take proper safeguards. By wearing protective clothing and standing behind a shield, however, risk can be effectively reduced. Kaplan and Garrick illustrated the relationship between risk and hazard as: Risk = Hazard/Safeguard (p. 12). This equation shows that risks may be reduced by increasing safeguards but they can never be reduced to zero. Both common sense and algebra will not allow it.

Risk perception

Risks are always relative. Suppose, for example, that two patients have been prescribed birth control pills. One has read an article implicating the pills as potential causes of blood clots, the other has not. For this reason, the latter person views the pills as quite safe while the former sees them as "risky." In other words, risk is not absolute; it varies with the observer. Many authors call an individual's perception of a situation "perceived risk"; we use this term as well. However, it is worthwhile noting that the term is somewhat misleading. As Kaplan and Garrick noted, calling something a "perceived risk" implies that there is some other sort of risk that is objective or at least "not perceived." In reality, however, all risks are relative to an observer; they must be perceived by someone. Even scientific estimates of risk are not entirely objective; they, too, require that judgment be exercised (Fischhoff et al., 1984).

To summarize, risk involves both uncertain decision outcomes and the possibility of loss. Risks arise from hazards but, depending on the safeguards taken, hazards may be made more or less risky (but the risk is never zero). Finally, risks are not absolute, objective properties of events; they depend on the actions one takes and one's knowledge about the outcome of these actions.

Factors Determining Perceived Risk

If the subjective perception of the risk involved in a decision affects preferences, it is worthwhile studying what factors in a decision situation affect perceived risk. Psychological research on this question has revealed that, to a great extent, risk perception is a function of the way in which judgment problems are presented. Consider, for example, a decision problem taken from Tversky and Kahneman (1981):

> Imagine that the USA is preparing for the outbreak of an unusual Asian disease which is expected to kill 600 people. Two alternative programs to combat the disease are proposed. Assume that the exact scientific estimate of the consequences of the program are as follows:
>
> If program A is adopted, 200 people will be saved
> If program B is adopted, there is a 1/3 probability that 600 people will be saved, and 2/3 probability that no people will be saved
>
> Which of the two programs do you favor? (p. 153).

Mathematically, the expected outcome of both programs is identical. That is, both are expected to result in 200 people being saved. Yet, when Tversky and Kahneman presented this problem to 152 people they found 72% preferred program A to program B. This preference can be explained if we assume that program B was perceived as riskier than A because its results were stated in terms of probabilities while the outcome of A was a sure thing. Tversky and Kahneman's subjects appeared to be avoiding risk by choosing a sure thing over a probability. A second group of 152 people was given the same problem as the first but with the following new alternatives to choose from:

If program C is adopted 400 people will die
If program D is adopted there is 1/3 probability that nobody will die, and 2/3 probability that 600 people will die

These two programs have the same expected outcome—400 deaths. This time, 78% of the subjects preferred program D to program C. It appears that when the sure thing is negative (400 dead rather than 200 saved), people prefer to take the "gamble."

These findings are important for medical decision making because they suggest that preferences for identical outcomes may change depending on whether negative or positive attributes of these outcomes are emphasized. A demonstration of this in a medical context was reported by McNeil, Pauker, Sox, and Tversky (1982), who asked people to imagine that they had lung cancer and to choose between two types of therapy. Everyone in the study received detailed descriptions of the two treatments, but half were told the probability of surviving for varying lengths of time with each treatment ("68 per cent survive 5 years," for example) while the other half were given the probability of dying ("32 per cent die within 5 years"). It was found that the way the numbers were presented determined therapy choice. Both laypersons and doctors had different preferences depending on whether the probabilities were stated in terms of death rates or survival rates.

Eraker and Sox (1981) performed a similar experiment in which subjects were required to choose between two drug therapies for each of three conditions (headaches, hypertension, and chest pain.) Their subjects read scenarios describing the various treatments. The outcome of one drug treatment was always stated with certainty while the other drug was always described as having two possible outcomes that could occur with stated probabilities. When the possible outcomes were stated as gains (blood pressure decreases, for example), subjects preferred the drug with a certain outcome even when the alternative had the potential to provide greater relief. When outcomes were described as losses (certain nausea versus some probability of nausea, for instance), people preferred the probabilistic alternative. This finding held true for patients suffering from the various conditions as well as randomly selected nonpatients. Eraker and Sox concluded that attitudes toward therapies depend on the manner in which they are presented. When two alternative treatments are available, doctors may produce different risk perceptions in their patients by emphasizing either their therapeutic effects or their negative side effects.

The preference for certain (100% probable) outcomes, when these are expressed as gains, was also demonstrated by Slovic et al. (1982a) in the context of a judgment concerning vaccinations. Two questionnaires were constructed. The first described a disease expected to affect 20% of the population and asked whether respondents would volunteer to receive a vaccine that is 50% effective against the disease. The second questionnaire stated that there were two mutually exclusive, and equally probable, strains of the disease and that each is likely to affect 10% of the population. The vaccine was said to be 100% effective against one strain and completely ineffective against the other. Although both forms of the questionnaire indicated that the vaccine reduces the risk of disease by 10%, those who received the second questionnaire were more likely to favor vaccinations than those who read the first one. Tversky and Kahneman would explain this finding as a result of "pseudodiagnosticity" (see Chapter 3). Since the second questionnaire described the vaccine as 100% effective, it was perceived as less risky than the 50% effective vaccine described in the first.

Because the outcome of a decision analysis often depends on how the problem is represented, there have been several attempts to develop aids to help decision makers structure problems so that they are suitable for decision analysis. Several of these aids are discussed in Chapter 5. For now, we wish to turn to the second step in risky decision making—assessing the probability of the various outcomes.

Assessing the Probability of Outcomes

Decision analysis requires that the probability of all likely outcomes be evaluated. Sometimes it is possible to estimate the likelihood of potential outcomes from available frequency data (the number of fatal anesthetic reactions in general surgery, for example), or from epidemiological studies (the relationship between smoking and disease, for instance). However, there are other probabilities that cannot be estimated from direct experience at all. Examples of the latter are the side effects of new drugs and the complications of new surgical procedures. These probabilities can only be estimated by analogy to earlier findings and by the introduction of subjective judgments. In this section, we are concerned with studies of how the *subjective assessment* of such probabilities is accomplished and where it may go wrong.

Measuring Subjective Probability

Risk analysis is a type of decision analysis in which the emphasis is on expected costs (disutilities) rather than expected gains. It involves the same steps described for risky decision making earlier in this chapter. When a risk analysis is combined with an analysis of benefits, the procedure is known as risk–benefit analysis. When risks are transformed into monetary estimates, this procedure is called cost–benefit analysis. Such analyses are discussed later in this chapter. Our present interest is solely on factors influencing the subjective probability of risks.

There are at least two ways to measure subjective probability—direct and indirect. As its name implies, the direct method simply involves asking the decision maker to provide a number from 0 to 1 corresponding to an outcome's probability: for example, "What is the probability that this patient's abdominal pains are the result of an inflamed appendix?" Sometimes, instead of probabilities, the physician is asked to provide odds (such as 10 to 1, 100 to 1, and so on). Odds can easily be converted to probabilities using the formula probability = odds/1 + odds. Thus, a doctor who gives odds of 10 to 1 against appendicitis is saying that the probability that the patient's symptoms are the result of appendicitis is actually only .091.

Indirect measures (also known as behavioral measures) require a series of judgments. For example, decision makers may be forced to choose between two bets: the probability of winning a lottery or winning a prize on the spin of a wheel of fortune. Two such bets are illustrated in Figure 4-8. The usual procedure is to begin with a small shaded area in the wheel and to ask the decision maker which wager is preferred. Generally, this will be the lottery. The size of the shaded area in the wheel is gradually increased (thereby increasing the probability of winning) until the wheel wager is preferred to the lottery. The shaded area is then

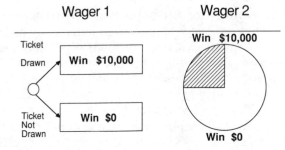

Figure 4-8 One way to measure probabilities is to compare a lottery (Wager 1) with a "wheel of fortune" (Wager 2). See text for details. Adapted from Wright (1984) with the permission of Penguin Books. Copyright © George Wright, 1984.

decreased until the decision maker is indifferent between the two bets. The ratio of shaded to unshaded portions of the wheel is taken to indicate the judge's subjective probability of winning the lottery. Note that this indirect method assumes that the wagers are identical. If an individual prefers the immediate payoff of the wheel to a lottery in which payoffs are delayed (until the end of the week, for example) then the indirect approach is invalid.

Although there has been little research on the relative reliability and validity of the two probability estimation methods, the available studies (see Slovic, 1962 and Slovic et al., 1977) appear to indicate that both approaches lead to fairly reliable estimates. Only when numbers are replaced with words ("very likely," "rare," and so on) does reliability fall below acceptable standards (see Chapter 2).

Judgment Bias in Risk Perception

As noted earlier, risks are always relative. Hazards appear more or less risky depending on who is making the judgment and the context in which the hazard is assessed. Since risk perceptions are relative, and mainly subjective, it is not surprising that they are susceptible to some of the judgment biases discussed in Chapter 3.

The availability heuristic exerts a particularly potent influence on risk perception because the ease with which an instance of an outcome can be called to mind is affected not only by its objective frequency but also by its emotional impact. This is why seeing films such as *Jaws* and *The China Syndrome* lead people to overestimate the risk of shark attack or nuclear power plant disasters (Slovic et al., 1982b). The availability heuristic may also explain why public discussion of the remote likelihood of contamination from new organisms created by recombinant DNA research has produced widespread overestimation of its risks (Slovic et al., 1981).

The influence of the availability heuristic is particularly striking in Slovic et al.'s (1979) study of the perceived lethality of various hazards (see Chapter 3). These researchers found that dramatic hazards (accidents, earthquakes, floods, tornadoes, homicides) were judged to be more common than they really are, while the probability of dying from an everyday killer such as diabetes, stroke, or asthma was consistently underestimated. Slovic et al. concluded that dramatic killers were more "available" than the less spectacular causes of death. In addition to its emotional impact, media coverage can also determine the perceived likelihood of a risk (Combs & Slovic, 1979). Among doctors, diseases have been found to be judged more prevalent the more attention they receive in medical journals (Christensen-Szalanski et al., 1983).

Reliance on the availability heuristic can also result in what appears to be a devil-may-care attitude toward everyday hazards. Svenson (1981), for example, found that just about everybody considers themselves less likely to have an automobile accident than the average driver.* Similarly, Weinstein (1980) found people to be unrealistically optimistic about their chances of escaping unpleasant life events. Most of his respondents believed they had a better than average chance to live past 80 and to escape heart disease. In yet another example, Irwin (1953) found that most card players expect to come out winners even in zero-sum games such as poker.

According to Slovic et al., (1982a) these attitudes result from the misinterpretation of everyday experience. Because most personal automobile trips end with our safe arrival at our destination, we believe that accidents are rarer than they really are. Reading about accidents in the newspaper only teaches us that they happen to others, not ourselves. In other words, when it comes to common risks, most people's attitude is "It can't happen to me." This is the same attitude expressed by the surgeons studied by Detmer et al. (1978), the majority of whom estimated overall surgical mortality as higher than the mortality of their own patients (see Chapter 3).

In addition to availability, anchoring and adjustment can also affect risk assessment. For example, Fischhoff and MacGregor (1980) asked people to estimate the likelihood of death from various hazards. The likelihoods produced depended on the elicitation format. When they asked how many people died from influenza last year, the average answer was 393 per 100,000 afflicted. However, when the subjects in this experiment were told that 80 million people contracted influenza last year, their estimates of its mortality averaged only 6 per 100,000 af-

* Our colleague, Paul Glasziou, pointed out to us that, although Svenson's subjects were probably being overoptimistic, it is worth noting that their responses may have been accurate. Consider, for example, 100 drivers 5 of whom have 20 accidents each during a year while the rest have none. The mean number of accidents in this group is 1, but a full 95% have a below-average number of accidents.

flicted. The anchoring effect produced by the 80 million figure changed the mortality estimate by a factor of 60!

As we discussed in Chapter 3, an important effect of the use of heuristics to estimate risk is overconfidence. One form of overconfidence with special importance for medicine is unjustified faith in the current status of scientific knowledge. The harmful effects of thalidomide, x-rays, and other procedures went unrecognized until their use had become very common. Overconfidence in the current state of scientific knowledge can lead to the stultification of progress and the unwarranted belief that today's technology will also be tomorrow's.

Quantifying Risk

To learn more about how people go about assigning numerical probabilities to risks, Fischhoff, Slovic, Lichtenstein, Read, and Combs (1978) asked educated laypeople and experts in engineering and technology to assign probabilities to 30 potentially life-threatening hazards. Their subjects were asked to give the least risky hazard a value of 10 and to assign ratings to the remaining hazards accordingly. Thus, a rating of 20 meant that a hazard was perceived to be twice as risky as the least risky hazard. Fischhoff, Slovic, Lichtenstein, et al. found marked differences between expert and lay judges. The experts viewed electric power, surgery, swimming, and x-rays as riskier hazards than the laypeople did. On the other hand, the experts rated nuclear power, police work, and mountain climbing as less risky than did the layperson.

Fischhoff, Slovic, Lichtenstein, et al. hypothesized that the differences they found between experts and laypeople were the result of the experts' basing their estimates on the actual frequency of the various hazards while the laypeople relied on judgment heuristics such as availability instead. To test this hypothesis, they correlated each subject's lethality ratings with the actual objective frequencies of the various hazards where these were available. For experts, the correlation between objective frequencies and risk estimates was .92. In contrast, lay judgments departed significantly from the objective frequencies. For laypeople, the average correlation between the two was only .56. Laypeople overestimated the risk to life posed by handguns and nuclear power plants while underestimating the risks of vaccinations and home appliances. Interestingly, when the experimenters asked lay subjects to estimate the objective frequencies of death from each hazard (the respective number of yearly fatalities), their fatality estimates failed to correlate with their risk estimates. Nuclear power, for example, was rated highest on risk and lowest on yearly fatalities of all hazards. For laypeople at least, the frequency of dying from a hazard and its risk are two separate things.

In an attempt to determine exactly why laypeople perceive some hazards as exceptionally risky (or safe), Fischhoff, Slovic, Lichtenstein, et al.

Table 4-1. Dimensions of Risk[a]

How well is risk known to science?
How clear are the risks to those who will be exposed?
Is the risk new or familiar?
Is the risk immediate or delayed?
Is exposure to the risk voluntary?
Can the risk be controlled or avoided by the individual?
Are the consequences certainly fatal?
Does the risk arouse strong emotions (e.g., dread)?
Is the risk catastrophic (many simultaneous deaths)?

---

[a] Adapted from Fischhoff, Slovic, Lichtenstein, et al. (1978). Reprinted with the permission of Elsevier Science Publishers.

devised a rating scale consisting of nine dimensions and asked people to rate each hazard on each dimension using a 7-point scale. For example, the first dimension assessed how well known the risk levels of a potential hazard were. Subjects had to assign a number from 1 (risk level precisely known to science) to 7 (risk level unknown) to each hazard. The procedure was the same for the remaining eight dimensions. The dimensions are summarized in Table 4-1.

It was found that the hazards perceived by lay subjects to be particularly risky produced different profiles on the nine dimensions from those perceived safe. Hazards believed to have great catastrophic potential and that produced strong feelings of dread were perceived as more risky than their objective frequencies warrant, whereas the risks of well-known hazards that claim lives chronically rather than all at once were underestimated. A time factor also appeared to be operating. Hazards with deferred consequences (many carcinogens, for example) were viewed as less risky than those whose effect is immediate. Voluntary activities (smoking, for instance) were perceived as less risky than those imposed by outside forces, such as pollution (see also Starr & Whipple, 1980). Factor-analytic studies by Slovic, Fischhoff, and Lichtenstein (1981) have confirmed these findings—dread, catastrophic potential, and voluntariness are the most important determinants of perceived risk.

In a discussion of these findings, Fischhoff, Slovic, Lichtenstein, et al. theorized that hazards such as nuclear power plant meltdown call forth vivid images of death and destruction. These images, in turn, produce dread and lead to overestimates of risk among laypeople. Experts, on the other hand, base their risk estimates on the actual number of fatalities produced by the various hazards. Since the main difference between experts and laypeople is their knowledge of these objective frequencies, it seems reasonable to assume that educating laypeople about them would lead to the laypeople behaving more like experts. Such an education program was undertaken in Sweden, where 80,000 people attended a 10-hour lecture series on nuclear power. Unfortunately, instead of turning laypeople into experts, the result of this lecture program was confusion, and in some cases, even higher estimates of the potential risk of nuclear accidents than before the program. It seems that those who attended the lectures had learned about the many things that could go wrong and this increased their dread. Doctors who believe that patients must be fully informed of every potential outcome, complication, or side effect of a course of treatment may unwittingly create similar dread when their purpose is just the opposite.

An important problem in assessing perceived risk, one touched upon in our discussion of problem representation, is the impact of "negative" as opposed to "positive" information. As we have seen, a treatment that saves 800 lives out of 1000 is preferred to one that sacrifices 200 out of 1000 despite the mathematical equivalence of the outcomes (see also Johnson & Tversky, 1984). This finding is important for medical decision making because government agencies such as the U.S. Food and Drug Administration (FDA) are requiring that information on a drug's risks and benefits be included in an increasing number of prescription drug packages. The rationale for such "package inserts" is that patients must be given the information necessary to judge whether the medication's benefits outweigh its risks. There is a danger in this practice—the format in which the information is presented can exert a powerful effect on risk perception.

Fischhoff (1980) studied the effect of package insert formats on risk perception. He had a group of laypeople read a package insert that had been prepared for prospective patients while another group read an insert prepared for doctors. Except for material that indicated that the drug was an oral contraceptive, Fischhoff removed nothing from the originals. After reading the inserts, the subjects completed a questionnaire dealing with the drug and its side effects. Although all of the subjects in this study felt that the information contained in the inserts was important and should be routinely available to patients, most felt that the risks were not explained clearly. Those who read the patients' insert felt that the drug was riskier than vitamin C, aspirin, or coffeee and about as risky as amphetamines. Those who read the doctors' insert felt the risks were greater than did those who read the patients'. Most readers of each form said they *would not* use the drug to relieve allergies, migraine headaches, *or as a contraceptive!*

Readers of the doctors' form estimated the frequency of blood clots (the major risk described) as 2.5 times as likely for those who use the drug than for those who do not. Readers of the patients' form felt that using the drug makes one 5.1 times as likely to get blood clots. In contrast, the overall incidence of side effects was judged to be 1 in 40,000 by readers of the patients' form and 1 in 2000 for readers of the doctors' form. The reason for the apparent inconsistencies appears to lie in the way the information was conveyed in the two forms. The patients' form actually provided representative death and mortality figures while the doctors' form did not.

Despite the best intentions of those who created the package inserts, the information they provided may not be leading to better patient decision making but to errors in judgment and improper conclusions. Perhaps part of the problem is that patient inserts are often produced by doctors who, because of their greater experience, usually view drug side effects as less serious than do laypersons (Keown, Slovic, & Lichtenstein, 1984).

A striking example of how subjects' risk perceptions may be easily distorted by small changes in the way problems are represented is provided by Fischhoff, Slovic, and Lichtenstein (1978). Their research required people to estimate probabilities using fault trees. A fault tree is similar to a decision tree, with each branch indicating a potential fault. One of their fault trees, describing the possible reasons a car will not start, appears in Figure 4-9.

The tree illustrated in Figure 4-9 plus pruned versions (in which branches had been eliminated) were presented to both laypersons and garage mechanics who were asked to state the probability that various factors were responsible for a car's failure to start. Assuming that all explanations for the car's failure to start are contained in the complete tree (the probabilities of the various faults total to 1), it should be obvious that removing a branch should either lead to an increase in the remaining probabilities or some mention that branches are missing. However, Fischhoff, Slovic, and Lichtenstein found that the probability assigned to one branch did not change significantly when earlier branches were pruned from the tree. Even the expert mechanics failed to mention the missing branches or to adjust their probabilities sufficiently for the missing data. In fact, when subjects were specifically alerted to focus on the tree's completeness, they still failed to compensate for the missing branches. Fischhoff, Slovic, and Lichtenstein dubbed this phenomenon "out of sight, out of mind." Interestingly, dividing a single branch of the tree into two branches increased its perceived importance even though no additional information was added.

These results suggest that one of the operational assumptions of SEU-based decision analysis—the probability of all potential outcomes must total to 1—may easily be violated. Kozielecki (1981) illustrated this with a clinically relevant example. He asked subjects to diagnose a patient on the basis of a set of symptoms. Since there were 21 possible diseases in his experiment, initially, at least, there were 21 possible hypotheses. Because subjects found it too difficult to consider all hypotheses simultaneously and to adjust the probability of each as new information about symptoms became available, many hit on the strategy of dividing the 21

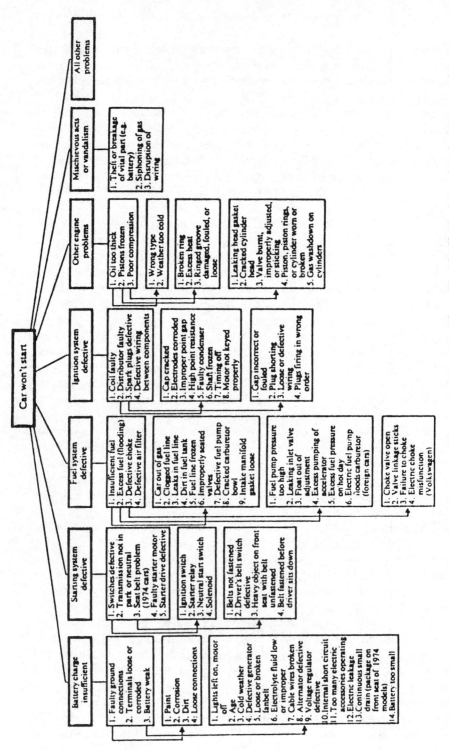

Figure 4-9 A fault tree for discovering why a car will not start. Reprinted from Fischhoff, Slovic, and Lichtenstein (1978) with the permission of the American Psychological Association and the author.

diseases into subsets. The first set consisted of the 3 to 6 hypotheses considered to be most likely on the basis of availability, representativeness, and other judgment heuristics, and the second set was a catchall category containing the remaining diseases. In effect, these subjects pruned a potentially large decision tree down to a smaller one. This strategy would probably work well in practice provided that the subjects remembered that pruning had occurred and that judgments must be checked against the diseases in the catchall set, but this is not what happened. Having pruned the hypotheses down to a small number, the subjects worked only with the reduced set and, consequently, made errors whenever the correct disease was a member of the catchall set.

Acceptable Risk

The concept of "acceptable risk" appears to have originated among engineers concerned with structural design (Green, 1979). To be "safe," buildings must be designed to withstand certain hazards (ice and snow accumulating on the roof, for example). The probability that a particular load will exceed a structure's resistance and result in its collapse can be determined from prebuilding stress tests. Usually, the only way this probability may be decreased is by building sturdier structures, but such structures are very expensive. At some point, those in charge (politicians, builders, consumers, and so on) will refuse to pay any more for increased safety. The probability of structural collapse that people are willing to accept for a particular outlay of money has become known as "acceptable risk." The concept spread quickly to other industries and eventually to technologies such as medicine (Fischhoff, Lichtenstein, Slovic, Derby, & Keeney, 1981).

There are at least two general approaches to measuring acceptable risk: revealed preferences and expressed preferences. The revealed preference approach relies on the idea that, over the years, we have arrived at a more or less optimum balance between the risks and benefits of any activity. Therefore, the acceptable risk of any new development can be measured by comparing it with those already in existence. A risk level is thought to be acceptable if it is no greater than that of existing activities offering similar benefits (Starr, 1969).

Starr (1969) examined the risks and benefits of a number of activities from which he derived what he called the "laws of acceptable risk." These include: greater risks are accepted for activities providing greater benefits, and greater risks are accepted from voluntary hazards (skiing, for instance) than involuntary ones (water pollution). The problem with revealed preferences is the underlying assumption that past behavior is a valid predictor of present preferences. After all, values do change. The reliance on past behavior may also fail to give sufficient weight to risks that take a long time to develop (carcinogens, for example).

The expressed preference method takes a more direct approach. Individuals are simply asked to indicate how much risk they are willing to tolerate for various activities. For many hazards, the expressed preferences agree with the revealed preferences, but researchers using the expressed preferences approach have shown that psychological variables such as the familiarity, controllability, and immediacy of a hazard can exert a strong effect on risk acceptability (Fischhoff et al., 1981).

A drawback to the expressed preferences approach is the finding that preferences can change depending on small changes in the way questions are asked (Johnson & Tversky, 1984). Although this is to be expected from the research on problem representation, it is nevertheless a difficulty for the expressed preferences approach.

Whenever tragedies such as the effect of thalidomide on babies hit the news, calls for zero-risk treatments are heard from politicians, laypeople, and some doctors. Although such treatments certainly sound very attractive, they are often impossible to achieve, If we choose to eliminate all risky treatments, then we must consider what they will be replaced with. It is possible that the alternatives (no treatment at all, in many cases) may actually be worse. This was the problem facing health authorities several years ago when consideration was being given to banning saccharin because of the possibility that it caused cancer. If diabetics who crave sweets cannot obtain saccharin they may turn to sugar—an even worse risk to their health than the saccharin. An insistence on zero-risk treatments may also stifle potentially beneficial new developments because, at least at the outset, their risks are unknown. Because it can retard progress and because it brings risks of its own, some writers have described a no-risk policy as, perhaps, leading to the highest risks of all (Wildavsky, 1979).

Is Risk Taking a Personality Trait?

We have all come across people we consider risk takers and other, more cautious, souls who avoid risk whenever possible. Indeed, attitude toward risk is one of the most important generalizations we make when describing someone's personality (he is timid and cautious, she is brave and daring). Common usage notwithstanding, there is actually very little evidence that people have a generalized tendency to avoid risk. Slovic, et al. (1980), for example, compared the scores of 82 individuals on nine risk-taking measures and found practically no consistency in risk taking across the settings tapped by the various tasks. People who were daring in one situation were found to avoid risks in another.

It is more likely that personality traits other than risk preference determine when someone will take risks. For example, someone with a high need for achievement may take risks when these may lead to advancement but not otherwise. It seems, however, that in real world decisions, the context in which a decision takes place (the problem representation) has a greater influence on the outcome than any personality traits (Kozielecki, 1981).

Problem Representations, Risk Assessment, and SEU

According to SEU theory, the product of the utilities and probabilities associated with various outcomes determines which of several alternative actions should be chosen. Provided its assumptions are met, SEU theory provides a powerful rationale for decision analysis. But what does it mean when the theory's assumptions are violated? In this section we have seen that probabilities and utilities are not always independent; under certain conditions, the probability of an outcome can affect its utility. We have also seen that decision makers are relatively insensitive to the omission of likely alternatives from a problem representation. They seem not to realize that the probability of the presented alternatives does not sum to 1. It would appear that SEU theory somehow fails to describe actual decision behavior.

From our discussion thus far, it would seem that one reason SEU may not always be descriptive is because it lacks any construct equivalent to perceived risk. Several attempts have been made to develop mathematical models of choice that do incorporate a risk parameter (see Coombs, 1975, for example), but so far such theories have not found widespread acceptance. One reason is the subjective nature of risk, itself. Because risk perception depends on the observer, even those theories that include it as a parameter are likely to be dealing with relatively unreliable data.

Of course, its failure to describe how people actually make decisions does not imply that SEU theory is not normative; it may still be the ideal way to reach decisions. We return to this point later in this chapter when we discuss cost–benefit analysis. For now, however, we continue our discussion of the steps involved in risky decision making by looking at Step 3, the measurement of utilities.

Utility Measurement

In several places in this and earlier chapters we have referred to the concept of utility, which we have defined as subjective value. Normative approaches to decision making such as SEU assume that decision makers' preferences for various outcomes are sufficiently consistent to be used to determine optimal decisions. In this section, we examine the concept of utility. We begin with several important definitions and a description of utility assessment methods. We then examine psychological research concerned with the measurement and meaning of subjective value. The implications of this research for medical decision making are discussed at the end of the section.

The Concept of Utility

According to Savage (1954), the first distinction between monetary value and utility was made by the 18th-century statistician Daniel Bernoulli (1954). Bernoulli's work was then taken up by the philosophers Jeremy Bentham and James Mill, who extended it far beyond its original boundaries.

Bernoulli's goal was to explain why people generally avoid risk and why risk avoidance decreases with increasing wealth. Bernoulli was particularly interested in situations in which people must choose between a certain gain (say, winning $800 with a probability of 1.00) and a gamble (say a .85 probability of winning $1000 and a .15 probability of winning $0). Assuming one can play many times, the expected gain of the gamble (.85 × $1000 = $850) is greater than that of the sure thing (1.00 × $800 = $800). Nevertheless, when given the choice, most people prefer the certain gain to the gamble. They forgo the higher expected monetary value in order to avoid the small risk of ending up with nothing at all.

Bernoulli argued that such preferences could only be understood if our choices do not depend on expected value but on the utility of the possible outcomes. He stated the relationship mathematically as follows:

$$u(\$800 \text{ win}) > 0.15 \ u(\$0 \text{ win}) + 0.85 \ u(\$1000 \text{ win})$$

where u is the subjective value, the utility, of the sum of money to the decision maker. It has become customary to refer to those who prefer a sure thing to a gamble with greater expected value as being *risk averse*. The concept of risk, as used here, is not exactly the same as the one introduced earlier. In the present context, risk is seen as consisting of two components: the likelihood of a loss and the utility of the loss, should it actually occur. The idea, introduced earlier in this chapter, that risk is something separate from probabilities and utilities, is not part of classical utility theory.

From Bernoulli's viewpoint, there are three possible relationships between choice and risk. People may be risk neutral, risk avoiding, or risk seeking. If your utility for money decreases with additional wealth, you are a risk avoider; if it increases, you are a risk seeker. If the two are unrelated then you are risk neutral. Figure 4-10 illustrates these three relationships.

Bentham and Mill extended Bernoulli's work and, in the process, turned the utility concept into a general theory of human nature. According to these philosophers, people behave in such a way as to gain pleasure and avoid pain. Since every decision outcome can be assessed for its pleasure-giving or pain-reducing properties, these assessments

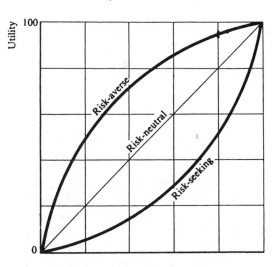

Figure 4-10   An illustration of the utility for money. If small amounts of money have relatively large utility, the individual is characterized as risk averse. The opposite pattern is called risk seeking. Those whose preferences fall along a straight line are risk neutral.

constitute an outcome's utility. Pleasure is measured in terms of positive utilities, pain by negative utilities. Bentham, and practically all philosophers and economists who came after him, assumed that a rational decision maker, faced with several alternative actions, would always choose the one "that leads to the greatest excess of positive over negative utility" (Edwards, 1954, p. 382). In other words, rational people behave so as to maximize expected utility.

Classical economists used Bernoulli's work and Bentham's extensions to develop models of consumer demand, culminating in what is known as the principle of diminishing marginal utility. In essence, the principle states that the more we have of a specific good, the lower our desire for more of that good. This principle is quite easy to illustrate. A consumer who does not own a car may have a strong desire to buy one. Once one has been obtained, the consumer may desire a second car, but less strongly than the first. The utility for a third or fourth car, even among those who could afford them, will diminish even further. Eventually, the utility for another car will reach zero. Assuming that it is possible to measure the utility for different outcomes in standard units, then the principle of diminishing marginal utility says that the utility of any good (not just money) is a monotonically increasing, negatively accelerated function of the amount of that good already possessed (this curve would look like the risk averse curve in Figure 4-10).

Table 4-2. E.W.'s Decision Problem

	Outcome	
Therapy	Mother	Child
Anticoagulants	Well	Well
	Well	Abnormal
	Well	Dead
No anticoagulants	Well	Well
	Dead	Dead

Even as far back as Bernoulli, it was obvious that the principle of diminishing marginal utility did not always hold. Savage (1954) gave the following example: A wealthy father may value even a small amount of additional money if he needs it in order to complete his son's ransom. Although economists have acknowledged that such cases exist, they are taken to be special exceptions to an otherwise widely applicable principle. The extent to which the principle of diminishing marginal utility applies to health decisions is discussed later in this chapter.

Utility Measurement Techniques

There are several utility measurement techniques currently in use, but the only one that actually follows from formal utility theory involves a choice between gambles or lotteries (see Raiffa, 1968). To understand how and why this technique is used, we apply it to one of the decisions facing E.W.—should she continue to receive anticoagulant therapy?

E.W.'s decision could lead to one of the four possible outcomes contained in Table 4-2. (Actually, this is a somewhat simplified statement of the true state of affairs, but sufficient for the present illustration.) To determine which treatment is preferable, E.W.'s doctors must know her utilities for the various outcomes. Furthermore, these utilities must be expressed as numbers so that they can be multiplied by probabilities. They must also be expressed on the same scale so that they can be compared. The best way to accomplish this is to measure utilities in terms of probability.

The procedure begins with the identification of the best and the worst potential outcomes. In E.W.'s case, Klein and Pauker (1981) decided, reasonably, that these were mother and infant both well and mother and infant both dead, respectively. These two outcomes become the end points of a utility scale in which the best outcome is assigned a value of 1.00 and the worst a value of 0. (Klein and Pauker actually used 100 and 0, but since the numbers are arbitrary the end points can be any numbers at all.) In E.W.'s case, the remaining two outcomes are presumed to be intermediate between the two extremes. One of these is mother well, infant dead. Suppose this outcome had a utility halfway between the two

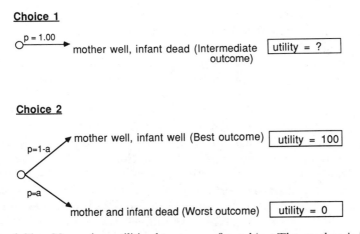

Figure 4-11   Measuring utilities by means of gambles. The mother is being asked to choose between a certain outcome with unknown utility and probabilistic outcomes for which the utilities are known (or assumed).

extreme outcomes, or .5. What would this mean? In probability terms, it means that if anticoagulation treatment had a 50–50 chance of leading to either the death of the mother and child or a perfectly well mother and child, E.W. would be indifferent between taking a chance on treatment and accepting with certainty that she will live while her child dies. If her utility for the mother well, infant dead outcome were .6, she would be indifferent between a treatment with a 60% chance of producing this outcome and the certainty that she would live but her child will die.

To determine utilities, then, it is necessary to ask E.W. to choose between certain outcomes and gambles. The certain outcome is the one for which utilities are being sought; the gamble is between the best and worst outcomes. E.W. must indicate which of the two she prefers. Specifically, to determine E.W.'s utility for the outcome mother well, infant dead, she must be asked to choose between this outcome occurring with a probability of 1.00 and a gamble between the best and worst outcomes in which the probability of each is less than 1.00. Once she has indicated her preference, she may be asked to choose again, but this time the probabilities associated with the gamble are altered. This procedure continues until E.W. shows no preference for either choice. This procedure is illustrated in Figure 4-11.

When the probability of the worst potential outcome is small (this is represented by a in Figure 4-11), E.W. will most likely prefer choice 2. When this probability is high, however, she may prefer choice 1. At some intermediate probability of the worst outcome, E.W. will be indifferent between the two choices. At this point, it is assumed that her utility for the two is identical and a utility can be assigned (see Lindley, 1975, 1977, for more on the rationale behind this technique).

Assigning utilities is a matter of straightforward arithmetic. Say E.W. has completed the gambling procedure and was found to be indifferent when the worst outcome in choice 2 had a probability of .10 (a = .10). The total expected utility of choice 2 in this case is equal to the product of the utilities and probabilities of the two possible outcomes. In this case, the probability of the best outcome is .90 and its utility is 1.00 and the probability of the worst outcome is .10 while its utility is 0. Thus, the total expected utility is .90 × 1 + .10 × 0 or .90. This is taken as equal to E.W.'s utility for the outcome mother well, infant dead. The same procedure can be repeated to determine E.W.'s utility for the fourth potential outcome, mother dead, infant well. In the end, each potential outcome will have been given a utility. These utilities can be multiplied by the respective probabilities to get an SEU. It should be emphasized that the utilities obtained by the gambling procedure are not absolute measures of subjective value. They are relative preferences that differ depending on the outcomes being compared.

The gambling procedure, while justified from the standpoint of formal utility theory, may, in practice, be quite difficult for patients to actually use. We have already shown that people often have difficulty thinking in probabilistic terms and few patients will find the task of choosing between gambles with similar probabilities (.8 versus .9, for instance) an easy one. For many patients, expressing preferences for different outcomes (maternal death versus fetal death) is distasteful, while for others it is impossible. For these reasons, some researchers have tried to devise more direct methods for assessing utility. Although there are several different direct approaches to measuring utility, all share the belief that people have a sort of table of values stored in their minds—a table that they consult whenever it is necessary to compare potential outcomes.

One direct utility measurement method was described by Gardiner and Edwards (1975). Their approach was to ask subjects to rank all potential outcomes of an action from best to worst and to assign an arbitrary utility value to the worst. Then, beginning with the second-worst outcome, decision makers were required to state how much they prefer the alternative outcomes to the worst one. For example, if the worst outcome in E.W.'s case (mother and infant both dead) was assigned a value of 10 and if the subjective value of the outcome mother well, infant dead was twice as large, it would receive a value of 20. An outcome with three times the utility would receive a value of 30 and so on. A similar approach begins with assigning a value to both the best and worst outcomes while the remaining outcomes are given values somewhere in between. A potential problem with this method is that most people tend to avoid the end points of the scale and the utility estimates tend to bunch up in the middle. (For more on direct methods for measuring utility see Kozielecki, 1981.)

Multiattribute Utility

The utility measurement techniques considered thus far look upon the various decision outcomes as unidimensional. However, in many decision-making situations, outcomes are not simple. Instead, each outcome can be described as the composite of a number of subdimensions. A new car, for example, can be described as a Ford or a Cadillac or it can be described in terms of a collection of attributes such as speed, style, economy, and so on. A surgical procedure can be described by its name (laryngectomy, tonsillectomy) or as entailing different degrees of pain, debilitation, increased life expectancy, and so on. In recent years, it has become quite common to decompose compound outcomes into their constituent attributes prior to evaluating their utility. In fact, an entire approach to decision making has evolved from the decomposition paradigm. This approach is known as multiattribute utility theory (MAUT) (see Gardiner and Edwards, 1975). Multiattribute utility theory consists of a set of assessment procedures and rules for making decisions; it is also a prescriptive rather than descriptive theory. Nevertheless, MAUT has affected psychological thinking and is therefore worth considering here.

Multiattribute utility theory is based on a decomposition approach to utility measurement. Each outcome is decomposed into its constituent attributes, which are valued separately. Next, each potential outcome is assigned a weight on each attribute and the outcomes are recomposed in such a way as to permit their multiattribute utility (MAU) to be determined. Recomposition can be accomplished in several ways, but the most common method is additive. That is, each outcome's MAU is simply the weighted sum of the utilities of the various attributes. This approach to MAUT is summarized by the following formula:

$$\text{MAU}_j = \sum_i b_i u_{ij} \tag{5}$$

where j represents a particular outcome, b_i is the relative importance of the ith attribute of outcome j, and u_{ij} is the utility of the jth outcome on the ith attribute. To make this formula concrete, let us go back to the car example. If u_{ij} is the relative importance of speed, u_{ij} would indicate how fast car j can go. Multiattribute utility theory's typical decision rule states that the action that leads to the outcome with the highest MAU be chosen.

The utilities of the decomposed variables can be measured either directly or indirectly. In this regard, MAUT utilities are no different from any other utilities. However, the way in which utilities are recomposed is important. Different recomposition methods can lead to different MAUs. Equation 5 requires that the attribute utilities be summed to calculate MAU. This is simply a mathematical description of the linear model discussed in Chapter 3. An alternative recomposition method would allow for configural relationships; that is, the weight assigned to one attribute can influence the utility assigned to another. For example, the pain produced by a surgical procedure may be disregarded if the operation makes a substantial improvement in the patient's quality of life. Trivial improvements, however, may not justify painful procedures. At present, there are few instances of decision analyses using configural decision rules; the linear approach is far more common.

Do the Various Utility Measurement Techniques Yield Comparable Data?

Since the indirect (gambling) method of measuring utilities and the direct methods are clearly different, it is not surprising that researchers have attempted to compare the two. Kneppreth, Gustafson, Leifer, and Johnson (1974) reviewed the literature but were unable to draw firm conclusions about which approach is better because studies have not been sufficiently systematic. Vertinsky and Wong (1975) compared direct and indirect methods and found the direct method more reliable and easier for most subjects, while the indirect methods yielded utilities that were better predictors of future choices. In a study directly concerned with medical decisions, Fryback (1974b) asked physicians and nonphysicians to evaluate the possible outcomes of kidney tests using both direct and indirect methods. He found the two approaches yield similar results. A more recent study by Llewellyn-Thomas, Sutherland, Ciampi, Etezadi-Amoli, Boyd, and Till (1984) required patients undergoing radiotherapy for laryngeal cancer to provide utility estimates for different aspects of voice function. These estimates were obtained holistically and for decomposed attributes at several occasions during treatment. The values they obtained were reasonably similar and equally stable over time.

Sometimes, in medical situations, it is more appropriate to think about outcomes in terms of regret rather than utility. Regret is measured by focusing on relative losses rather than relative gains. Consider, for example, a situation in which there are three potentially effective treatments, T^1, T^2, and T^3. The utilities for these treatments are ordered $u_1 > u_2 > u_3$. This means that T^1 is the "best" treatment and administering either T^2 or T^3 will lead to a suboptimal outcome. Let us assume, however, that for some reason, T^2 or T^3 is chosen. The result, so far as the patient is concerned, is a loss. The amount of this loss is the difference between the utility of the optimum treatment and the one actually selected ($u^1 - u^2$ or $u^1 - u^3$). This loss is known as regret. If we use regret

rather than utility to characterize treatment outcomes, then regret mini-
mization rather than utility maximization becomes the most common
decision rule. A study by Le Minor, Alperovitch, and Knill-Jones (1982)
found that direct and indirect methods of measuring regret yielded very
similar results.

Utility and regret estimates may not vary greatly from one elicitation
method to another, but subtle changes in the way problems are presented can make a big difference. Changing the presentation emphasis
from gains to losses (from lives saved to lives lost), providing anchors,
presenting information in different orders, and so on can affect utilities
just as strongly as these factors affect probability estimates (Kahneman &
Tversky, 1979).

Problem representation has a particularly powerful effect on utility
assessment when people are unfamiliar with the potential outcomes (Fischhoff, Slovic, & Lichtenstein, 1980). This finding has important implications for medical decisions because patients are often ignorant about
the outcomes of the various potential courses of action. Could E.W.
really be expected to know what life would be like with an abnormal
child? It is entirely possible that if she were permitted to observe families
with handicapped children her utilities would change. Ignorance about
the precise consequences of medical decisions can be dispelled to some
extent by fully informing patients about likely outcomes, but doctors
must be careful not to bias patients by giving them incomplete information or by seeming to favor particular actions. There is, after all, no
particular reason why a patient's utilities should mirror his/her doctor's
(for more on this point see Elstein & Bordage, 1979).

Since utilities are simply subjective values, we cannot ask, as we did for
probabilities, whether an individual is well calibrated. We expect individuals' utilities to differ, and it makes no sense to say that a person's
utilities are right or wrong. This does not mean that any numbers produced by any direct or indirect measurement method can simply be
plugged into the appropriate parts of a decision analysis. Decision analysts make several strong assumptions about the nature of utilities. If
these assumptions fail to be met, then the whole basis of SEU theory and
decision analysis may be called into question.

Formal Utility Theory

A formal theory of utility was formulated by von Neumann and
Morgenstern (1944). Their theory is composed of a number of axioms
from which the rationale for SEU theory can be derived mathematically.
If these axioms are accepted, then it follows that SEU is a normative
theory. Savage (1954), expanding on von Neumann and Morgenstern's
work, identified four axioms as being of primary importance:

1. *Decidability (Connectivity).* The decision maker must be able to say whether one outcome is preferred to another or whether two or more outcomes are equally preferred.
2. *Transitivity.* If outcome A is preferred to outcome B and B is preferred to C then A must be preferred to C as well.
3. *Dominance.* Decision makers prefer the action that leads to the overall best outcome.
4. *Independence (Sure Thing Principle).* If two alternative actions share a common outcome, preference for one or another should not be influenced by that outcome. For example, choosing between two operations for baldness (punch grafts or scalp reduction) should not be influenced by the possibility of an antibaldness drug coming on the market because this will affect both choices equally (see Edwards, Lindman, & Phillips, 1965, for additional examples).

These four axioms, along with several others, ensure that utilities constitute an interval scale with arbitrary end points but with ratios preserved (a utility of 20 is twice as large as a utility of 10). It also follows from these axioms that maximizing utility is the optimal decision rule. In the discussions that follow, we review research on how well these axioms describe human behavior. In the process, we show that people often behave in ways contrary to those demanded by formal utility theory. The implications of these findings for medical decision making are discussed.

Decidability and transitivity

According to SEU theory, decision makers must be able to say whether one outcome is preferred over another (decidability) and their preferences must be transitive. On the surface, at least, these two axioms are not controversial. Indeed, decidability and transitivity are the very essence of rational thought. If outcome A is preferred to outcome B and B is preferred to C then consistency and common logic demand that A be preferred to C. This makes it all the more surprising that, when people are actually asked to order their preferences for three outcomes, intransitivity may sometimes occur.

For example, Papandreou (1953) asked people to choose between several sets of tickets to sporting and theatrical events. The sets were arranged so that each contained four tickets to two types of events (three plays and one football game, two plays and two football games, and so on). Papandreou presented the ticket sets three at a time and asked subjects to arrange them in order of preference. He found that about 5% of preference orderings were intransitive—the subjects were inconsistent in their preference orderings.

Papandreou considered the 5% of intransitive preference orders too rare to pose a serious problem for formal utility theory, but other studies have found intransitivity to occur more frequently. In one such experiment (May, 1954), males and females were asked to choose between potential boyfriends and girlfriends each of whom was described using three dimensions: intelligence, attractiveness, and wealth. Each dimension was given a weighting on a 3-point scale in which 1 indicated the lowest and 3 the highest possible value. Thus, a very attractive, highly intelligent, rich candidate was described as a 3,3,3. May provided his subjects with several pairs of such descriptions and asked them to indicate their preference. May found that about 25% of preferences were intransitive. For example, suppose a female subject was given descriptions such as the following:

	Intelligence	Attractiveness	Wealth
A =	3	1	2
B =	2	3	1
C =	1	2	3

Some females respond that they prefer A to B, B to C, and C to A! May explained intransitivities of this sort as the result of a cognitive strategy or, to use the present terminology, a judgment heuristic. Specifically, when comparing each pair of males, the female judges may use the rule of always preferring the person with higher ratings on the majority of dimensions. Thus, A is preferred to B because he is more intelligent and wealthier, B is preferred to C because he is more intelligent and attractive, but C is preferred to A because he is more attractive and wealthier. In other words, what appears to be a relatively sensible judgment rule can lead to the violation of one of the fundamental axioms underlying SEU theory.

May's experiment was criticized on methodological grounds by Edwards (1954), who pointed out that May's subjects were not permitted to be indifferent; they were forced to always make a choice. If this choice was made randomly, then they would be expected to be intransitive 25% of the time, just as May found. Although this argument clearly has merit, other researchers have found intransitive preferences even when indifference was a permissible choice (Tversky, 1969).

Intransitivity of preferences can be demonstrated in a medical situation using, as an example, three potential heart bypass operations. Each operation has been rated for its effect on life expectancy and its ability to reduce pain. These ratings are expressed on a 10-point scale where 1 is the lowest rating and 10 the highest. The three operations are described as follows:

Operation	Life Expectancy	Pain Decrease
A =	1	10
B =	2	6
C =	5	2

When presented in pairs, one way to choose between these operations is to weight each according to the perceived importance of the various dimensions. For example, a decision maker who considers life expectancy more important than pain relief will begin by examining the life expectancy increase expected with the various operations. If possible, a decision will be made on the basis of this dimension alone. A possible decision rule might be, "if an operation's life expectancy rating differs from another by 3 or more points, choose the one that leads to the longest increase in life expectancy regardless of its ability to relieve pain." This means that pain decrease ratings will only be considered for those operations that fall within 3 points of one another in life expectancy ratings. In such cases, preference will be determined by which operation leads to the greater pain decrease. A decision maker who uses such a strategy will prefer operation A to B and B to C but will prefer C to A. In such a case, intransitivity is not only possible, but apparently quite reasonable.

Although intransitivity can sometimes result from the use of what appear to be reasonable judgment strategies, it can also result from misunderstanding of the task, laziness, and sheer stupidity. In practice, it is often difficult to decide which of these is responsible. For this reason, the interpretation of research findings demonstrating intransitive preferences is controversial (see Pitz & Sachs, 1984, and Slovic, Fischhoff, & Lichtenstein, 1977, for reviews). No one denies, however, that formal utility theory and most decision analyses require transitivity of preferences. If, for whatever reason, preferences are intransitive, the validity of a decision analysis is thrown into doubt.

Of course, it is always possible to test the effect of intransitivity of preferences (or any other SEU parameter) through sensitivity analysis. An example was presented in Klein and Pauker's (1981) analysis of E.W.'s case. In a sensitivity analysis, one or more parameters is allowed to vary. If the final decision is unchanged, the analysis is considered insensitive to changes in that parameter.

Sensitivity analysis is a valuable technique, but, as Fischhoff et al. (1980) pointed out, it does not really solve the important problems associated with violations of SEU axioms. Sensitivity analysis does nothing to avoid the biases created by problem representations and, when changes in a parameter do lead to shifts in preferred actions, the sensitivity analysis does not tell us which action is "correct."

Dominance

The dominance axiom of formal utility theory requires that the action that maximizes expected utility be preferred over all others. This sounds quite logical. Yet, in practice, it is quite easy to create situations in which the dominance axiom is violated.

For example, Coombs & Huang (1974) asked people to choose between three gambles; A, B, and C. A had the smallest expected value, C had the highest, and B was somewhere in between. They found many of their subjects to prefer gamble B, a clear violation of the dominance axiom. Edwards (1955) also found that preferences for gambles were not necessarily determined by expected value. Many of his subjects expressed definite preferences for long-shot bets in which large amounts could be won and little lost over bets with better odds but smaller payoffs. This was true even when the latter bets had greater expected value. Lichtenstein et al. (1969) confirmed Edwards' finding and showed that explaining the concept of expected value to subjects did not change their preferences. When gambling, at least, people do not necessarily choose the action that maximizes expected utility.

Whether or not the dominance axiom is violated depends partly on how decision problems are represented. This was demonstrated by Lichtenstein and Slovic (1971), who asked gamblers on the floor of a Las Vegas casino to either choose which of two gambles they would prefer to take or to bid for the chance to play one of two gambles in a kind of auction. They found that the two procedures resulted in different preference orderings. Moreover, people adhered to these different preference orders even when their inconsistency was pointed out.

Subjective expected utility theory assumes that rational individuals act to maximize expected utility. Psychological research indicates that this is not always the case. Does this mean that people are irrational? Not necessarily. We have already seen that some decisions are perceived as "riskier" than others. Preferences for actions with lower "risk" can hardly be characterized as irrational despite their violation of the norms of formal utility theory.

Independence

Savage's (1954) independence axiom states that outcomes that are not differentially related to the possible actions should have no effect on the decision maker's choice of one action over another. This axiom is important to SEU theory because, if choices are affected differently by outcomes with the same utility, multiplying utilities by probabilities would be pointless.

The most famous demonstration of the violation of the independence axiom is the one provided by the French economist Allais (1953). Allais' demonstration, known as Allais' paradox, requires a choice between two gambles, 1 and 2. These gambles are illustrated in the top part of Table 4-3. Gamble 1 is relatively simple. Anyone who chooses it is certain to win $10,000. Gamble 2 is more complicated; there are three possible outcomes: a .10 probability of winning $50,000, a .89 probability of winning $10,000, and a .01 chance of winning nothing at all. According to Allais, the majority of people prefer Gamble 1 to Gamble 2. That is,

Table 4-3. Allais' Paradox[a]

Pair	Probability of Winning	Amount ($)
Gamble 1	1.00	10,000
Gamble 2	.10	50,000
	.89	10,000
	.01	0
Gamble 3	.11	10,000
	.89	0
Gamble 4	.10	50,000
	.90	0

[a] Adapted from Wright (1984). Reprinted with the permission of Penguin Books. Copyright © George Wright, 1984.

they prefer a certain $10,000 to the small chance of winning nothing in Gamble 2.

Now consider Gambles 3 and 4, illustrated in the bottom of Table 4-3. Gamble 3 consists of a .11 probability of winning $10,000 and a .89 probability of winning nothing while Gamble 4 consists of a .10 probability of winning $50,000 and a .90 probability of winning nothing. Allais claimed that when given a choice between Gambles 3 and 4, most people prefer Gamble 4, which has similar probabilities to Gamble 3 but offers a much bigger prize.

Although neither the preference for Gamble 1 over Gamble 2 nor the preference for Gamble 3 over Gamble 4 are remarkable in themselves, but taken together they are very interesting indeed. To see why, imagine that the gambling choices were restated algebraically. Preferring Gamble 1 to Gamble 2 implies that SEU Gamble 1 > SEU Gamble 2. This means that:

$$u \, \$10,000 > .10u \, \$50,000 + .89u \, \$10,000 + .01u \, \$0$$

If we do some algebra and subtract $.89u \, \$10,000$ from both sides of the equation we are left with:

$$.11u \, \$10,000 > .10u \, \$50,000 + .01u \, \$0 \qquad (6)$$

Now let's look at Gambles 3 and 4. A preference for Gamble 4 over Gamble 3 implies that SEU Gamble 4 > SEU Gamble 3. Thus,

$$.11u \, \$10,000 + .89u \, \$0 < .10u \, \$50,000 + .90u \, \$0$$

If we do some algebra and subtract $.89u \, \$0$ from both sides of this equation, the result is:

$$.11u \, \$10,000 < .10u \, \$50,000 + .01u \, \$0 \qquad (7)$$

Equations 6 and 7 directly contradict one another, yet they describe most people's preferences, hence the "paradox." According to Allais, the

Table 4-4. Allais' Paradox and the Independence
Axiom[a]

Pair	Ball Numbers		
	1	2–11	12–100
Gamble 1	10,000	10,000	10,000
Gamble 2	0	50,000	10,000
Gamble 3	10,000	10,000	0
Gamble 4	0	50,000	0

[a] Adapted from Wright (1984). Reprinted with the permission of Penguin Books. Copyright © George Wright, 1984.

paradox arises because SEU theory does not take riskiness into account while decision makers do. Gamble 1, which offers a certain win, is perceived as less risky than Gamble 2. Gamble 4 is preferred to Gamble 3 because its payoff is much larger for almost the same "risk." To see why such preferences violate the independence axiom, it is necessary to restate the gambles in more concrete form (Slovic & Tversky, 1974).

Imagine that 100 numbers, each representing a different probability, were individually printed on a set of 100 golf balls. The 100 balls are placed in a barrel where they can be drawn randomly one at a time. The four gambles are illustrated in Table 4-4. In Gamble 1, which corresponds to Allais' Gamble 1, you win $10,000 no matter which ball is drawn. In Gamble 2, as in Allais' Gamble 2, you win nothing if ball number 1 is drawn, $50,000 if any of the balls marked 2 to 11 is drawn, and $10,000 if any other number is drawn. Gambles 3 and 4 correspond to Allais' Gambles 3 and 4 and are illustrated similarly. When the gambles are represented this way, Table 4-4 indicates that the information contained in balls 12–100 is irrelevant to the choice between Gambles 1 and 2 because, no matter which is chosen, the outcome for these balls is identical. The same is true for Gambles 3 and 4. Nevertheless, Allais' paradox illustrates that people do change their preferences on the basis of the information contained in balls 12 through 100, thereby violating the independence axiom.

It is true, of course, that most people are not sufficiently sophisticated mathematically to have ever heard of the independence axiom. It is possible, therefore, that their "paradoxical" behavior is merely the result of ignorance. This possibility was studied by MacCrimmon (1968) using a sample of businessmen training for top management positions. MacCrimmon's technique involved giving the executives decision problems specially designed to test their acceptance of the axioms of formal utility theory. The executives were asked to give their initial (untutored) answers to these problems and then they were provided with arguments favoring the axioms or conflicting with them. The executives were asked

Table 4-5. A Hospitalization Insurance Decision

| | Outcome | |
Decision	Hospitalized	Not Hospitalized
Insure	No loss[a]	Small loss (premium)
Do not insure	Large loss (hospital charges)	No loss

[a] Because the premium is not reimbursed, this outcome may also be considered to be a small loss.

to critique these axioms and to indicate which they believed to be "most logical." As if all this were not enough, each executive also participated in a 30-minute discussion centered on what constitutes the "correct" answer to each of the problems presented initially. The results were as follows: the executives initial answers to the problems contained frequent violations of the axioms of formal utility theory (40% of their initial choices violated at least one axiom), and many executives did not even perceive these axioms as logical. However, after the discussion, they were able to see the error of their ways and accept the axioms, including the independence axiom, as logical and correct.

Exactly what MacCrimmon said to the executives during these discussions is not known. This is unfortunate, as other psychologists who have tried to replicate MacCrimmon's procedure have found that their subjects persistently violate the independence axiom even after it is carefully explained to them (Slovic & Tversky, 1974). Moskowitz (1974) used a number of different presentation formats, including lectures and tree diagrams, to try to get people to accept the independence axiom, also without much success. MacCrimmon himself has had second thoughts and has suggested that SEU theory may require reevaluation (MacCrimmon & Larsson, 1976).

Violation of SEU axioms in medical situations

It is not necessary to look for unusual examples to show that the axioms of formal utility theory may be violated; it happens every day. Consider hospitalization insurance. Table 4-5 indicates the possible outcomes of an insurance decision. As can be seen, those who are insured and not hospitalized lose their premium (small loss) while those who fail to insure and are hospitalized incur substantial hospital charges (large loss). The remaining outcomes lead to little or no loss.

Following the line of reasoning underlying SEU theory, a risk-neutral individual should consider insurance to be a worthwhile purchase when the annual premium equals the probability of hospitalization multiplied by the potential loss:

$$\text{premium} = P(\text{Hospitalization}) \times \text{Hospital Charges}$$

Risk avoiders, on the other hand, should prefer to buy insurance when the utility of the small loss represented by the yearly premium is greater than the utility of the larger loss of hospitalization multiplied by the probability of hospitalization plus the utility of no loss multiplied by the probability that no hospitalization will occur, or:

$$u(\text{premium}) = P(\text{Hospitalization}) \times u(\text{Hospital Charges}) + P(\text{No Hospitalization}) \times u(\text{No Charges})$$

In other words, a risk-averse individual may be willing to pay an insurance premium slightly higher than the risk-neutral individual, particularly when the cost or probability of hospitalization is high.

Observations of actual insurance buyers (Kunreuther, 1976) and experimental simulations of insurance purchases (Tversky & Kahneman, 1981) have found that people are reluctant to buy insurance even when premiums are set to levels that directly reflect their utility for money. Many even decline to buy government-subsidized insurance in which the premiums are so low that buyers are effectively in a "can't lose" position. Such behavior violates the dominance axiom because it means that people are not choosing the action that maximizes utility. Instead, they use a set of informal heuristics such as availability ("I don't need insurance since I have never been hospitalized"). These findings also suggest that people are often risk seeking when it comes to losses; they are willing to chance a loss even when they can insure against it. This behavior contrasts with the evidence from gambling reviewed earlier, in which most people were found to be risk averse.

The possibility that attitudes toward risk change depending on whether potential losses or gains are involved was studied by Eraker and Sox (1981) in a medical context. They used the direct gambling method to measure patients' utilities for different drug treatments. Patients were asked to choose between two drugs, one with a certain, moderately successful outcome and the other with two extreme outcomes. When the outcomes were stated positively (70% of patients improve), most people preferred a drug with a certain intermediate outcome to one that could produce either a large favorable effect or no favorable effect at all. When outcomes were specified negatively (30% experience adverse effects), preferences reversed. The drug that offered at least some possibility of no adverse effect was preferred to the one with a certain, but intermediate, adverse effect. Attitudes toward risk, then, are not constant properties of individual decision makers; they can change with presentation context. This finding also agrees with those obtained by the studies of insurance buying; people appear risk averse when it comes to gains and risk seeking when it comes to losses.

As we have noted many times before, the way in which a problem is represented can have important effects on judgment—it can even determine utilities. For example, Llewellyn-Thomas, Sutherland, Tibshirani,

Ciampi, Till, and Boyd (1984) presented people with different descriptions of states of health (these are similar to treatment outcomes). These descriptions were presented either in narrative form or simply by indicating each person's most severe problem. Utilities for the various states of health were solicited by either the indirect gambling method or by direct ratings. The manner in which the states of health were presented, the method by which utilities were solicited, and even the sequence in which the descriptions were read affected the obtained utilities.

In a related experiment, Sutherland, Dunn, and Boyd (1983) asked ambulatory patients to rank five scenarios describing states of health in order of preference. They found several scenarios ranked worse than death by a significant portion of patients. They then asked the patients to rate each state of health by placing a mark somewhere along a 10-centimeter long visual scale. The ends of the scale were marked 1.0 (perfect health) and 0 (death). This procedure was repeated with the end points of the scale marked with intermediate states of health ("marked disability" and "little disability"). They found the ratings assigned to the various states of health varied with changes in the end points of the rating scale. Two aspects of this study are especially significant. First, it shows the effect of anchoring and adjustment on measures of preference. Second, it indicates that for some patients there are outcomes worse than death. E.W.'s doctors may have been wrong to assume that the outcome mother dead, child dead has a utility of zero. This study and the one by Llewellyn-Thomas, Sutherland, Tibshirani, et al. (1984) and Llewellyn-Thomas, Sutherland, Ciampi, et al. (1984) demonstrate that preferences for various health outcomes can change with changes in elicitation methods. Given such instability, violations of the dominance and transitivity axioms are inevitable.

Preferences can also change with a patient's state of health. As Elstein and Bordage (1979) pointed out, a patient in severe pain may produce different preference orderings when pain decreases. Similarly, a recovered patient may have different preferences from one who is acutely ill. Christensen-Szalanski (1984) examined the changes that occur over time in attitudes toward pain avoidance and anesthesia in childbirth. He found that women preferred to avoid anesthesia prior to active labor but preferred to avoid pain (by receiving anesthesia) during childbirth. One month after delivery, their preferences once again turned against anesthesia. Clearly, preferences measured at any particular time need not remain static (see Sjoberg, 1983, for another example).

The time dimension has received considerable attention by students of medical decision making not only because utilities may change over time but also because of what economists call the "discount function." This term refers to the empirical finding that an outcome's utility tends to diminish (be discounted) with time. (For example, most people prefer to win $100 today to $125 six months from now.) Discounting applies not only to positive consequences but to negative ones as well. Smoking and drinking are well-known causes of physical disability, but their consequences are so far in the future that their negative utilities are substantially diminished (Kozielecki, 1981).

In a widely cited study, McNeil, Weichselbaum, and Pauker (1978) elicited utilities for extra years of life using the direct gambling technique. They found a decreasing marginal utility for additional years. Thus, the value of an additional year of life is not constant; it varies depending on when in life it occurs. An extra year of life starting from today is worth more than an extra year 30 years from today.

The utility of an extra year of life also depends on its quality. McNeil et al. (1981) found that approximately 20% of their subjects preferred radiation treatment to surgery for cancer of the larynx because the former treatment preserved speech quality. Since radiation treatment has a higher mortality than surgery, their subjects were, in effect, trading off life expectancy for improved life quality. Similar findings were reported by Sutherland, Llewellyn-Thomas, Boyd, and Till (1982).

Since life quality influences the utility of surviving extra years, a fair amount of attention has been directed at measures of life quality. The pitfalls and successes of this work are reviewed by Kaplan (1982; Kaplan and Bush, 1982). An interesting finding of these efforts is that previous events can affect the utilities of future ones. For example, a patient who has already undergone a series of medical tests may refuse to undergo further testing even when such testing has the potential to yield important information. In economic terms, the time, effort, and money spent on earlier tests are "sunk costs" that cannot be recovered and that should not influence future decision making. Yet, the research suggests that they often do (see Arkes & Blumer, 1985).

Measuring utilities for future years of life assumes that patients really can make the judgments required of them. Writers have criticized this assumption on several grounds. Bursztajn and Hamm (1982) argued that fear and denial can affect such judgments, particularly for patients who have only recently been diagnosed. Fearful or denying patients may be unable or unwilling to appreciate the implications of choosing between longer or better lives. Bursztajn and Hamm also noted that some patients may assign utilities to an increased life span by considering the effect on their families (caring for an invalid and so on) while others may consider only themselves. Still others may consider religious or moral strictures more important than personal values. We might add to these problems that the task itself is fairly ambiguous. How, exactly, is a patient who is asked to choose between 4 years of survival with a handicap or 2 years of survival with fairly good health supposed to interpret the choice? Is survival guaranteed for 4 years followed by certain, and im-

Table 4-6. Variables Affecting Utility Judgments

Problem Representation

The manner in which the options are defined.
The number and specificity of the options given to the decision maker.

Measurement Technique

The way in which utilities are elicited.
The labels given to the consequences.
The sequence in which options are presented.
Amount and specificity of the information provided.

mediate, death?* Does the question mean, "at least 4 years?" Such ambiguities can result in unreliable findings.

Up to this point we have assumed that doctors should use their patients' utilities when making decisions. This is the position favored by most writers (Kassirer, 1983; Kaufman, 1983). There are times, however, when someone else's utilities are relevant. Such a situation arises when scarce resources must be allocated to specific patients (organ transplants) and when patients cannot make the necessary judgments (infants, the mentally incompetent). There are also decisions that are best made by therapeutic teams. In the latter case, it would be useful to have some measure of group utility. Unfortunately, utilities cannot simply be averaged across individuals—they are relative, not absolute measures. Various negotiation procedures have been developed to help group members "trade off" differences (Keeney & Raiffa, 1976). These negotiations take time, however, and in medical decision making time is usually not available. Instead, some consensus among clinicians is achieved informally. Research indicates that most doctors' utilities are so similar that such informal consensus procedures probably produce equivalent results to the more formal ones (Krischer & Dixon, 1982; Theodossi, Spiegelhalter, McFarlane, & Williams, 1984).

Problems in Interpreting Utility Assessment Studies

Taken as a whole, the research reviewed in this chapter suggests that utility assessment is far from an exact science. Small changes in context and elicitation techniques can have large effects on utilities. The factors known to affect utility assessments are summarized in Table 4-6.

Our discussion has been based on a specific interpretation of the experimental findings: we have inferred that a failure to behave as SEU

---

* Jorgen Hilden of the University of Copenhagen captured the ambiguity inherent in giving people a choice that includes 4 extra years of life with the following query: Does this mean that the patient can enjoy skydiving without a parachute for the next 4 years?

theory expects means that the theory fails to describe actual behavior. This interpretation is not the only one possible. As Fischhoff, Goitein, and Shapira (1979) pointed out, it is possible that subjects in these experiments are behaving as the theory predicts but that experimenters have just failed to notice it. Take the dominance axiom, for instance. We have interpreted the research findings to indicate that people sometimes fail to choose the action that maximizes utilities, as this axiom requires. However, it is always possible that subjects are actually maximizing their utilities and we have simply omitted some of the relevant actions from consideration. In Fischhoff et al.'s words, "with sufficient ingenuity, we can always find something that a particular decision maker has maximized in a particular situation" (p. 3). It is also possible that some variation of SEU theory can account for the behavioral data (see Quiggin, 1985, for example).

One particularly clever way to ensure that SEU theory survives unscathed from any encounter with apparently disconfirmatory data is to assume that evaluating alternatives and assigning probabilities—decision making itself—is an activity with negative utility (see Shugan, 1980, for example). The best way to reduce this negative utility is not to do so much thinking. Thus, when decision makers select what appears to be a suboptimal action, they may still be maximizing their utility by minimizing the negative utility produced by thinking through to the best action. Acceptance of this argument ensures that the dominance axiom is not experimentally testable. The axiom is always correct; researchers who appear to find differently have just failed to look at all the possible utilities (see Schoemaker, 1982, for more on this).

The essential unfalsifiability of the axioms of formal utility theory theory has also been mentioned by Dowie (1985), who noted that studies porporting to demonstrate violations of SEU axioms assume that their subjects are perfectly calibrated probability judges. This assumption is necessary because, without it, a failure to elicit reliable utilities may result simply from misunderstanding about probabilities. Consider, for example, the so-called "certainty effect." Given a choice between an action that will save 45 lives with certainty or an action that can potentially save 100 lives (with .5 probability) but may wind up saving no lives (also with .5 probability) most people prefer the action that leads to the certain outcome. From the standpoint of formal utility theory, such behavior is peculiar because the expected gain is higher for the action with uncertain outcomes.

Tversky and Kahneman (1981) concluded that actions leading to certain outcomes have higher utility than those leading to uncertain outcomes. If true, this means that people are violating one of the important operational assumptions of SEU theory—the assumption that utilities are not influenced by probabilities. As Dowie (1985) pointed out, however, Kahneman and Tversky's interpretation assumes that people understand that a probability of 1.00 means certainty and that they also know that a probability of 1.00 is twice as great as a probability of .5. If people do not know these things, they may believe a .5 probability to be less than one-half of 1.00 and, therefore, their preference for the certain outcome may be justified. As things stand, it is impossible to decide which of these two explanations for the certainty effect is valid.

The effect of criticisms like these on the field of decision making is to throw into question not the results of studies on utility measurement but their interpretation. Those writers who believe that SEU theory is not descriptive of human decision making take the research findings to show a need for new, descriptive theories. Those who view the research as inconclusive argue that apparent violations of SEU axioms demonstrate the need for formal decision analyses since peoples' intuitions clearly cannot be trusted. As Pitz and Sachs (1984) put it, faced with those who violate formal utility axioms, the latter writers would try to talk them into accepting them while the former writers would try to come up with a theory consistent with their behavior (see Klein, 1983, for several possibilities).

Utility Assessment: Summary

Beginning with Bernoulli's work in the 18th century, the concept of utility or subjective value has become a common part of economics and decision theory. Classical economists and most judgment and decision making researchers assume that rational choice involves comparing the utility of all possible outcomes and choosing the action that leads to the outcome with highest utility.

Measuring utility requires that the subjective values for various outcomes all be expressed on a similar scale. This is accomplished using a gambling procedure in which utility is expressed in terms of probability. This gambling procedure can be time consuming and difficult, so some researchers have attempted to measure utility directly. Still others have suggested that complicated outcomes be subdivided into simpler attributes whose utilities are measured separately and then aggregated. Although the evidence is not entirely clear, it does seem that the various methods for eliciting preferences produce fairly similar utilities provided that problems are represented in a similar manner. However, subtle changes in the way outcomes are described can exert a profound influence on expressed preferences, particularly when the decision maker has only partial information about the various potential outcomes.

Unlike probability calibration, which may be validated by comparing subjective estimates with real world frequencies, utilities cannot be validated—they are simply value judgments. This does not mean that any old utilities will do. Formal utility theory makes important assumptions about the mathematical relationships among subjective preferences. For example, they are assumed to be transitive and to obey the dominance and independence axioms. Psychological research conducted in both the laboratory and the clinic has revealed numerous violations of these axioms. It is difficult to escape the conclusion that SEU theory is not always descriptive. Whether this means we need to teach people to accept SEU axioms or to develop more descriptive theories is a controversial question. It comes up again in the next section of this chapter when we discuss how financial considerations are—and how they should be—incorporated into medical decision making.

Comparing Costs and Benefits

Thus far, we have viewed medical decision making as a matter of comparing probabilities and utilities and choosing the action producing the greatest expected utility. Except indirectly, we have not considered the cost (in dollars and cents)* of the various alternatives.

In one sense, this neglect may be justified. Most people, at least in western countries, have some form of government or private health insurance. Since insured individuals pay only a small part of the costs involved in their own health care, they have little reason to include them in their decision making. Doctors, too, are often reluctant to allow costs to influence treatment management, particularly when it appears that a "suboptimal" treatment may be chosen purely on economic grounds. After all, the argument goes, how can you put a price on someone's life?

But it remains true that hospital beds, equipment, drugs, doctors, nurses, and technicians all cost money. They can only be provided if someone (either other insured persons or society as a whole) agrees to pay. Thus far, many wealthy societies have been willing to spend whatever it takes to give patients a free choice of health care alternatives. Societies have responded to the increasing demand for health services by increasing the amount they spend: more doctors have been trained, more equipment purchased, and more hospitals built. However, even in rich countries such as the United States, spending cannot be expected to continue increasing forever. Sooner or later, the money will run out. When it does (and this has already begun to happen in many places around the world), hard choices will have to be made. Expenditures on medical care will have to be justified in the light of the various alternative ways that public funds may be spent.

The present section is concerned with this justification process. Specifi-

---

* Although the term "costs" is sometimes used to refer to any negative consequences resulting from a medical decision, including pain and discomfort as well as death (see Pauker & Kassirer, 1975, for example), we shall use it only in its narrow, financial, sense.

cally, we discuss cost–benefit analysis and cost-effectiveness analysis, two techniques for deciding how best to allocate scarce resources.

Cost–Benefit Analysis

In the abstract, cost–benefit analysis sounds a bit like financial accounting, the field from which it is derived (Mishan, 1976). One of its earliest advocates was Benjamin Franklin, who, in a letter to Joseph Priestly, described the process as follows:

> In the affair of so much importance to you, wherein you ask my advice, I cannot, for want of sufficient premises, advise you what to determine, but if you please, I can tell you how. When those difficult cases occur, they are difficult, chiefly because while we have them under consideration, all the reasons pro and con are not present to the mind at the same time; but sometimes one set present themselves, and at other times another, the first being out of sight. Hence the various purposes or inclinations that alternatively prevail, and the uncertainty that perplexes us. To get over this, my way is to divide half a sheet of paper by a line into two columns; writing over the one Pro, and the other Con. Then, during three or four days consideration, I put down under the different heads short hints of the different motives, that at different times occur to me, for and against the measure. When I have thus got them all together in one view, I endeavor to estimate their respective weights; and where I find two, one on each side that seem equal to some two reasons con, I strike out three. If I judge some two reasons con, equal to some three reasons pro, I strike out the five; and thus proceeding I find at length where the balance lies; and if, after a day or two of further consideration, nothing new that is of importance occurs on either side, I come to a determination accordingly. And, though the weight of reasons cannot be taken with the precision of algebraic quantities, yet when each is thus considered, separately and comparatively, and the whole lies before me, I think I can judge better, and am less liable to make a rash step, and in fact I have found a great advantage from this kind of equation, in what may be called moral or prudential algebra (cited by MacCrimmon, 1973, p. 27).

As Franklin's letter shows, the technique involves forming a balance sheet of costs and benefits. All possible adverse consequences of an action are identified and the probability and magnitude of each is calculated. Each outcome's cost is multiplied by its probability to determine its expected cost. The sum of the various expected costs constitutes the total expected cost of the action. So far, the process is identical to risk analysis, but there is another step; the benefits of the action must be estimated as well. The procedure is analogous to the one followed for costs. All positive consequences are identified, weighted, and multiplied by their respective probabilities to obtain each consequence's expected benefits. The sum of these benefits represents the total expected benefits of the action. The difference between the total benefits and total costs is the action's net benefit. If this difference is positive, the action should proceed; if it is negative, it should not. Since costs and benefits are compared directly, they must be expressed in the same unit. Usually, this unit is money.

Consider, for example, a cost–benefit analysis applied to a decision affecting many people: Should high-risk persons receive influenza vaccinations? In such situations, the cost of the proposed medical program includes the money required to pay the necessary personnel and obtain the other required resources (drugs, equipment, and so on) necessary to carry out the program. The benefits of the program are the reduction in mortality and morbidity (as well as the increased productivity) it is expected to produce (Pliskin & Taylor, 1977). Since each illness cured or prevented eliminates society's need to spend money, reductions in mortality and morbidity must also be expressed in monetary terms. That is, the benefits of any proposed medical program are equal to the total costs of the illness it was designed to prevent (or cure) plus the increases in economic productivity generated by allowing otherwise sick people to return to work (see Table 4-7 for a simple example.)

Sometimes, benefits are divided into two categories: direct and indirect (Weinstein & Fineberg, 1980). The direct benefits of a medical program (the money saved that would otherwise have gone toward expenditures on health care) are easy to estimate from commonly available health statistics. Indirect benefits, such as the value of increased life expectancy and economic productivity, present a bigger measurement problem. The monetary value of a human life has been equated to an individual's expected future earnings, to the amount awarded by courts to accident victims and their families and to the salaries paid to workers in risky occupations (Fischhoff, 1979). Howard (1978) has suggested that a person's private value for their own life can be measured by asking questions such as: How much money would you want for swallowing a pill that has a .001 chance proving fatal? The various methods of measuring the value of a life yield different results, and choosing one rather than another involves serious ethical judgments (Bishop & Cicchetti, 1973).

Since medical procedures may produce (or reduce) pain and discomfort, they too are indirect results of medical treatment that may also be expressed monetarily. Once again, there are several ways to do this: court judgments and insurance company payouts to accident victims are two, the revealed preferences approach discussed earlier is a third. However, none of these methods is without its critics, and when the methods produce different results it is difficult to choose among them (Pliskin & Taylor, 1977).

A complication affecting the assessment of both direct and indirect costs is the time dimension. Today's action has immediate costs while its benefits may be far in the future. For example, the goal of a screening

Table 4-7. Cost–Benefit Analysis

A hypothetical mass immunization program is proposed to prevent a major outbreak of lamb flu. Without the program, the disease is expected to affect 50% of the 50 million citizens in the high-risk categories (the aged, children under 2, and those with pulmonary disease). Of those who catch lamb flu, 2% are expected to die. The immunization is not 100% effective, but it should prevent about 75% of cases that would otherwise have developed.

Aside from its manufacturing and administration costs, the drug is also known to cause fatal allergic reactions in 1% of those who receive it. The following simplified cost–benefit analysis looks at a decision to immunize all 50 million high-risk people. The analysis assumes a value of life of $500,000 dollars regardless of the age of the patient. We also assume that those patients who become sick but survive will require $100 worth of medical services.

Benefits

First, there will be a 75% reduction in the expected number of cases. Instead of 25 million, we now expect only 6.25 million. Of the 18.75 million prevented cases, 2% (375,000) would have died. The benefits of saving these lives amounts to $185.75 billion. The remaining 18,375,000 prevented cases do not have to spend $100 each on medical services, a total of $1.838 billion. Total benefits = $187.588 billion.

Costs

The manufacture of the drugs and their administration costs $100 million ($2/person). One percent of those who receive the drug will have a fatal allergic reaction; a total cost of $250 billion. Total costs = $250.1 billion.

Balance

Since the costs exceed the benefits, the project should not go ahead. However, note, that a small change in the number of allergic reactions (from 1% to, say, 0.75%) could swing the balance in the opposite direction.

program may be to prevent future cancers. According to economists, and the research discussed earlier, future benefits are valued less than present ones. Does this mean that future benefits such as cancer prevention should be "discounted?" If so, by how much? Should the possibility of inflation also be considered? At present, there is no generally agreed upon answer to these questions (see Swets & Pickett, 1982, for more on the problem of the effect of changing circumstances on cost–benefit analysis).

Proponents of cost–benefit analysis emphasize its versatility. Because benefits and costs are expressed in similar units, programs with different purposes may be compared. For example, the state health budget for dental care may be 30 million dollars. Cost–benefit analysis may be used to decide whether this money should be spent on fluoridation, school dental clinics, or public advertising campaigns (or some combination of all three). The costs and benefits of the programs may be compared and money allocated to achieve the greatest net benefit across all individuals (the greatest good for the greatest number).* There is no requirement that the programs being compared are related. Since costs and benefits are expressed in the same units, a school dental program may be compared with an influenza immunization program or even with a proposal to build a new road. The philosophy behind cost–benefit analysis is that society has only a limited amount to spend and that the maximum excess of benefits over cost (for the most people) is generally the best way to make spending decisions.

It should be obvious that cost–benefit analysis is really a type of decision analysis in which both positive and negative utilities are taken into account (Fischhoff, 1977). Consider, for example, the analysis of the benefits, risks, and costs of pertussis vaccinations as conducted by Koplan, Schoenbaum, Weinstein, and Fraser (1979). They began by estimating the number of extra whooping cough cases that would be expected if routine immunizations were discontinued. The number of cases they estimated would increase by a factor of 71 and the number of expected deaths would increase by 400%. The vaccinations themselves can cause encephalitis, so these cases must be considered a negative aspect of a vaccination program. The costs of a vaccination program are substantial but much less (69% less) than the costs of the illness. The bottom line—continue the vaccination program.

Because they are so similar, it is probably not surprising that the problems facing cost–benefit analysis are the same as those we have discussed in relation to decision analysis. Specifically, misunderstandings about probability, difficulties in measuring utility, incomplete specification of all possible consequences, a failure to accept the axioms underlying the decision rule, and the like can affect the validity of a cost–benefit analysis in the same way that they affect a decision analysis.

A special problem facing cost–benefit analysis is its failure to address how costs and benefits are distributed among the population (Fischhoff, 1977; Fischhoff et al., 1981). There are programs that result in some individuals paying the costs while others receive the benefits. This is certainly the case for many medical programs in which patients, physi-

* In some circumstances, other decision rules make more sense. For instance, when all outcomes involve only costs, the best strategy is to choose the action that results in minimum cost.

cians, and insurers may have quite different perspectives on what constitutes an acceptable level of costs and benefits. Although it is sometimes
possible for those who receive the benefits to compensate those who pay
the bills (tax deductions for charitable contributions, for example), this is
rarely the case when it comes to medical programs.

As in the case of decision analysis, the uncertainties inherent in a cost–
benefit analysis may be examined using sensitivity analysis. In the cost–
benefit analysis contained in Table 4-7, for example, small changes in
the assumptions could tip the balance in the opposite direction. In contrast, if the outcome remains unchanged, despite changes in a parameter, then it is fair to say that the analysis is insensitive to reasonable
changes in that parameter. Of course, the limitations of sensitivity analysis noted earlier (what data to test, how to decide on realistic ranges) also
apply.

Despite these problems, cost–benefit analysis remains an important
tool for making decisions when resources are scarce. It has been success-
fully applied to several types of medical problems (Bunker, Barnes, &
Mosteller, 1977; Drummond, 1980; Warner & Luce, 1982).

Although it may be used to evaluate decisions affecting a single patient, cost–benefit analysis has been applied primarily to decisions affecting large-scale health programs and many patients (Bunker et al., 1977).
However, there is a variant, called cost-effectiveness analysis, that is
suitable for evaluating decisions that concern small groups of patients or
even an individual (Weinstein, 1981). We discuss this technique in the
next section.

Cost-Effectiveness Analysis

Cost-effectiveness analysis is concerned with the efficiency of resource
allocation. In such analyses costs are generally expressed in economic
terms, although they can be stated in other ways (hours of physician's
time, days in hospital). Benefits are typically expressed in terms of the
number of cases detected (for screening programs) or increased longevity (for treatment or prevention programs). Because longevity alone may
not always be perceived as a benefit—when the patient is severely disabled, for instance—a better measure may be the "quality" of the life
extended by the treatment or prevention program. Although such a
measure sounds good in the abstract, it is not easy to devise. As we have
already seen, the way in which preferences are elicited can affect patients' judgments (see Kaplan & Ernst, 1983, for example). However,
several sophisticated instruments for measuring life quality have been
developed specifically to be used in analyses of cost effectiveness (Kaplan, 1982; Kaplan & Bush, 1982).

The output of a cost-effectiveness analysis is the ratio of costs to benefits, as in the cost per case detected or the cost per quality-adjusted year

of life saved. If there are several alternative programs, these can be ranked according to the size of their respective cost–benefit ratios. Programs may then be implemented starting with the highest ratio and working downward until resources are exhausted or until some cutoff point is reached where the cost–benefit ratio exceeds the willingness to pay. Setting this cutoff point is a matter for policymakers and clearly depends on their utilities and the level of available resources.

Although there is obvious overlap between cost–benefit and cost-effectiveness analysis, the two techniques do use different data and tend to be applied in different circumstances. For example, since cost-effectiveness analysis uses a direct measure of program effectiveness (number of cases detected, for example), it only permits programs using the same measure to be compared. Screening programs designed to detect cases, therefore, cannot be compared with, say, those designed to prevent pregnancy or reduce smoking. Cost–benefit analysis, which values everything in monetary terms, can compare any two programs, regardless of their purpose.

A particularly valuable aspect of cost-effectiveness analysis is its ability to estimate marginal costs—the incremental cost for every unit of extra benefit. The use of cost-effectiveness analysis for this purpose is illustrated by the following example, adapted from Weinstein and Fineberg (1980).

Costs and benefits of five screening strategies for colon cancer

In a population of men between 60 and 80 years of age, one in every 1000 examined has colon cancer ($P = .001$). Thus, in a hypothetical sample of 100,000 men, 100 will have cancer. There are three common screening methods for colon cancer: a manual examination of the rectum (digital exam); examination with an instrument called a sigmoidoscope (sigmoidoscopy); or examination of the stools for small traces of blood (hemoccult test). The costs of the three screening approaches (including equipment, instruments, materials, labor, and so on) for the three tests in 1980 dollars is (from Weinstein & Fineberg, 1980):

Digital exam: $2.00
Sigmoidoscopy: $25.00
Hemoccult: $.50

Not only do the three methods differ in cost, they also differ in their ability to detect cancer. The hemoccult test only picks up those cancers that bleed (about 80%); digital exam explores only the lower end of the colon, where only 10% of cancers occur. Sigmoidoscopy examines more tissue than a digital exam; it picks up 85% of cancers whether they bleed or not. Weinstein and Fineberg (1980) assumed that digital exam and sigmoidoscopy have minimal false-positive rates, whereas the hemoccult test has a false-positive rate of 10%. They also assume that patients with postive hemoccult tests will receive a definitive follow-up test, a barium enema. The barium enema costs $80.

Weinstein and Fineberg calculated the cost effectiveness of the three screening techniques plus some strategies that used combinations of the various techniques. They began by first determining the overall costs and the number of cases detected by each screening approach. For example, the expected cost of a digital examination alone is $200,000 (100,000 × $2). Since a digital examination can be expected to pick up only 10% of tumors, the expected number of cancers identified this way is 10.

Like digital exams, the expected cost of hemoccult tests is equal to the cost per test ($.50) times the number of tests (100,000), or $50,000. However, since all positive tests will be followed up with a barium enema, the costs of the follow-up test must also be considered. The hemoccult test picks up 80% of the 100 true cancers, but it also produces a positive result for 10% of those who do not have cancer. Thus, the total number of positives is $(.8 \times 100) + (.10 \times 99,900) = 10,070$. If each person with a positive test result receives a barium enema, the expected cost is $805,600 plus $50,000 for the hemoccult tests or a total of $855,600. Eighty cancers will be detected this way.

Following a similar logic, Weinstein and Fineberg calculated the expected costs and the number of cases detected for various combinations of screening tests. They also looked at the costs of administering the tests in different sequences. They found that each successively more expensive strategy detects more cases of cancer. For example, the digital exam alone costs $200,000 and is expected to detect 10 cancers. The hemoccult test plus barium enema follow-up on positive cases costs $855,600 and detects 80 cases. Combining the two strategies raises the cost to $1,054,960 but allows 82 cases to be detected, and so on. Weinstein and Fineberg found that no strategy was completely dominant. That is, no screening technique may be completely eliminated because it costs more and yields fewer benefits than another.

Weinstein and Fineberg then looked at marginal (incremental) costs. Their technique was to compare each strategy with the next most expensive. The least costly strategy is to do no testing at all. Of course, such a strategy will result in no cases being detected. The second-least costly option is the digital exam, which has a total cost of $200,000 and is expected to detect 10 cases of cancer. The difference between these two options is an expenditure of $200,000 and 10 detected cases. The ratio of these differences is $200,000/10 or $20,000. Thus, the marginal cost per additional case of cancer found for the digital examination is $20,000.

Now let us compare the digital exam with the next-most expensive option, the hemoccult test (plus follow-up barium enema for positive cases). The latter strategy's costs were estimated at $855,600 and the former's were $200,000. The difference is $655,600. The increment in the number of cancer cases detected is 70. This means that for an expenditure of an extra $655,600 we can detect 70 more cases of cancer, a marginal cost of $9366 per case. The reader will note that, although the hemoccult test plus follow-up is more costly than the digital exam, its marginal cost per case detected is actually lower.

Weinstein and Fineberg repeated the calculations for the marginal costs per additional cancer case detected for sigmoidoscopy and each of the possible screening strategies (by themselves and in various sequences and combinations). These were ordered from lowest to highest marginal cost. Which approach is eventually adopted depends on the available resources. The more money available, the more cases of cancer that will be detected (but at higher marginal cost).

In another example, Weinstein and Fineberg showed how cost-effectiveness analysis may be used to decide whether coronary bypass surgery should be administered to men suffering from angina and reduced cardiac output or whether the money should be used instead to treat men in the same age group for hypertension. In this case, life expectancy rather than cases detected is the variable of interest. Weinstein and Fineberg began with the cost of the surgery which is multiplied by the expected increase in life expectancy to produce a cost per year of life saved. The cost per year of life saved by the medical management of hypertension was calculated to be less than surgery. Weinstein and Feinberg concluded that it is more cost effective to treat hypertension than to perform the surgery. However, life expectancy was not adjusted for life "quality." The side effects of antihypertensive drugs may have a negative effect on life quality, while surgery may greatly improve it. When life quality was taken into consideration, the results of the analysis changed. Surgery became a more cost-effective option than the treatment of mild (but not more severe) hypertension. The important effect of life quality measures on the outcome of cost-effectiveness analyses is also discussed by Kaplan and Bush (1982).

The literature contains many examples of the application of cost-effectiveness analysis to medical decisions (Bunker et al., 1977; Churchill, Lemon, & Torrance, 1984; Elliot, Watts, & Reuler, 1983; Read, Pass, & Komaroff, 1982; Weinstein, 1981), but the technique has its critics as well (Fischhoff et al., 1981, for example). Like cost–benefit analysis, cost-effectiveness analysis assumes that all possible significant outcomes can be predicted in advance. It also assumes that the probability and magnitude of these outcomes may be measured and that widely different costs can be compared. Often, all of these conditions cannot be met. For example, the long-term side effects of a new drug may not be known.

In some cases, outcomes may be known but not their likelihood. This is particularly true for the side effects of many medical interventions whose probabilities are rather small. When uncertainties about outcomes or their magnitude exist, there is no option but to rely on expert judgment to fill in the gaps. As we have seen, these judgments may be biased. Since a cost-effectiveness (or a cost–benefit) analysis is only as good as the data upon which it is based, there is good reason to worry about the findings of such analyses. Ultimately, the acceptability of cost–benefit and cost-effectiveness analysis boils down to a matter of judgment.

Summary

Building on Chapters 2 and 3, which were concerned with gathering and interpreting clinical data, the present chapter reviewed the research on how actions are chosen. We began by reviewing the steps involved in making decisions when the outcomes are not perfectly predictable— risky decision making. We presented an example of risky decision making based on SEU theory. The power of the approach was illustrated but so, too, were some of its drawbacks. The first problem is to structure the decision task so that the problem is adequately represented. Decision analysts often take it for granted that decisions are represented adequately and that all likely consequences have been identified. Psychological research indicates that people are often insensitive to missing consequences and often fail to recognize that decision problems have been poorly represented.

One of the most important findings of researchers in the area of risky decision making is that people do not always behave as normative theories such as SEU say they should. There have been several attempts to explain why this should be so. One school of thought holds that people are irrational; indeed, they sometimes are. However, in many situations, the reason they violate SEU axioms has more to do with perceptions of risk than with irrationality. Risk perception turns out to be a complex function of how risks are presented, their predictability, and their "voluntariness." We seem to tolerate risks that we bring upon ourselves (smoking, skiing) but not those that are out of our control (nuclear energy accidents). We also seem to be greatly influenced by the way in which problems are presented. Two hundred deaths out of 600 patients sounds worse than 400 people saved out of 600. The decision heuristics that can lead to biased estimates of probability and riskiness also affect our choice of outcomes.

Although utility is an integral aspect of decision analysis, it too is not easy to measure. The gambling techniques required by SEU theory are often difficult for patients to use. Alternative, direct methods are easier to apply, but are theoretically unjustified. Perhaps even more worrying than measurement problems is the common finding that people routinely violate the axioms underlying formal utility theory. Once again, subtle changes in the way that problems are phrased can exert an important effect on measured utilities. Even relatively objective economic analyses such as cost–benefit and cost-effectiveness analysis are subject to the same biases and problems facing any form of human judgment.

Despite these problems, there is still merit in trying to formalize decision making. There is no evidence that suggests that intuitive decision making is superior to the formal approach and quite a lot that suggests it is not. Perhaps what is needed is a new sort of educational program. In the next chapter, we examine how decision makers learn from experience and whether such learning can be taught. We also look at the effectiveness of decision-making courses and the value of decision aids.

5

Learning, Feedback, and Decision Aids

Our conduct is influenced not by our experience but by our expectation of life.

George Bernard Shaw

The first four chapters of this book were concerned with the importance of decision making for medicine. In them, we described research on how doctors gather information, generate hypotheses, and make patient management decisions. Although this research is interesting in its own right (it helps us to understand a great deal about how people think), it has a definite practical purpose as well. This purpose is the development of new teaching methods. It is a commonly expressed belief that once we understand how people make judgments, we should be able to teach them to make better ones (see Kepner & Tregoe, 1965; Schrenk, 1969). Unfortunately, despite its importance for professional training, relatively little research has focused on the best way to make doctors better decision makers. This chapter describes attempts to train people, especially doctors, to be better decision makers. Also reviewed are educational programs, computer expert systems, and other approaches to improving decision making.

Traditionally, medical education has been divided into two parts. In the first, the basic sciences curriculum, students are exposed to biology, chemistry, anatomy, and other sciences. The major goal of this aspect of medical training is to teach students the relevant scientific "background" of clinical medicine. The goal of the second part, the clinical curriculum (which may be conducted simultaneously with the first), is to provide students with the clinical acumen, the expertise, of experienced doctors.

Becoming an expert clinician requires that the student learn several skills. The novice physician must first learn what the salient problems are (disease categories, for example) and the relevant dimensions (signs and symptoms) on which these problems are evaluated. The doctor must then learn how to evaluate patients on these dimensions, the relative importance of the various dimensions, and, finally, the optimum combination rule for making management decisions. Substantial learning is required in each of these stages.

In an attempt to describe on a theoretical level the mechanisms by which students learn to make expert judgments, Shanteau and Phelps (1977) discussed three possibilities. The first, and simplest, is that students learn on the basis of feedback. That is, they make judgments and observe what happens. This type of learning requires a fair amount of trial and error because feedback from good and bad outcomes eventually leads to improved judgments.

A second method for gaining expertise is to learn to match a model or ideal decision rule. Students are given the "optimum" decision rule for a particular situation and must learn to apply it. (For example, when the probability of pneumonia is greater than 50%, order an x-ray.) Superficially, at least, training by rules appears to be a more efficient way of gaining expertise than simply relying on trial-and-error feedback, but, of course, the technique requires that the optimum rule be known in the first place.

Shanteau and Phelps' third method of gaining expertise is to learn to match an expert judge ("learning at the master's knee"). This is the method employed in clinical training. For this method to be effective, we must first identify who the experts are, the nature of their expertise, and the best way of transferring their expertise to students. At present, expertise is thought to be gained by working alongside experienced physicians and observing their methods. Exactly how such observations lead to the transfer of skills from the expert to the student is rarely discussed. It is generally assumed that simply observing an expert is sufficient.

This chapter is divided into five parts. The first is concerned with measuring doctors' performance. Before we can develop effective educational procedures, we must know how we want physicians to behave in the first place. For this reason, we begin the chapter with a review of both quantitative and qualitative attempts to evaluate clinical judgment.

Because doctors are frequently called upon to make probabilistic judgments, it is no surprise that some educators have suggested that training in decision analysis will improve medical decision making. The direct, classroom approach to teaching medical decision making is not meant to be a substitute for clinical training but rather an adjunct to more traditional experiences. The content of decision-making courses, their effectiveness, and some alternatives to classroom-based instruction (teaching clinical algorithms, teaching specific judgment skills) are also reviewed in the second section.

The third part of this chapter is concerned with expertise itself. Among the questions addressed are: Is expertise simply a matter of knowing more about a particular topic, or do experts actually learn different ways of thinking (heuristics)? and Does experience always improve expertise?

The fourth section looks at the mechanisms by which expertise is gained. Two singled out for special attention are those emphasized by Shanteau and Phelps: learning from feedback and learning to match optimum rules. As we have noted several times, many, if not all, medical judgments involve probability. Symptoms have a probabilistic relationship to diagnoses, and treatments have a probabilistic relationship to outcomes. This section reviews the psychological literature on how people learn probabilistic relationships on the basis of feedback or rule matching.

The fifth and final section of this chapter is concerned with conveying the results of decision analyses without actually requiring doctors to perform such analyses themselves. For example, decision analyses may be conducted by biomedical researchers and their findings translated into specific rules about what actions are optimal given certain patient management situations. These rules, often called algorithms, may then be applied by doctors when they encounter similar situations. Algorithms are easily translated into computer programs (many are computer programs); these programs can function as automatic decision makers. However, there are some drawbacks to algorithmic programs that have led some researchers to prefer a rather different approach to automating clinical expertise—knowledge-based "expert systems." Both types of clinical computer systems are discussed in section five.

Measuring Doctors' Performance

Mention performance reviews and most physicians think of large-scale studies of the frequency with which various medical and surgical procedures are used. Typically, these studies involve examining official records such as hospital charts, bills, insurance reimbursements, or public health statistics. Eisenberg and Nicklin (1981), for example, analyzed doctors' use of diagnostic procedures by examining bills submitted for reimbursement to a government health insurance program. Their study included over 55,000 patient visits to more than 300 physicians. In addition to some relationships between the number of tests ordered and medical specialty (internists ordered more tests than general practitioners), they also found a negative relationship between years of experience and the number of laboratory tests ordered (more experienced doctors ordered fewer tests). They even found a relationship between the number of tests ordered and the type of medical school the doctor graduated from (public or private). Reviews of other public records have found regional differences in the application of surgical procedures and other interesting correlations (see Kelman, 1980, for the results of several such reviews).

Although these findings are interesting, and suggest important hypotheses that are worth following up (are private medical schools teaching doctors to be wasteful, or are public schools teaching them to be neglectful?), they do not tell us much about the performance of individual doctors. Are the doctors who order many tests making more accurate diagnoses? Are their patients receiving better care? What are the thought processes, the heuristics, underlying doctors' selection of tests? The answers to these questions require that individual doctors' patient management decisions be studied. Several attempts to do this are reviewed in this section.

General Performance Reviews

According to Kelman (1980), the first systematic study of doctors' performance was conducted 30 years ago by Peterson, Andrews, Spain, and Greenberg (1956). Peterson et al.'s method was based on the observation of physicians in their own clinics. Specifically, Peterson et al. recruited a group of university-based physicians to observe a sample of 88 general practitioners and to rate their performance in evaluating and managing patients. Performance ratings were made on a 5-point scale in which a rating of 1 was best and a rating of 5 worst. As might be expected, the largest number of doctors were rated 3 (average) and most of the rest were rated either 2 or 4. However, 16 of the 88 physicians evaluated received the worse possible rating of 5 while only 7 were given the best possible rating of 1.

The judges in Peterson et al.'s study based their ratings on several aspects of doctors' performance (manner, thoroughness, and so on), but major emphasis was placed on the data-collection process. Doctors rated in the lowest category were described as performing "sketchy" physical examinations, ignoring important problems, failing to order appropriate laboratory tests, and neglecting potentially serious complaints.

The judges also found even above-average physicians to be poor at managing some conditions, particularly anemia and hypertension. Doctors often failed to explore the reasons for anemia and, in the case of hypertension, frequently recommended only an antihypertensive drug without giving much attention to weight loss or low-sodium diet (of course, knowledge about alternative treatments for hypertension was limited in 1956.)

Peterson et al.'s results were largely confirmed by another study using a similar method (Morehead 1962; cited by Kelman, 1980). Morehead reported that 43% of the patients seen by doctors in the survey sample received less than "optimal" treatment. When these cases were characterized as to type of deficiency, more than half were found to involve inadequate data-collection procedures. This study, and Peterson et al.'s, suggest that there may be a tendency among some doctors to treat superficial symptoms while making only a minimal attempt to identify the precise nature (and extent) of the underlying pathology.

Additional performance reviews have been conducted over the years (see Kelman, 1980). Although they attempt to study individual doctors, the information gained from them is fairly limited. The problem is the superficial nature of the research itself. The methodology of these studies does not permit any insight into why doctors' performance is sometimes suboptimal. They leave unanswered several important questions: Were the doctors ignorant? Were they constrained by econimics? (Perhaps some of their patients were unable to bear the expense of diagnostic tests.) What about hospital policy toward "excessive" diagnostic procedures? Before we can say that doctors are using faulty heuristics we need to know the answers to all of these questions. To do this, we must study physicians' thinking in a more direct fashion. First, we need some way to measure clinical thinking.

Measuring Medical Thinking

One of the first attempts to measure the cognitive processes underlying doctors' clinical judgment was reported by Williamson (1965). His subjects, 252 doctors, were required to read simulated case histories of patients suffering from either hypertension, congestive heart failure, or a pulmonary embolism. The case-specific information provided included presenting symptoms and relevant history. The doctors were also given a list of possible diagnostic procedures. Their task was to select the procedure they would order first for such a patient. They could obtain results simply by erasing a special patch alongside the procedure's name (the results were hidden underneath). The doctors in this study could "order" as many procedures as they liked. Once they were satisfied that they understood the patient's case, the doctors were asked to choose, from a number of therapies, the one they believed optimal for the particular patient. (For all cases, optimal treatments had been preestablished by expert cardiologists.)

Williamson found that his subjects performed very well at choosing the proper (defined as most useful) diagnostic procedure, but they had a great deal of difficulty choosing the optimal therapeutic course. These findings conflict with the results of the general performance reviews. The common finding of the former studies was that suboptimal performance is mainly a matter of poor data collection rather than the selection of suboptimal treatments. In part, the discrepancy may have been the result of the way the two studies were conducted. General performance reviews are carried out by observing physicians in the real world of the clinic, whereas Williamson's study involved hypothetical cases and a "paper-and-pencil" task. It is possible that the same doctors may behave one way in the clinic and another way in the laboratory if they perceive problems differently in the two situations. For example, it is possible that some therapies, antibiotics, for instance, are perceived to be so safe and effective that they are prescribed for some conditions (sore throats, coughs) without first obtaining bacteria cultures. The same physician may, when given a paper-and-pencil test, order the culture because it is the "correct" thing to do, knowing full well that it may not be the most "practical" option. The psychological literature contains several references to experts behaving differently in the laboratory from the way they behave in the "real world" (see Ebbeson & Konecni, 1980, for example). Such differences make it very difficult to generalize paper-and-pencil findings to actual clinical practice.

Another problem with Williamson's approach was its *ad hoc* nature. To be of any value, a measure of physician thinking must be reliable (free from measurement error) and valid (it must actually measure medical judgment uninfluenced by extraneous factors such as economic constraints or hospital policies). Producing reliable and valid measures is difficult unless we are quite specific about the skills we are attempting to assess.

Illustrative attempts to devise measures of the cognitive processes underlying medical judgment were reported by Balla (1980) and Wright, Stanley, and Webster (1983). Balla's subjects consisted of medical students at various stages in their education as well as expert clinicians. Each subject was given a questionnaire to complete. The questionnaire was divided into seven parts, each designed to tap a different aspect of what Balla called "logical thinking." The tasks included making diagnostic judgments based on varying amounts of positive and negative data, combining prior probabilities with case-specific information, organizing anatomical information in a clinically useful way, and formulating hypotheses on the basis of limited data. Balla found that experts and students at various levels of training experienced similar difficulties performing the required tasks. All subjects had a particular problem using "negative" characteristics (the absence of a sign) to make diagnostic judgments, and many also appeared confused about how prior probabilities should be combined with case-specific information to reach diagnostic judgments (see Eddy, 1982, for more on this last point). Balla found that expert clinicians were superior to students in generating hypotheses from clinical data, an ability that seemed to develop slowly with training.

Although the skills Balla measured certainly appear to be important ones, he made only minimal attempts to examine the reliability of his scale, and his finding that experts often performed no better than students on measures of logical thinking suggests either that his scale was not a valid measure of expertise or his "experts" were not very expert. Wright et al. (1983) also devised a scale to measure medical thinking, but they did attempt to determine its reliability and validity. They began by enumerating the cognitive abilities their scale was designed to measure. These included:

1. Observation (noting important patient characteristics and any changes in a patient's condition).
2. Communication (understanding and conveying clinical information).
3. Hypothesis formation and verification (forming hypotheses and searching for confirmatory or disconfirmatory data).
4. Diagnosis (reaching a conclusion based on an evaluation of relevant data).
5. Management (formulating treatment plans and following up treatment results).
6. Review (evaluating and learning from the total clinical situation).

Wright et al.'s measure consisted of a series of short-answer clinical problems designed to tap each of these skills. The final measure showed a high degree of interrater reliability. They also found that the ability to perform well on one cognitive skill did not necessarily ensure that performance would be equally good on another skill. This suggests that the various skills are independent. Although the authors concluded that their test is valid, they did not present any evidence that better physicians score higher on their test. Nevertheless, measures such as theirs are a necessary first step in the design of useful tests of physicians' cognitive skills.

Patient Management Problems

One of the most promising developments in the evaluation of physicians' thinking is the creation of standard patient management problems (PMPs) (Hubbard, 1971; McGuire, Solomon, & Bashook, 1976). The typical PMP is an elaborate simulated case study specially designed to tap the cognitive processes underlying typical patient management decisions. Patient management problems may be presented in printed form (Allen et al., 1984), via computer (Johnson, Moller, & Bass, 1975), or via tape recordings or videotape (acted out). For a particularly high-fidelity simulation, the decision problem can be acted out using actors (or real patients) in the various roles (see Berry, 1961 and Elstein, et al., 1978). The most common format, however, is printed.

The typical PMP begins with the patient's chief complaint and includes information on the patient's history. This is generally followed by sections dealing with the physical examination, diagnostic procedures, and attempted therapies. Each of these sections presents the physician with a series of decision options, and feedback (laboratory findings, for example) is provided to the doctor as it would be in normal clinical practice. (An exception to this is the result of any therapeutic intervention, because this could give away the most likely diagnosis.) The number of correct management decisions, diagnostic accuracy, and the appropriateness of therapeutic choices may all be evaluated and scored. Examiners can also follow the doctor's line of thought by observing the decision sequence (see Elstein et al., 1978, for an example).

Although the idea behind PMPs is not new (similar techniques formed the basis for Williamson's research in 1965), substantial effort has been devoted to improving the psychometric qualities of modern PMPs in an attempt to make them reliable and valid assessment devices. Wolf, Allen, Cassidy, Maxim, and Davis (1983) found that performance on PMPs correlates with performance on other tests of medical competence such as Part I of the American National Board of Medical Examiners' test. They also found that performance on PMPs improves after a course on medical problem solving. These results seem to support the validity of PMPs as measures of clinical competence.

Despite these findings, there are still some controversies in the literature. These controversies are worth examining not only for what they tell us about PMPs but also because they illustrate the difficulties involved in developing adequate assessment devices.

A problem discussed by Newble, Hoare, and Baxter (1982) relates to what earlier researchers (McCarthy, 1966, for example) called the "cueing" problem. Simply, the problem is this: doctors tend to chose more options (more tests, for example) when the choices are listed for them—as in the typical PMP—than when they must make the choices without a list of options to choose from (as in the typical clinical situation) (see also Goran, Williamson, & Gonella, 1973).

Another problem, also pointed out by Newble et al., is that the correlation between years of clinical experience and performance on many PMPs is fairly weak (they actually found it to be negative). Wolf (1984), in a reanalysis of Newble et al.'s findings, also found no statistically significant PMP performance differences between doctors with different levels of experience. It is difficult to see how a test can be considered a valid measure of competence if inexperienced doctors (and students) perform as well as experienced clinicians (the same problem was noted for Balla's scale as well).

The cueing problem, and the failure to find the expected correlations between experience and performance, are not the only difficulties noted with PMPs. There is also the problem of intraindividual inconsistency. Elstein et al. (1978) and Allen et al. (1984) found little relationship between performance on one clinical problem and performance on another dealing with a different clinical situation. This suggests that the problems are tapping knowledge about particular diseases (or particular tests) rather than characteristic thinking processes.

Patient management problems and the other assessment devices discussed here share the underlying assumption that medical expertise can be validly and reliably measured. Another assumption shared by medical educators is that decision-making expertise may be taught. Attempts to teach courses in decision making to medical students and expert doctors are discussed next.

Training in Decision Making

Why a Course in Decision Making?

As Elstein (1982) pointed out, the medical curriculum has always been crowded and precious little time is available for adding new courses. The introduction of a new topic into the curriculum, therefore, requires substantial proof that it will improve patient care. Elstein argued that medical decision making is one such topic. He believes it warrants addition to the medical curriculum because it deals with questions of uncertainty and value, questions doctors face every day.

A similar argument is made by Weinstein and Fineberg (1980, see also, Fineberg, 1984) in their widely used book on clinical decision analysis. They note three additional reasons why doctors should learn formal methods of decision analysis. First, decision analysis provides the physician with a vocabulary, a way of talking about uncertainty and value, that is more rigorous and less ambiguous than common terminology. Second, decision analysis offers a systematic method for structuring problems; it allows the doctor to focus on one aspect of a complex problem at a time. Third, decision analysis can clarify medical controversies by making clear exactly where disagreements lie.

The research reviewed in the first four chapters of this book makes it fairly clear that, without special training, both novice and expert physicians are likely to have trouble thinking probabilistically and may sometimes reach suboptimal decisions. Unfortunately, training people to become better decision makers has received scant attention in the psychological literature. In 1973, Nickerson and Feerher attempted to write a review of all controlled studies on how best to train people to make decisions under uncertainty. They found none. As recently as 1977, an extensive review of the decision making literature by Slovic et al. also included no references to training. In the last few years this situation has begun to change, but there are still few good studies on training decision makers. This dearth of literature on training is not for lack of advice about how such training should be conducted. There is plenty of advice available. The problem is that few researchers, or educators, have bothered to test this advice for its usefulness and practicality.

In this section, we review several approaches to training decision makers and the evidence, if any, for their effectiveness.

Classroom-based Approaches

According to surveys conducted by Elstein (1981, 1985), only one-fourth of the 80 responding institutions (medical schools and hospitals in North America and Mexico) offered some type of training in medical decision making. These courses were aimed mainly at medical students, medical faculty, and hospital house staff. Clinical practitioners were generally perceived as "less interested in formal approaches to clinical decision making than those who train them" (Elstein, 1983, p. 71).

Since Elstein's survey, interest in medical decision making has increased, and a number of new courses are now being offered (see Elstein, Rovner, & Rothert, 1982, for example), computer-assisted courses in judgment and decision making have been developed (see Bisseret, Redon, & Falzon, 1982, for an example), and a series of television films on medical judgment and decision making are in production in the United Kingdom (Dowie, 1984). Although Fryback and Thornbury (1978) found that just thinking about problems within a decision theory framework (without applying the actual mathematics) improves clinical judgment, most modern courses tend to emphasize the explicit application of formal decision analysis to clinical problems. An example of a fairly typical course is described by Cebul and his colleagues (Cebul et al., 1984).

The general course described by Cebul et al. involves 16 3-hour class meetings (half lecture, half workshop), a "coursebook" of materials specially designed to accompany the lectures, and a selective reading list. The course covers four main topic areas:

1. Selecting and interpreting tests
2. Decision tree analysis
3. Cost–benefit and cost-effectiveness analysis
4. Critical review of the medical literature (from the viewpoint of decision analysis)

Each section of the course introduces the decision concepts relevant to the particular topic. For example, probability revision and receiver operating characteristic (ROC) analysis are discussed as they relate to evaluating tests, and utilities are discussed in the section dealing with decision trees. The topics covered in this course are representative of those offered by other decision making courses.

Cebul et al. used several techniques to evaluate their course. Questionnaires were administered after each class section. These questionnaires asked the participants to indicate what new skills they believe they acquired, the clinical and educational relevance of the material presented, and the adequacy (clarity, coherence) of the presentation. Informal feedback to instructors from participants was also invited. In addition, each participant was evaluated using an examination designed to test their knowledge of decision analysis. To determine how much the participants had learned, this examination was given both before the course began and after its completion. Participants were also required to submit an independent research project that formed part of their final assessment.

A version of the general course was provided separately for medical students, postgraduate physicians, and physicians working at a community hospital. The three courses were not identical. The postgraduate course consisted of only three sessions, for example. Overall, the course was favorably received by the various audiences and, judging by the substantial improvement from pre- to posttest on the decision-making examination, most participants learned something as well.* Shanteau, Grier, Johnson, and Berner (1981) reported a similar improvement in nurses' decision skills following a course in decision making. The only dark cloud in all of this is Cebul et al.'s finding that 64% of the physicians rated the course's relevance to their clinical work as inadequate or merely adequate.

Elstein (1984), describing his experiences teaching medical decision making to medical students, reported a similar outcome. He also found students to be interested in the subject but, like Cebul et al., he could provide no evidence that those who complete his course actually use decision analysis in practice. Indeed, Elstein seemed to feel that a course in decision analysis, by itself, is unlikely to win any converts.

Cebul et al. hypothesized that the perceived lack of relevance of decision analysis to clinical practice may have been the result of the heterogeneous sample of their participants. What is relevant to doctors in one specialty may be irrelevant to doctors in another. Another possibility discussed by Cebul et al. is that experienced physicians already have their own way of making clinical decisions, which may make it difficult for them to see how to incorporate formal decision analysis into their everyday work. The discrepancy between how physicians think and formal decision analysis has also been suggested as one of the reasons computer-assisted diagnosis has not made greater headway. We deal with the point in more detail later in this chapter when we discuss computerized "expert systems."

Not all attempts to improve decision making by instruction have involved courses in formal decision analysis. Instead, some educators and psychologists have advocated teaching clinicians how to avoid the judgment biases and errors described in Chapters 2 through 4 without necessarily requiring that they understand the mathematical underpinnings of normative decision theories. Examples of this approach to training are discussed next.

---

* This conclusion must be considered tentative because only a minority of practicing physicians actually completed the posttest.

Improving Judgment Skills

As we have already noted, psychologists have found it extremely difficult to change peoples' judgment biases. Faulty judgment heuristics are not eliminated by informing decision makers about them; in fact, people tend to deny their existence even after being shown how they work (Fischhoff, 1982a). Being an expert in a field is also no guarantee that judgments will not be biased (Arkes & Blumer, 1985). Some authors (Nisbett, Krantz, Jepson, & Fong, 1982, for instance) have argued that decision makers must learn a new set of accurate "statistical heuristics" to replace (or use alongside) the judgment heuristics described in Chapter 3 (representativeness, availability, and so on). Several other writers have suggested teaching decision makers techniques for avoiding and correcting judgment biases (Kahneman & Tversky, 1982a). However, attempts to teach people to use these techniques to produce normatively correct judgments have met with only mixed success (see Fischhoff, 1982a, for example).

An alternative to statistical training is to teach people qualitative techniques designed to help them avoid common judgment errors. The goal of this training is to produce judges with "educated intuition" (Slovic, 1982). An example is the work of Gaeth and Shanteau (1984), who described how training can improve the judgments made by soil analysts. Soil analyses are performed routinely prior to road, dam, and other types of construction and as part of agricultural development. Although soil analyses may be carried out in the laboratory, this is often too time consuming and expensive for practicality. Instead, a soil judge is called in to determine the texture of a soil sample (the relevant percentage of sand, silt, and clay) simply by sifting some through his/her hands. In judging soil, the presence of any material other than sand, silt, or clay (rock fragments larger than 2 millimeters, for example) is irrelevant. So too is the soil's moisture content. Empirical research has found, however, that judges frequently allow these irrelevant factors to influence their analyses (see also, Shanteau, 1980).

Gaeth and Shanteau's subjects were a sample of soil judges who, on a pretest using several different soil samples, were found to be influenced by irrelevant information. Gaeth and Shanteau devised two training procedures. The first involved a lecture on relevant and irrelevant cues. In the second training method, labeled "interactive," the judges were given hands-on experience with soil samples in which the amount of irrelevant materials was systematically varied. Judgments of these materials could be immediately corrected by the instructor (hence the term "interactive"). A posttest administered after the lecture found only a minimal improvement in judgment, whereas the same test given after the interactive training showed a marked improvement. Interactive training led to a significant decrease in the influence of irrelevant information on the soil judges and an increase in the accuracy of their analyses. The effect of interactive training remained apparent when the soil judges were examined 1 year later.

Gaeth and Shanteau demonstrated that training can improve judgment under certain specific conditions, but learning to ignore irrelevant information is not the only problem facing decision makers. A more common source of errors is neglecting relevant information. Ignoring prior probabilities, for example, is a frequent source of error in clinical judgment (see Chapter 3). Fischhoff and Bar-Hillel (1984b) attempted to train judges to attend to all relevant information, including prior probabilities, when making statistical judgments. Their training employed what they called "focusing techniques." They described four such techniques. The first, "minimal focusing," simply involved asking judges to attend to all relevant information. The second technique, "subjective sensitivity analysis," required that decision makers consider what difference it would make to their judgment if an ignored item of information (prior probability) was not only included in their deliberations but also allowed to assume several different values. "Balanced subjective sensitivity analysis" required subjects not only to consider the effects of changes in prior probability but also to think about the effects of changes in other variables that were not ignored. The fourth focusing technique, "isolation analysis," required that judgments be made separately (on single items of information) prior to forming an overall judgment based on all of the available information.

Fischhoff and Bar-Hillel found that both subjective sensitivity analysis and isolation analysis improved judgment by focusing attention on the otherwise neglected prior probabilities. Simply asking judges to attend to all the relevant information also helped a little. Nevertheless, Fischhoff and Bar-Hillel did not declare focusing techniques an unqualified success. The reason? They found that focusing techniques served not only to direct attention to previously ignored relevant information but also to irrelevant information as well. They concluded that focusing techniques do not actually improve peoples' understanding of the importance of prior probabilities; they just encourage the use of more information. The implication of these findings is that unless "mechanical" techniques such as focusing are combined with knowledge about normative decision making they may be inappropriately applied. What appears to be necessary is training in formal decision making as well as training in specific judgment skills.

The difference between the successful training reported by Gaeth and Shanteau and the rather less successful findings reported by Fischhoff and Bar-Hillel is probably the result of the different skills each was trying to teach. It may be easier to learn to ignore irrelevant data than to learn to attend to relevant data.

There have been several attempts to improve the subjective probability estimates and the utility estimates used in decision analyses (Politser, 1981; Slovic et al., 1977). Although success has been reported for some techniques and some problems, the problems discussed in the first four chapters of this book remain largely unresolved. The mixed findings indicate the difficulty educators have in designing procedures to improve judgment. Although specific skills (and new statistical reasoning heuristics) may improve performance in specific judgment situations, there is always the possibility that, without the appropriate background knowledge in formal decision analysis, the techniques may be misapplied.

Given the difficulties involved in training clinicians in decision analysis and even in improving judgment skills, some writers have advocated teaching doctors ideal decision-making strategies for specific clinical situations. Teaching these strategies, called algorithms, to doctors is discussed next.

Clinical Algorithms

There is a substantial gap between textbook descriptions of diseases and their management and the daily life of a busy doctor. Textbook readers can think over the implications of what the author has written, they can reread whatever was unclear, and they can look ahead to see how the present information relates to future topics. In addition, patients described in textbooks are generally fully worked up, usually clear-cut cases; test results are rarely uncertain. In other words, the textbook reader is not constrained by time or circumstance in the same way as the clinician. The clinician must actively seek our information that is generally received sequentially, rather than all at once. Patient management, as we have seen, is typically a matter of making sequential decisions, each one based on the information gained thus far.

Computer scientists have long represented their programs graphically in the form of flow charts. Since programs, like patient management, involve sequences of decisions, some educators have suggested that flow charts might also be useful ways to illustrate the steps involved in managing patients. Over the years, these flow charts have become increasingly precise; many have sufficient detail to be called clinical algorithms (Komaroff, 1978; Lusted, 1968). Clinical algorithms, also known as "protocols," are precise descriptions of the appropriate steps involved in managing a case. They cover history taking, diagnostic procedures, and treatment selection. Where specific patient factors can affect diagnosis or treatment outcome (age, past illnesses, and so on), algorithms include choice points (branches) that permit management to be tailored to the specific case. Although they are typically presented in the form of flow charts, algorithms may sometimes be written as decision tables (see Holland, 1975) or computer programs (the latter are covered in greater detail in the final section of this chapter).

Algorithms were first used to train physician assistants and nurse practitioners (Sox et al., 1973). These "new health practitioners" were taught to use clinical algorithms to guide their interactions with patients, only calling in the physician when expert judgment or intervention was required (to write a prescription, for example) or to verify the assistant's observations. This system is designed to cut the costs involved in having every patient see the doctor as well as provide a rationale for patient management. Surveys have shown that patients have generally been satisfied with the service provided by nurses and assistants using protocols (Greenfield, Komaroff, & Anderson, 1976).

Early algorithms were designed to be as "complete" as possible; consequently, they required many laboratory tests and lengthy physical examinations. However, experience soon revealed that many of these procedures were unnecessary and the algorithms were simplified (see Wood, Tompkins, & Wolcott, 1980, for instance). The result has been that, instead of increasing the number of tests, algorithms have been found to decrease the cost of patient care (Christensen-Szalanski, Diehr, Wood, & Tompkins, 1982; Orient, Kettel, Sox, et al., 1983). Algorithms have been developed for the management of both acute and chronic diseases, emergencies, x-ray interpretation, and many other clinical problems (Komaroff, 1982). They have also been used for the evaluation of clinical performance and for setting standards of care (Margolis, 1983; Sox et al., 1973). In addition to the development of new algorithms, old ones are constantly being updated in the light of scientific and technological developments (Komaroff, 1982).

Preparing a clinical algorithm is clearly a large-scale undertaking. In their book on the subject, Lewis and Horabin (1979) listed seven steps:

1. Identify the precise performance required of the clinician (say, emergency room triage).
2. Clarify the set of problems (recognizing levels of seriousness).
3. Decide who will solve the problems (nurses, doctors).
4. Determine whether the algorithms will be used for teaching, as an aid in decision making, or both.
5. Begin with a rough outline.
6. Revise the algorithm on the basis of feedback from users.
7. Continue to test and revise until learning or performance criteria (specified in step number 4) are met.

Lewis and Horabin pointed out that algorithms are not mere lists of symptoms or diagnostic procedures but logical flowcharts or decision tables designed to help clinicians make decisions in the clinical context. An example appears in Figure 5-1.

Evidence from a variety of fields, not just medicine, confirms that

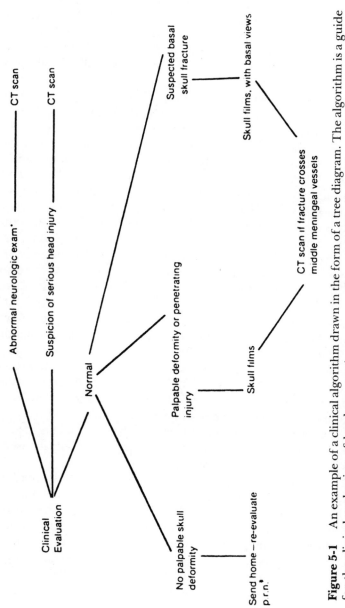

Figure 5-1   An example of a clinical algorithm drawn in the form of a tree diagram. The algorithm is a guide for the clinical evaluation of head trauma (p.r.n. means "as required"). Taken from Vydareny, Harle, and Potchen (1982) and reprinted here with the permission of Lippincott Publishers.

algorithms are an effective teaching tool. They have been found to convey more information in a shorter time and lead to better comprehension and retention than traditional textbooks (Margolis, 1983; Merrill, 1977). These findings have encouraged authors to produce textbooks that present information in algorithmic form (Eiseman & Wotkyns, 1978). Algorithms have also been used to teach patients how to look after some of their own health problems (Sehnert & Eisenberg, 1975).

Unlike decision analyses, algorithms may not typically specify probabilities and utilities. Instead, they often assume that the outcomes of various actions are known with certainty. Their recommendations take the following form: IF X IS TRUE THEN DO Y. Margolis (1983) believes that algorithms and decision analyses have different uses. Algorithms, he argued, are best used in common clinical situations in which treatments are largely either helpful or useless, but benign, and for which generally agreed-upon management protocols have been worked out. He reserved decision analysis for more difficult cases and when some actions may potentially result in harming the patient. However, there really is no reason why the algorithms and decision analyses cannot be used together, and some researchers have attempted to do just that. Komaroff, Pass, and McCui (1978), for example, used decision analysis to determine the probabilities for various diagnoses that then formed the basis for an algorithm designed to help clinicians manage urinary tract infections.

Despite their successes, algorithms have always created some uneasiness among those who believe they may lead to rigidity and mindless rule following (see Ingelfinger, 1973, for example). Of course this is possible, but thus far, at least, the available evidence suggests precisely the opposite happens (Margolis, 1983). Doctors taught to use algorithms become expert at noting which cases do not fit the standard profile and learn to adjust their management strategies accordingly. Also, because they make explicit the reasoning process involved in making management decisions, algorithms may be continuously tested and revised on the basis of experience with diverse cases.

Algorithms are obviously not a substitute for decision analyses, and learning them does not mean that doctors do not have to be taught to improve their judgment and decision making. Since algorithms involve gathering and interpreting data, they are as prone to judgment bias as any other clinical technique that depends on human perception and cognition. Without good judgment skills, doctors will be unable to employ even the simplest algorithm. The main virtue of algorithms is their explicit nature. Komaroff (1982) put it this way:

> a great virtue of algorithms is that, by making an explicit recommendation, they invite challenge and help focus the debate . . . they serve as a device for integrating information . . . to *organize* decisions, to clarify our knowledge and to recognize our ignorance. They can help us to demystify the

practice of medicine, and to demonstrate that much of what we call the "art" of medicine is really a scientific process, a science which is waiting to be articulated. (p. 11)

Objections to Training Doctors in Decision Making

In a recent symposium on the teaching of decision making, Elstein (1984) discussed some of the difficulties that he and others have had in teaching formal decision analysis and related topics to medical students (see also Elstein, 1983). As part of his talk, Elstein summarized the objections raised by his students to decision analysis. Some of these (the difficulty in measuring the utility of future health states and the frequent lack of appropriate prior probabilities) have already been discussed in the earlier chapters of this book. Other objections pertain to the specific atmosphere in which doctors work. For example, decision analysis is often seen as time consuming and therefore inappropriate for the clinic, where experts must render instantaneous decisions. These objections may all be termed "practical" ones. They suggest that decision analysis, as generally taught, is perceived as interesting, even important, but not very practical. Elstein (1983) took up this point directly:

> The problem here is that an experienced clinician may feel that decision analysis inherently simplifies a complex problem. No problem should be so simplified that crucial aspects of clinical reality are lost. . . . On the other hand, if actual clinical dilemmas are selected, the situation is unquestionably real and the clinical connection is clear, but the decision analysis may be so complex that learners give up. (pp. 283–284)

Some writers have found "hidden ethical problems" in decision analysis. Brett (1981), for example, argued that, when alternative actions lead to small differences in outcome, doctors should make their choice not on the basis of which outcome is "best" in decision-analytic terms, but on "ethical" grounds. He provided a hypothetical example. Diseases X and Y produce similar superficial symptoms and cannot be distinguished until they have run their course. In the population of patients who display the relevant symptoms, 20% turn out to have disease X, which has a 60% mortality rate unless treated with surgery, which itself has a mortality rate of 10%. The 80% of symptomatic patients with disease Y always recover without treatment. Brett claims that from a decision-analytic viewpoint, the optimal action is to operate on all patients with symptoms because this procedure yields a lower total mortality (10% versus 12%).

Despite its higher mortality, Brett argues for choosing the nonsurgical strategy. He bases his case on the following reasoning: if all symptomatic patients undergo surgery, the majority of those who die will be suffering from disease Y; these patients would have lived if they had not undergone the operation. If no one receives the operation, only those suffering from disease X would die. In other words, Brett seems to prefer slightly more deaths from "natural causes" to fewer deaths when some of the latter are iatrogenic and he believes that decision analysis leads to the opposite course. But Brett's description of a decision analysis omits what for most people is the very essence of the process—patient utilities (an omission he, himself, recognizes). Since surgical death is immediate, as opposed to the more likely *but delayed* death caused by disease, many patients may prefer the nonsurgical strategy. If these preferences are strong, they will outweigh the small mortality difference between the two strategies and the decision analysis will arrive at the same recommendation as Brett. Brett has not really discovered a hidden ethical dilemma in decision analysis, but his belief that he has is important because it probably reflects the view of many doctors and is therefore, one reason for resisting decision analysis.

Perhaps the most challenging objection to the decision-making training reported by Elstein (1984) is the perception among some doctors that decision analysis, with its reliance on numbers, is "dehumanizing" (see also Bursztajn, Feinbloom, Hamm, & Brodsky, 1981). Some doctors fear that adopting a decision analysis perspective would regiment medical care and remove all clinical "art." Elstein explained this reaction to decision analysis by suggesting that there is a need among doctors to appear "artful" and that this need is enhanced by maintaining an air of vagueness and mystery about how medical decisions are reached. When formal decision analysis is used, vagueness and mystery largely disappear. Dealing with this objection presents an important challenge to medical educators because the reaction appears to be largely psychological. One way to meet this objection is to study experts themselves. Understanding the nature of medical expertise should serve to demystify it and, at the same, allow new teaching methods to be developed. The nature of expertise in general and medical expertise, specifically, is discussed next.

The Nature of Medical Expertise

Acknowledged experts—financial advisors, petroleum geologists, academics, and of course, physicians, to name a few—often earn their livelihood in environments that can be characterized as containing uncertain information. Experts represent recognized talent in their respective fields; their superior ability is the result of intensive training, hard work, practical experience, and professional dedication.

Researchers have tried to understand how experts comprehend, remember, and use information in their chosen specialty. In this section, we review some of this research to show how experts differ from beginners. The goal is to gain an appreciation of the thought processes that

underlie complex cognitive activity. First, we review psychological studies of experts in several non-medical fields. Next, expertise in medicine
is discussed. Because it is the best researched area, we have decided to
focus on only one representative area of medical expertise—radiological
diagnosis and the differences between qualified radiologists and trainees
in the types of errors they make, the visual search patterns they use, and
the thought processes underlying their diagnostic judgments. After
these examples, we discuss the application of expert reasoning to computer-assisted medical decision making.

Experts and Novices

The experimental method of comparing experts to "novices" (usually
operationally defined as those with less experience) is of particular interest to cognitive psychologists because experts are assumed to be "better"
thinkers than novices. By comparing the two groups, psychologists can
gain some idea of the cognitive changes that occur as one acquires expertise. Adriaan de Groot is the researcher widely credited with giving
impetus to this approach. Working in the late 1930s and early 1940s, de
Groot had the opportunity to study some of the best chess players of the
time, players whose performance he compared to those less proficient.

In de Groot's (1965, 1966) studies, chess players with different levels
of expertise were shown a chess board with pieces distributed as if a
game were in progress and asked to consider their next move. The
players were asked to "think aloud" while they did this. De Groot's
findings did not support the intuitively plausible notion that chess masters ponder more possible moves and explore the consequences of those
moves deeper into the game than their less expert opponents. In fact,
chess masters did not consider more moves than other players, nor did
they analyze moves deeper into the game. Chess masters did, however,
spend more time thinking about "good" moves while weaker players
spent more time on "bad" moves. (Moves were defined as "good" or
"bad" according to their impact on the outcome of the game.) For chess
masters, then, optimal moves seem to come readily to mind; bad moves
are filtered out and never even considered. Collecting "thinking aloud"
data produced only a starting point for de Groot's understanding of
chess expertise. He was also interested in the cognitive abilities of expert
chess players. Measuring these required experimental methods.

Using a visual memory task, de Groot noticed that after only a brief
exposure to a chess board (5–10 seconds), chess experts were able to
recreate chess positions almost perfectly. Weaker players could not do
this. Can this ability be attributed to superior short-term memory?
Short-term memory ordinarily has a capacity of about seven items of
information; perhaps chess masters can remember more. Chase and
Simon (1973b) addressed this question by asking chess masters and novi-

ces to recreate chess boards on which the pieces were arranged randomly. Chess masters were no better at this task than less skilled players. Their short-term memory, therefore, does not appear to be superior. Instead, their memory appears to be specialized for recalling meaningful chess positions.

De Groot's visual memory task, which involves only a short exposure to the chess board, does not allow time for complex cognitive processing. Therefore, the chess masters' superiority must rely on fast perceptual recognition processes. The precise difference between the recognition processes of masters and other players was the subject of further work by Chase and Simon (1973a,b). They used two procedures to investigate the way patterns of chess pieces are reconstructed. The first was simply to record the chess players on videotape as they recreated a chess board from memory. The second procedure again required players to recreate chess positions; however, this time the original board was in plain view and the positions were recreated on an adjacent board. Head turns between the two boards were recorded on videotape.

Chase and Simon found that board reconstruction was done in bursts punctuated by pauses. The pieces placed down in the bursts were found to consist of highly familiar stereotyped patterns that were determined by both the spatial orientation of pieces and their function (attack or defense). Of interest here is that, while all levels of players produced about the same number of patterns, the masters included many pieces in their patterns (about six patterns of six pieces). Novice players produced patterns consisting of only single pieces. The same characteristic patterns were also evident when masters recalled whole games after briefly seeing chess positions. Superior pattern recognition processes were demonstrated during the "Knights Tour Puzzle" in which a knight is moved over a prescribed path using legal moves; masters perceive squares available to the knight very quickly. Chess masters, therefore, are not endowed with superior short-term memory capacity (that is, their memories hold the same number of patterns, or "chunks," as other players), but each of their chunks contains more chess-specific information.

These studies led Chase and Simon to conclude that chess masters have a large repertoire of chess patterns (possibly as many as 50,000) stored in long-term memory that they can quickly match to patterns on the board and that are associated with good moves. Merely good players have fewer patterns (about 1000), and the novice cannot recognize any patterns at all. The intuitive notion of the master player as a deep and systematic thinker is belied by these findings—the chess master is a superior recognizer rather than a deeper thinker.

How does fast pattern recognition aid the chess master? One explanation is that pattern recognition substantially reduces cognitive load. The best moves are immediately available in long-term memory, thus eliminating the need to search for them. Fast pattern recognition also explains the remarkable ability of masters to defeat many weaker players simultaneously. When they return to a game, they do not have to remember the course of each but simply recognize patterns of positions to generate good moves. Rapid access to good moves has been termed "chess intuition." It has also been found to be an important skill in other games such as go, gomoku, and bridge (see Chase & Chi, 1981).

Another area of expertise that has received considerable attention is physics problem solving (Chi, Feltovich, & Glaser, 1981; Chi, Glaser, & Rees, 1982; Larkin, McDermott, Simon, & Simon, 1980). It turns out that "physical intuition" is similar to "chess intuition." Experts have the ability to solve physics problems rapidly with little conscious deliberation. Physics experts group problems around principles (Newton's Second Law, for example) while novices respond to the physical entities in the problem (a spring or inclined plane problem) (Chi et al., 1981). The same is true of mathematical problem solvers (Sweller, Mawer, & Ward, 1983). Like chess masters, expert physics problem solvers have a rich store of problem types that they rapidly access. Generating solutions from principles is called "top-down" processing in contrast to the "bottom-up" processing (also called means–end analysis) relied on by novices. As in chess, the experts' knowledge organization is crucial to efficient problem solving.

> The fact that the expert physicist has a more coherent, complete, and principle-oriented representation of physics knowledge necessarily implies that his or her initial understanding of the physics problem must necessarily be better, leading more easily to correct solution. (Chase & Chi, 1981, p. 117)

Psychological research on chess players and other experts has found that expertise is not a matter of having a larger capacity memory or being a deeper thinker. Instead, experts are distinguished from novices mainly by their ability to use their knowledge of a field to generate likely hypotheses (top-down processing) and their ability to perceive quickly the important aspects of a problem. We now turn to expertise in medicine. Some of the questions that are addressed are: What factors distinguish expert doctors from less experienced ones? Are the best doctors those who can make judgments quickly? Does their skill resemble chess or physical intuition—the ability to perceive patterns quickly and with little deliberation? Do expert doctors reason in a way similar to expert physics problem solvers, using top-down processing, or do they reason from the bottom up?

Expertise in Medicine

Medical textbooks and journals are replete with advice by expert doctors about the "what" and "how" of medical procedures in various circumstances. However, there is not a remarkable amount of systematic research into the cognitive nature of medical expertise. As already noted, sound medical practice is thought to be achieved simply by observing experts (some sort of osmotic process must be implied here). This, of course, begs the question: What, exactly, is learned with experience?

Studies of medical expertise have three possible motives. The first motive is scientific. Medicine is studied because it is a high-level cognitive skill and is *ipso facto* of interest. The second motive is more practical. Attempts are made to understand expertise so that teaching the requisite skills can be approached with more confidence and with improved results. It seems pedagogically sound to know the skill being taught as thoroughly as possible. Finally, the study of expert medical decision making is undertaken to construct computer-based decision aids such as expert systems, which are discussed later in this chapter.

Although medical examples are not numerous, there is enough material for us to construct a picture of expertise in radiology (examples from other areas of medicine are also given where appropriate). The greater concentration of studies of expertise in radiology is due, in part, to empirical work by psychologists attracted by its perceptual nature and the relatively constrained task environment of the radiologist. Radiology also proves to be an adequate case study because all doctors, and many laypeople, have some familiarity with x-rays.

Expert Radiological Diagnosis

The sick patient is at the very heart of the radiological process, which is initiated by a request for a radiological consultation on a patient who is either known or presumed to be ill. This request reflects the physician's need for further information in order to solve a diagnostic problem (Abrams, 1981, p. 122).

A radiographical image is used to tell what organ or tissue is abnormal, where to cut, what to biopsy, and where to treat. The radiologist today has at his/her disposal a wide range of imaging modalities. Each one, to a greater or lesser degree, provides interpretive problems because of the similarity in appearance of some normal and abnormal structures (for example, blood vessels viewed end-on can simulate pulmonary nodules) (Gale, Johnson, & Worthington, 1979). The inherent difficulty of the task is largely the result of the lack of depth cues. In normal pictures, such as photographs, the forwardmost objects occlude those further back. This cue tells us which objects are behind others, and, therefore, further away. There are no such overlap depth cues in a radiograph because a pattern on the film is determined by all the tissues the beam passes through from the source to the x-ray plate. Bone, for example, blocks the beam and thus appears white on the film; but it will also appear white whether soft tissue is in front of or behind it or absent altogether. For this reason, both front and side views are required to locate a lesion accurately. Moreover, simply distinguishing organ contours, which overlap in the two-dimensional film, often requires considerable practice.

Signal detection theory (SDT) has often been the basis for studies of image interpretation (Lusted, 1984). Using its terminology we can state the radiologist's task as detecting a visual "signal" in a background of visual "noise." We have already discussed SDT and its performance measure (the ROC curve) in Chapter 2. The same terminology is used in this section to discuss radiological expertise.

Studies in radiology can be broadly separated according to two main goals: those that concentrate on the influence of image type and quality on diagnosis (see, for example, Abrams, 1981; Gray, Taylor, & Hobbs, 1978; Kundel, Revesz, Ziskin, & Shea, 1972; Rossman & Wiley, 1970; Swets & Pickett, 1982), and those that seek to understand the perceptual and cognitive processes employed by the radiologist. Our interest lies with the latter category.

Errors in radiology are by no means rare. A consistent finding of many studies, which underlines the inherent difficulty of the task, is that 30% of positive (abnormal) chest films are classified as normal (Forrest & Freidman, 1981; Garland, 1959; Guiss & Kuenstler, 1960; Herman et al., 1975; Herman & Hessel, 1975; Smith, 1967; Tuddenham, 1962; Yerushalmy, 1969). Moreover, these findings do not apply only to subtle signals but also include many lesions that are obvious in retrospect. Errors of omission [variously called misses, false-negatives (FNs), or underreading] are far more common than errors of commission [false alarms, false-positives (FPs), or overreading]. Garland's (1959) figure of 2% of films being overread is well supported, while other authors set the FN to FP ratio at about 80 : 20 (Herman & Hessel, 1975; Herman et al., 1975; Rhea, Potsaid, & De Luca, 1979). Variability, both inter- and intraobserver, is about 20% (Chikos, Figley, & Fisher, 1977; Gale et al., 1979; Garland, 1959; Herman et al., 1975; Smith, 1967).

Comparisons between these studies are hazardous because of the different subjects, materials, and methods used.* The above findings, however, do appear robust. It is hardly surprising, given these results, that studies have concentrated on understanding the detection and omission of lesions.

---

* The reader of these articles is struck by the large differences in experimental methodology. Materials differ in type, complexity (the number of lesions per film), quality, patient population, and the relative proportions of negative and positive films. Data are gathered directly, by having doctors look at x-rays, or indirectly, from patient records. The amount of clinical information, in addition to the x-rays, available to the doctors varies and so too does the significance of the lesions (minor or major). Finally, the criterion of accuracy is sometimes objective (i.e., agrees with biopsies or autopsies) or subjective (i.e., agrees with another radiologist.)

Accuracy and Experience in Radiology

The error rates in radiology certainly suggest that there is no room for complacency, but how does accuracy relate to experience? Herman and Hessel (1975) gave eight radiologists of different degrees of experience 100 chest films to read. Although significant individual differences in accuracy were found, there was no consistent pattern related to the duration of training beyond the first year of residency. They concluded that, once an individual's radiology education had progressed beyond a fundamental level, unspecified individual reader characteristics overshadowed experience in the accuracy of chest film interpretation.

Herman and Hessel (1975) used a SDT-type classification of errors (FPs and FNs), but did not complete a ROC analysis because their films contained multiple abnormalities and, thus, rendered ROC analysis very difficult. Films that would be amenable to ROC analysis may, according to these authors, be unrealistic. (Actually, ROC analysis can be applied to multiple signals; see Metz, Starr, & Lusted, 1976a).

In contrast to Herman and Hessel's findings, other studies have found that inexperienced film readers make different errors from the more experienced. The most common finding is that the former make more FP errors than the latter (Herman and Hessel's data hint at this, but they do not emphasize the point). Sheft, Jones, Brown, and Ross (1970), for example, found that, when reading chest films, radiology technologists had favorable true-positive (TP) rates when compared to residents and staff radiologists, but their FP rates were often twice as high. Radiology technologists have also been found to perform creditably, when compared to radiologists, in scanning mammograms, but their TP rates were achieved only at the expense of true-negative (TN) rates (Alcorn & O'Donnell, 1969; Alcorn, O'Donnell, & Ackerman, 1971). Likewise, in the interpretation of radionuclide liver images, a higher incidence of FP readings was associated with inexperienced observers (Nishiyama, Lewis, Ashare, & Saenger, 1975). A ROC analysis found staff physicians more accurate than fellows or residents, thus indicating greater sensitivity to the signals (liver diseases). Staff physicians had higher TP and lower FP rates than the other groups (equivalent to a greater "sensitivity" in a full ROC analysis, (Nishiyama et al., 1975). Seltzer, Hessel, Herman, Swensson, and Sheriff (1981) found that, as residents gained experience, they were corrected less often by reviewing staff radiologists and also made fewer FP errors.

These studies suggest that less experienced x-ray readers adopt a more "pessimistic" decision criterion than more experienced ones. That is, they are more likely than staff physicians to call a film "abnormal" when they are uncertain. Less experienced readers may, of course, be more uncertain than the more experienced, and this would suggest a more "noisy" environment (greater overlap of the signal and signal–

noise distributions). Experienced radiologists may also be more aware of normal anatomical variation and the costs associated with subjecting a well person to medical procedures by making a FP error (see Chapter 2 for more on decision criteria). Unfortunately, the effect of experience on sensitivity and bias remains unclear.

In a slightly different vein, Chikos et al. (1977) found a relationship between experience and accuracy among subjects required to assess heart chamber size from chest radiographs. Chikos et al. concluded that experience is especially helpful in evaluating subtle changes and resolving conflicting findings.

Experience and Search Strategies

Some researchers have attempted to find the causes of radiology errors. One fruitful avenue has been the study of the perceptual and cognitive processes that underlie radiological diagnosis. We now turn to the perceptual search strategies used by radiologists.

Search strategies have been studied in two main ways. One is to experimentally manipulate the areas of the film that can be searched, the time available to search the film, and the available information. Another way is to record eye movements made during film reading. A combination of eye movement recordings and experimental manipulations can also be used. The rationale behind recording eye movements is that attention is focused on the part of the film held in foveal vision (peripheral vision is also used during search but is widely held to guide foveal attention). The recording that is produced is a trace of the perceptual–cognitive processes employed by the x-ray reader. Process tracing methods, such as eye movement recordings and having decision makers talk aloud, mark a shift from simply observing errors to a focus on underlying cognitive processes.

The search (or scanning) strategy that a film reader employs has been found to be influenced by experience. Kundel, Nodine, and Carmody (1978) dissected experience into three categories—object knowledge, background knowledge, and sampling distributions. The first category, object knowledge, is awareness of what normal and abnormal structures actually "look" like; that is, the size, shape, and density that make objects distinctive. Object knowledge serves to limit the number of possible two-dimensional patterns that compete for attention and classification. Background knowledge is a more advanced understanding of the relationship between normal (noise) and abnormal (signal) patterns.

One feature of x-rays that makes them difficult to read (and also leads to an example of the relationship between experience and object knowledge) is that the boundaries between structures are unclear. This may lead the less experienced to perceive an abnormality as either too large, by incorporating some background, or too small, by confusing part of

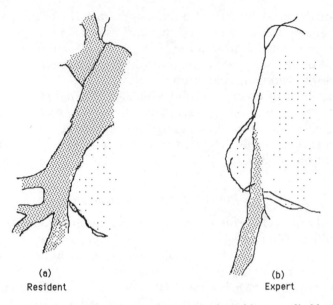

(a)   (b)
Resident   Expert

Figure 5-2   Sketches of the lung structures seen by subjects studied by Lesgold (1984b). Residents tended to "use up" the high-density region by drawing a large pulmonary artery. Experts, on the other hand, depicted the region accurately (it contained only a small collateral of the pulmonary arterty). Reprinted from Lesgold (1984b) with the permission of the author and the Psychonomic Society.

the abnormal structure with background noise. An example of the second type of error is provided by Lesgold (1984a, 1984b).

Lesgold asked radiologists and residents to trace the outline of an abnormality on a chest film. The film showed a collapse of the middle lobe of the right lung that was represented by a large sail-shaped wedge in the part of the lung near the heart (a collapse causes increased density of the lung material). Even though this abnormality is relatively common, it may be confused with certain tumors and several other disorders that can look similar. Figure 5-2 shows the tracings of the sail-shaped region drawn by experts and residents.

While experts saw only a small collateral of the pulmonary artery (shaded area) entering the region of high density, the residents tended to follow various bits of noise and thereby recruit much of the critical region into their representation of the pulmonary artery. These representations left experts with a region that could be explained by a collapsed lung. Residents, however, left with only a small, high-density area to be explained, tended to call if a tumor.

Experience is also reflected in the order in which different parts of the radiograph are visually sampled by observers. So-called sampling distri-

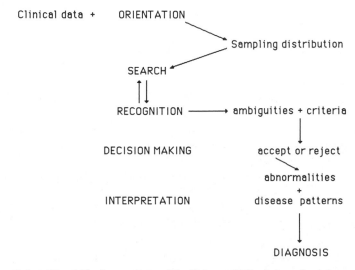

Figure 5-3   Kundel's five-step model of the radiologist's task. Adapted from Kundel et al. (1978) and reprinted with the permission of the authors and Lippincott Publishers.

butions, in this sense, embody the experts superiority in "knowing where to look." For example, a clinical history that directs a reader to expect to see a particular disease will influence the search strategy used (Kundel & Wright, 1969; Kundel et al., 1978; Schreibner, 1963). Experience suggests strategies in the same way that prior information serves to select a particular strategy (Gale et al., 1979). Eye movement recordings have been used to capture the sampling distributions of experienced and inexperienced radiologists. Whereas inexperienced observers use a localized central scan, a more circumferential scan is employed by the more experienced. A circumferential scan is a general survey of the radiograph that is usually followed by a detailed examination, whereas a localized search pattern immediately focuses on suspect regions of the film (Kundel & Wright, 1969). The circumferential scan appears to evolve with training (Kundel & La Follete, 1972). The visual sampling distributions of experienced radiologists have also been found to approximate estimates of the probability of finding abnormalities in chest films (Kundel, 1974). That is, they tend to examine those areas of the film that are most likely to contain abnormalities.

Kundel et al. (1978) and Kundel and Nodine (1978) have proposed a five-step model to describe the radiologist's task. These steps are found in Figure 5-3, and it is useful to discuss them here. (A similar model is offered by Gray, et al., 1978.) The first stage is orientation to the radiograph as a whole. An experienced radiologist can extract a substantial amount of information from a film in an initial glance (200–300 milliseconds) (Carmody, Nodine, & Kundel, 1980a; Kundel & Nodine, 1975; 1983; Swensson, Hessel, & Herman, 1982). In fact, obvious abnormalities appear to be detected almost instantaneously by comparing patterns with a previously learned representation of "normal" held in memory (Christensen et al., 1981). Not surprisingly, these authors discovered that experienced readers found more abnormalities in a short time than less experienced readers. The amount of search required depends on whether a lesion is obvious or subtle and, as one becomes more experienced, more lesions become obvious. Berbaum, Franken, and Smith (1985) have demonstrated that the concept of "normal" is better developed in experienced observers. Indeed, according to Hillard, Myles-Worsley, Johnston, and Baxter (1985), the concept of normal is so highly developed in experienced radiologists that they do not consciously process normal features but attend directly to abnormal ones. In this way, they are similar to chess masters who ignore most "bad" moves, leaving them free to concentrate their energies on good ones. In Berbaum et al.'s study, detection performance for reading pediatric chest films was improved for beginning residents by supplying normal x-rays for comparison with abnormal ones. More advanced residents did not benefit greatly from comparison x-rays. It would seem that early visual information provides a kind of orientation that, along with the three categories of experience (object knowledge, background knowledge, and sampling distributions), influences the remaining stages of information processing.

Search strategies are determined by recording the area of the film covered by a "useful visual field" (Kundel, Nodine, & Toto, 1984). Much work has been done to find out which search strategies are best. Is it helpful, for example, to direct a reader's attention to a particular type of lesion or area of the film most likely to contain a lesion, or is it better to allow the reader to search the film freely and report any abnormalities seen? Unfortunately the answer is equivocal. Some studies report that directed search (of area or type of lesion) is better than free search while other studies reach the opposite conclusion.

Free search has been found to be superior to directed search by type of lesion by Swensson, Hessel, and Herman, (1985) (although peer comments following this article raise some questions about the methodology used). Free search has also been found superior to directed search by film location (Carmody, Nodine, & Kundel, 1980b; Swensson, Hessel, & Herman, 1977, 1982). Under directed search conditions, errors of omission are reduced but at the expense of an increase in FPs. That is, a less stringent reporting criterion is used. Carmody et al. (1980b) suggested that allowing a reader to search only certain segments of a film denies the use of comparisons between normal and abnormal structures within the film. However, Gale and Worthington (1983), whose subjects were *trained* to use a comparison search strategy, also found a shift in criteria.

Another study that directed search to areas of the radiograph, but also allowed comparisons with the rest of the film, found directed search to be better than free search (Parker et al., 1982; see also Carmody, 1984).

Eye movement recordings have also shown that comparisons are made between lesions and anatomical structures, and that subtle lesions receive more comparisons (Carmody, 1984; Carmody, Nodine, & Kundel, 1981). It is reasonable to suggest that as object and background knowledge improve, along with expected sampling distributions, comparisons become more efficient and normal and abnormal structures are compared both to learned prototypes in memory and to contextual information contained in the film.

An efficient search strategy will increase the probability that an abnormality will pass through the useful (central) field of vision. However, a lesion may be covered by the scan but not necessarily recognized as such. The third stage in radiological diagnosis is the recognition of a potential abnormality. A lesion may be recognized but not perceived as a strong enough "signal" to be classified as abnormal. Making a decision about whether an abnormality is genuine is step four in the model. Finally, interpretation is a higher level of decision making and leads to a list of diagnostic possibilities.

Using this model, errors can be designated as the result of faulty scanning (a lesion is not viewed in central vision), faulty recognition (a lesion is covered but not recognized), or faulty decision making (an abnormality is recognized but not called a lesion). Radiologists in the Kundel et al. (1978) study searched for simulated lung nodules. Their FNs were 30%, 25%, and 45% for stages two, three, and four, respectively (the first and last stages were not included for error analysis). In the absence of empirical evidence, it is interesting to speculate how errors may change as a function of experience. It is appealing to think that, as a radiologist learns his/her profession, errors will be more likely to occur at later stages in the five-stage process. That is, beginners may make more scanning errors but, once scanning and recognition skills have developed, the decision making and interpretation stages will be the sources of most errors.

Gale et al. (1979) saw perception as a dynamic process in interaction with the stimulus information [as in Neisser's (1976) "perceptual cycle"]. They postulated an anticipatory schema (or cognitive strategy), roughly similar to Kundel's orientation stage and open to the same influence by experience, that directs exploration of the x-ray. This initial exploration affects selective visual sampling of the stimulus information, which, in turn, modifies the schema. Experience serves to select useful schemata, in the same way that clinical information does, whose anticipatory nature allows the observer to rapidly disregard the normal radiological anatomy and concentrate on the abnormal. The concept of schemata also explains why obvious abnormalities are sometimes missed; even a missing arm or breast occasionally go unnoticed (see Gale et al., 1979). That is, the possibility is not contained in the schema. As is discussed in the next section, with experience the resident will enlarge and refine his/her repertoire of schemata.

Much of the research on radiological expertise suggests that experienced radiologists have a rich memory store of representations of abnormalities to which they compare features of the film under review. These comparisons are often made rapidly and in this aspect radiologists are similar to the chess masters discussed earlier. We now turn to the question: How do radiologists reason when making diagnoses, and do they share other qualities with experts in other fields?

Expert Radiological Reasoning

Evidence from the search studies just mentioned and from analyses of verbal protocols converges to form a clear picture of how experienced and less experienced radiologists differ. Lesgold and his colleagues (Lesgold, 1984a, 1984b; Lesgold, Feltovich, Glaser, & Wang, 1981) have used verbal protocols, recorded during x-ray diagnosis, to study the reasoning involved in expert radiological diagnosis. It is their work that is summarized here.

Before we continue, however, it is appropriate to say more about verbal protocols. The most valid method of collecting verbal data is to ask the subject to "think aloud" while performing a task, as opposed to asking, "What did you do?" (retrospective protocols) (Ericsson & Simon, 1980). The former method was used by de Groot to study chess players. Transcripts of the recorded thinking-aloud protocols can be coded into knowledge states (medical facts, physiological concepts, and diagnostic hypotheses) and processes (attention to information, information search, hypothesis generation, comparisons, and evaluation) (Newell & Simon, 1972). This approach is typically referred to as a process tracing because the analysis is assumed to identify a temporal "trace" of the processes underlying judgment. (For more on the validity of verbal data and details of process tracing, see Ericsson & Simon, 1980, 1984; Fidler, 1983; Hayes, 1982; Nisbett & Wilson, 1977; Payne, 1980; Svenson, 1979).

From Lesgold's work, it seems that experts have two main advantages over novices in the field of radiological diagnosis. First, they have rich and flexible disease schemata that they can call upon to resolve incongruities in clinical data. According to Lesgold (1984b) rich schemata permit experts to engage in "opportunistic planning." Novices, on the other hand, are tied to classical schemata, the application of which can lead to unresolved or even unnoticed incongruities (see also Feltovich, Johnson, Moller, & Swanson, 1984). Second, experts know where to look

Table 5-1. Expert Diagnostic Performance[a]

Something is wrong, and it's chronic:
"We may be dealing with a chronic process here . . ."
Trying to get a schema:
"I'm trying to work out why the mediastinum and heart is displaced into the
   right chest. There is not enough rotation to account for this. I don't see
   displacement of fissures."
Experiments with collapse schema:
"There may be a collapse of the right lower lobe but the diaphragm on the right
   side is well visualized and that's a feature against it . . ."
Does some testing; schema doesn't fit without a lot of tuning:
"I come back to the right chest. The ribs are crowded together. . . . The crowd-
   ing of the rib cage can, on some occasions, be due to previous surgery.
In fact, . . . the third and fourth ribs are narrow and irregular so he's probably
   had previous surgery . . ."
Cracks the case:
"He's probably had one of his lobes resected.
It wouldn't be the middle lobe.
It may be the upper lobe.
It may not necessarily be a lobectomy.
It could be a small segment of the lung with pleural thickening at the back."
Checks to be sure:
"I don't see the right hilum . . . [this] may, in fact, be due to the postsurgery
   state I'm postulating . . .
Loss of visualization of the right hilum is . . . seen with collapse . . ."

---

[a] Reprinted from Lesgold (1984b) with his permission and the permission of the Psy-
chonomics Society.

and what to see and engage in a recursive interaction with the film in
which both bottom-up and top-down reasoning are equally employed.
This contrasts with Kundel and Nodine's (1978) model, which largely
involves bottom-up reasoning (see Figure 5-3). In this respect, Lesgold's
verbal data support Gale et al.'s (1979) speculations about the cognitive
processes used by radiologists mentioned toward the end of the last
section.

As an example of flexibility of expert reasoning, Lesgold (1984b) provided an excerpt of thinking-aloud data (see Table 5-1). The comments
refer to a chest film of a patient who was currently healthy but whose
right upper lung lobe had been removed 10 years earlier. Abnormal
features will be observed because organs shift to occupy the lobe space
and produce unusual densities. Some experts and most residents quite
reasonably concluded that the film showed disease-induced lung collapse. Other residents said that the patient suffered from congestive
heart failure. Obviously, a correct assessment would lead to no action
and each incorrect diagnosis would lead to a different treatment.

As shown in Table 5-1, the recognition of the possibility of a chronic complaint came very quickly (within 2 seconds). The expert then followed up by trying to explain some features by rotation (that is, the patient was not correctly facing the plate) and then considered the collapse schema. However, the expert was not satisfied with this schema and further hypothesis testing led to the "cracking" of the case. Even at this stage, schema testing continued. As Lesgold stated: "Throughout, the expert displayed flexibility, the ability to push, tune, and retreat from a schema that was guiding his thinking" (1984b, p. 82). Expert radiologists are not always correct. The same flexibility in reasoning is still evident, however, even when their conclusions are wrong (see Lesgold et al., 1981, for examples).

In contrast to flexible expert reasoning, less expert residents tended to hold onto schemata. For example, even when they were told that the patient was now healthy, that a similar film had been taken 1 year previously, and that the patient had had a lobectomy performed many years before the film, some still preferred their diagnosis of congestive heart failure. Lesgold concluded that they were "unable to test the schemata or the specific hypotheses they had invoked or to take account of the new data we provided" (p. 84).

Feltovich et al. (1984) also noted the ability of expert doctors to tune their schemata. These researchers were interested in the development and application of medical knowledge in pediatric cardiology. Patient data from histories, physical examinations, x-rays, and electrocardiograms were presented to specialists, residents, and students from which they made diagnoses of different types of congenital heart disease. The correct diagnosis was only one of a set of plausible alternatives that, together, formed a logical competitor set (LCS) of possible diagnoses. Verbal protocols were collected and examined. Feltovich et al. concluded that, while less experienced physicians reasoned along the lines of classical categorizations of the members of the LCS, experts were more flexible. They were able to reorganize disease categories to accommodate important radiological features. Figure 5-4 illustrates one such example.

As can be seen in Figure 5-4, the expert created a category that crossed over the original classical set of diseases. The less expert doctors focused on the "classical" hypothesis of partial anomalous pulmonary venous connection, and never once considered the correct disease, *total* anomalous pulmonary venous connection, a disease that is very similar, even in name. The explanation is that the less expert subjects became stuck in a LCS with which the correct diagnosis was not associated. Experts had at their disposal an overlapping disease category with "increased blood flow on the right side" as its defining feature.

A similar observation was made by Pauker, Gorry, Kassirer, and Schwartz (1976). Expert doctors were able to "tune" their initial hypothesis, which was generated very early during taking a patient's history, by

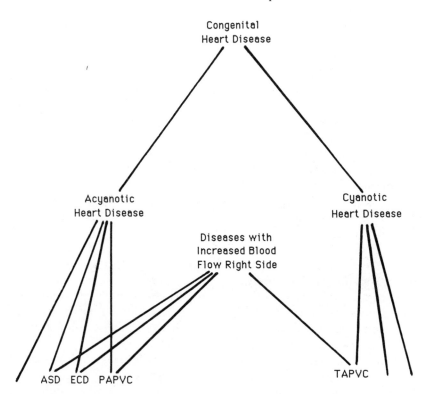

Figure 5-4   Experts can often create new "subcategories" to classify atypical patients. In this example, the *outsides* represent the classical categorization of heart disease, and the *inside lines* represent the expert's regrouping. (*TAPVC* = total anomalous pulmonary venous connection; *PAPVC* = partial APVC; *ASD* = atrial septal defect; *ECD* = endocardial cushion defect.) Taken from Feltovich et al. (1984) and reprinted here with the permission of Dr. P. E. Johnson.

calling to mind other hypotheses with which it may be confused (for example, multiple pulmonary emboli are often confused with cardiomyopathy). The expert's LCS is more refined than the medical student's because the student knows fewer such relationships. Pauker et al. suggested that, because the less experienced doctors do not tune their hypotheses effectively, early hypotheses generated by these doctors produce the risk of serious errors. They also noted, however, that junior doctors counter this limitation by using highly structured, methodical approaches to diagnosis.

The development of rich and flexible schemata may, however, be associated with a temporary cost. Lesgold (1984a, 1984b) noted that, at least for difficult films, residents in their mid-residency years perform less accurately than experts *and* less experienced residents. According to Lesgold, this finding may be associated with a change from diagnosis

using classically learned disease sets to the reasoned diagnosis characteristic of experts. Newer residents try to fit their classical schemata to the
case at hand, which is similar to a high-probability guess. As skill develops, however, the resident sees complexities and uses deeper analysis
of details that do not fit the classical picture. Although the more complicated approach is potentially more accurate, it imposes a temporary
increase in conscious processing (at least until expertise develops) and
this load may adversely affect performance.

Experienced radiologists, as we have already mentioned, rapidly access good schemata. Lesgold's work confirmed this (Lesgold, 1984a,
1984b; Lesgold et al., 1981). For example, when viewing a film showing
chronic lung disease, experts are much more likely to mention findings
that are consistent with the film. Residents, on the other hand, more
frequently mention findings inconsistent with, or neutral for, the correct
diagnosis of chronic lung disease. After the chronic lung disease schema
is "triggered," the expert engages in top-down reasoning, exploring and
making statements about the lungs and pleurae. Not surprisingly, residents tend not to follow up with statements about the lungs. The diagnostic process, then, has both a bottom-up component (early triggering
of schemata) and a top-down component. Top-down reasoning is remi-
niscent of how expert physicists solve problems.

Top-down reasoning was also found by Johnson, Hassebrock, Duran,
and Moller (1982) to be characteristic of expert clinicians. Using a problem similar to that of Feltovich et al. (1984) (i.e., diagnosis of congenital
heart disease) and collecting verbal protocols, they concluded that expert clinicians were more likely to notice data incongruities and then use
lines of reasoning that reflect a global control of knowledge so that
resolution of immediate data incongruities would not result in unantici-
pated errors. Less expert clinicians had a limited control over their problem solving knowledge so that their lines of reasoning were data driven,
applying only to the resolution of apparent data incongruities.

Similarly, Kassirer and Gorry (1978) analyzed the tape recordings of
experienced clinicians during "taking the history of the present illness"
from simulated patient data. The overall strategies used were a focused
approach, a systematic exploration method, and a chronological technique. Clinicians outside the relevant specialty (nephrology) tended to
use systematic exploration while nephrologists were likely to employ a
focused approach.

To conclude this section, we summarize the differences between expert and less expert radiologists. One difference is in the type of errors
made. The less experienced make more FP errors than do experts.
Differences were also found in three components of experience in
search strategies—object knowledge, background knowledge, and sampling distributions. A five-stage model of the radiological process was
used to discuss search strategies, and we also mentioned on several occa-

sions the ability of the expert to recognize x-ray patterns very rapidly. A review of search studies led Gale et al. (1979) to postulate a dynamic process with stimulus and observer in constant interaction. This idea is supported by Lesgold's (1984a, 1984b; Lesgold et al., 1981) studies using thinking-aloud techniques. The x-ray triggers a schema (bottom-up processing), at which time reasoning becomes schema driven (top-down processing). Also noticed by Lesgold and others are the rich and flexible schemata available to the expert. These schemata are "tuned" with experience. Novices, on the other hand, are tied to classical schemata, which sometimes provide correct diagnoses but may not always do so. In reviewing radiological expertise, similarities with other areas also became apparent. In particular, rapid recognition of radiological patterns and the top-down processing characteristic of expert reasoning have been observed in chess masters and expert physics problem solvers, respectively.

At the beginning of this section on experts, we mentioned that the popular notion of the chess master as a deep thinker is not supported by the empirical evidence. Pauker et al. (1976) have this to say about the expert physician:

> Our study clearly illuminates an important difference between the expert in practice and the expert as often pictured in literature or folklore. The epitome of the expert in fiction is the detective who, through superior deductive powers and by sheer force of logic, organizes the facts at hand in a way that they lead to a single, inevitable conclusion. (p. 995)

The empirical evidence presented here suggests an alternative view of the expert physician: not someone with greater intelligence or logical ability but one whose knowledge is organized in such a way that relevant data may be quickly retrieved and put to use. But if this is what an expert is, then it is reasonable to ask, how does one learn to organize knowledge in the optimal (expert) way? Is it simply something that "happens" with experience, or can it be taught? This is the subject of the next section.

Learning from Experience

As we have shown in Chapters 2 and 3, medical judgment often involves testing one or more clinical hypotheses (Elstein et al., 1978). Typically, the process requires that: (1) information be gathered from a variety of sources (laboratory tests, physical examinations); (2) the various items of information be weighted for their importance, and (3) the weighted information be integrated into some overall judgment. Normally, this process involves dealing with probabilities (a particular diagnostic sign has only a probabilistic relationship to a diagnosis, a treatment has only some probability of success). In the psychology literature, judgments that require several data items to be used to predict a criterion to which each item bears a probabilistic relationship are called "multiple-cue probability judgments." Learning how to make such judgments is known as "multiple-cue probability learning" (MCPL; Todd & Hammond, 1965).

The Role of Outcome Feedback in MCPL

Psychological investigations of MCPL frequently make use of "diagnostic" tasks. A subject in these experiments is given a set of cues (symptoms, for example) and asked to make a diagnosis or some related judgment. The outcome of the judgments (correct or incorrect) is made known to the subject, who is then asked to try again with a new set of cues. The process is repeated until the subject reliably makes the "optimum" diagnostic judgment. (The optimum judgment is established either by consulting experts or on theoretical grounds such as how closely it approximates the judgment suggested by SEU theory.)

The reason for the focus on feedback is simple. Most psychological learning theories (Skinner, 1938, for example) assume that it is environmental feedback about the consequences of our actions that signal whether our decisions are good or bad. Actions that lead to desirable consequences (positive feedback) are good; those that elicit negative feedback are bad.

Feedback is also viewed as a way to change undesirable behavior. For example, one popular method of motivating doctors to contain costs involves sending them copies of their patients' hospital bills. Chart audits follow a similar logic. Although some positive feedback programs have led to behavioral changes (see Eisenberg & Williams, 1981, for a review), the most successful programs are those in which doctors can expect negative consequences for failure to conform (withdrawal of hospital privileges, for instance).

In theory, at least, feedback may also be useful in teaching new skills. For example, feedback on judgments, in the form of a faculty review of residents' radiograph interpretations, has been suggested as the most effective way to improve radiological skills (Seltzer, Doubilet, Sheriff, & Katz, 1984). Sufficient experience with actions and their positive and negative outcomes should also permit people to induce specific decision heuristics. These heuristics take the form: In situation A, take action B, because this will lead to positive consequence C. Although the logic sounds plausible, psychological research has not shown that outcome feedback always leads to the induction of appropriate decision rules. Summarizing the results of many studies that failed to find much evidence that outcome feedback leads to effective learning, Brehmer (1980) concluded:

> These results, taken as a whole, strongly suggest that people simply do not have the cognitive schemata needed for efficient performance in probabilis-

tic tasks. . . . People do not learn optimum strategies from experience, even if they are given massive amounts of practice. (p. 233)

Why should it be so difficult to induce optimum decision rules from outcome feedback? Several reasons have been suggested. One possibility is that feedback on successes and errors alone ignores the continuous character of the probability of a diagnosis as it is generally understood in the clinic. Scoring rules for providing continuous (probabilistic) feedback have been developed (Hilden, Habbema, & Bjerregaard, 1978), and such feedback has been shown to improve diagnostic performance (De Dombal, 1979; Habbema & Hilden, 1981).

Taking a rather different tack, Einhorn and Hogarth (1978) laid part of the blame for the poor showing of outcome feedback on MCPL tasks on the one-sided nature of outcome feedback. Typically, the real world decision maker receives only partial feedback, a situation that can lead to inductive errors. We illustrated the problems that partial feedback can cause in Chapter 3 when we discussed Bushyhead and Christensen-Szalanski's (1981) demonstration of the "illusion of validity." They showed how a doctor can gain an erroneous idea about the relationship between rales (diagnostic chest sounds) and pneumonia when only patients in whom rales are detected receive x-rays. The doctor never receives x-ray feedback on those patients for whom rales are not detected and may wind up believing that rales are significantly related to pneumonia even when they are not.

The need to attend to multiple sources of information (Shaw, 1982) and misperceptions of task structure may also make it very difficult to learn from outcome feedback. Consider the following problem, which is adapted from one described by Einhorn (1980).

A physician is seriously concerned about a patient who has had a positive result on laboratory test Z. The reason the doctor is so concerned is that, in his experience, every patient with such a result has turned out to have condition A and 75% of the time sufferers from condition A require major surgery. The doctor wishes to give the patient some idea of the probability that she will require major surgery. What should he tell her?

The most common answer to this question is 75%. To see why this answer is misleading, let us restate the problem in terms of conditional probabilities. The information available is as follows:

P(Surgery Required/Condition A) = .75
P(Condition A/Positive Test Z) = 1.00

The probability the physician wishes to give the patient is: P(Surgery Required/Positive Test Z) but, the information available is not sufficient to calculate this probability. Part of the difficulty lies in the relationship between laboratory text Z and condition A. While it appears to be true that a positive result implies that condition A is present, the opposite relationship has not been demonstrated. That is, the P(Positive Test Z/

Condition A) is unknown. If only a small number of patients with condition A produce positive results on Test Z, then it is entirely possible that the probability that this patient requires surgery is much lower than 75%; it may even be 0. An intuitive way to see this latter possibility is to imagine that lab test Z only picks up the 25% of sufferers from condition A who do not require surgery. The doctor who has received feedback only on the probability of Condition A given a positive result on test Z can easily be led to an overly pessimistic conclusion.

It appears that outcome feedback alone may not be the best way to teach doctors how to perform MCPL tasks. What about other types of feedback? Shanteau and Phelps (1977) suggested teaching people optimal rules as a way of helping them to learn in MCPL tasks. Research contrasting the rule-based and outcome feedback approaches is discussed next.

Lens Model Approaches to MCPL

Researchers interested in examining the role of decision rules in MCPL have generally looked at the task from the viewpoint of Brunswick's (1956) lens model (see Figure 1-2, Chapter 1). As noted in Chapter 1, the lens model construes the judgment process as analogous to a convex lens in which a judge's perception (the judgment) and the "true" state of the environment (the criterion) are mediated by a set of cues that are probabilistically related to both. Since the actual criterion can never be perceived directly, judges have no option but to base their judgments on the mediating cues. According to the lens model, what needs to be learned in a MCPL situation is how important each of the various cues are and how the cues may best be combined (Hammond, 1971).

Experiments based on the lens model typically contrast three types of feedback (Rappoport & Summers, 1973):

1. *Outcome feedback.* As already described, subjects are told, after each judgment (or set of judgments), whether they were successful.
2. *Prior set.* This is really a type of "feedforward." Subjects are told the ideal weights for each cue before making any judgments. Their task, then, is simply to learn to apply these weights properly. In some experiments, prior set is combined with outcome feedback.
3. *Lens model feedback.* As its name suggests, this type of feedback involves giving subjects an idea of how they are using the cues. The typical approach is to have subjects make a number of judgments and then to provide them with information about their own judgment "model." This information includes the importance weights they have assigned to the cues as well as the functional relationship between each cue and their overall judgments (linear, curvilinear, and so on). At the same time, they are also given the "ideal model" (the one with the best weights) for comparison. Thus, lens model feedback consists of spe-

cialized feedforward and feedback information. The goal is to provide subjects with information sufficient for them to alter their individual judgment models to conform with the ideal one.

Although there are many ways to convey lens model information, graphic displays such as the one appearing in Figure 3-3, Chapter 3 appear to be easiest for subjects to understand (Hammond, 1971).

There have been a number of laboratory studies of MCPL (Hoffman, Earle, & Slovic, 1981, Slovic & Lichtenstein, 1971, and Slovic et al., 1977, review many of these experiments). In addition to feedback, these studies have manipulated such variables as the number of relevant cues, the diagnosticity of the cues (how well they predict the criterion), the form of the cue–criterion relationship (linear or nonlinear), and the relationships among the cues themselves. The findings of these studies may be summarized as follows: (1) subjects can learn to use probabilistic cues to predict criteria, (2) linear relationships are easier to learn than nonlinear ones, and (3) people are generally insensitive to relationships among the cues.

As far as type of feedback is concerned, research results generally favor lens model feedback. For example, Todd and Hammond (1965) compared performance for subjects who received outcome feedback alone with those who received lens model feedback and with those who received a combination of both. They found no difference between the two lens model groups. Both were superior to the outcome feedback group, which hardly learned anything at all (see also Deane, Hammond, & Summers, 1972). Similar results were reported by Hammond and Boyle (1971) and Hoffman et al. (1981). It would seem, then, that the most efficient training procedure in MCPL tasks is one that combines feedforward of the optimum rule with lens model feedback.

An example of the relevance of this research for medical training comes from an experiment conducted by Shiels (1981). Her specific task concerned the side effects of various cortisone preparations. Certain illnesses (chronic bronchial asthma, for example) require long-term cortisone therapy, which, in turn, may produce side effects. Six side effects are most common: weight gain, hypertension, Cushing face (puffy face), gastric ulcers, hirsutism (excess hair growth), and myopathy. Alternative cortisone derivatives produce these side effects with different frequency and severity. Previous research by Aschenbrenner and Kasubek (1978) established the side effects patterns of seven common cortisone drugs. Expert physicians were used to determine which combination of side effects was "least evil," second-least evil, and so on. Using multiattribute utility theory, Aschenbrenner and Kasubek also estimated the importance weights for each side effect. Shiels' goal was to teach subjects these importance weights as well as the ideal method for combining them to choose between cortisone therapies.

Shiels' method was to present hypothetical cortisone preparations to her subjects in the form of a bar graph (similar to the one in Figure 3-2, Chapter 3) and ask them to evaluate each one as to the overall pattern of side effects. Feedback consisted of either outcome feedback, feedforward of the ideal decision rule, or lens model feedback, and the subjects were either doctors, medical students, or non-medical professionals. Shiels found that only doctors benefited from simple outcome feedback, and the non-medical professionals only learned the optimum rule when given lens model feedback. Interestingly, all three groups learned at about the same rate when given lens model feedback.

Shiels' finding that doctors can learn from outcome feedback appears to be at variance with the findings reported earlier. Her results suggest that outcome feedback can be effective when subjects have some prior familiarity with the learning task. Most of the earlier MCPL experiments, which found little learning on the basis of outcome feedback, used highly artificial tasks guaranteed to be unfamiliar to their subjects. However, the superiority of lens model feedback in all groups suggests that it is the preferable approach in teaching both physicians and non-physicians how to perform MCPL tasks.

Despite the difficulties experienced by researchers trying to teach subjects how to perform MCPL tasks, we know that performance outside the laboratory, on real world tasks, is not always bad. People have learned to predict the weather, the economy, medical treatment outcomes and other probabilistic events, sometimes with great accuracy. Surely, when it comes to natural MCPL learning, some of us are doing something right. Klayman (1984) has suggested that the laboratory studies present an artificial environment where learning depends entirely on information provided by the experimenter. In contrast, learning in the natural environment requires that "students" take a more active role in searching for and discovering important cues and using these cues to build elaborate judgment models.

Instead of feedback about their judgment policies and feedforward of optimum rules, some researchers have suggested that what doctors need is a decision "assistant" to help them make the optimum judgment in MCPL situations. Such an assistant can come in many different guises, but what most people have in mind is a computer decision maker. Attempts to computerize medical judgment are discussed next.

Automatic and Algorithmic Decision Making

Clinical decisions may be characterized along a repeatability dimension that goes from routine, everyday problems to unique, once-in-a-lifetime choices. As noted earlier in this chapter, common decisions are probably best taught using clinical algorithms while unique problems generally require some form of decision analysis. To assist the clinician (doctor or paraprofessional), standardized protocols allow the relevant patient data to be entered into specially designed forms that guide the user to the appropriate conclusion. Studies of physicians and professionals using protocols have generally shown that they are effective aids to improving the quality of patient care (Margolis, 1983). Because of their explicit nature, clinical algorithms can be computerized. The computer can then become an aid to decision making (MacDonald, 1977). However, computerizing nonalgorithmic aspects of clinical judgment is not as straightforward as it might first sound. Automating rationality requires that rational thinking be clearly understood in the first place, and we are a long way from that.

Over the past 20 years, there has been an increasing interest in representing expert knowledge and reasoning in the form of computer programs. These programs were once called "consultation programs" because they mimic an expert specialist who is asked to provide advice (diagnosing an illness, recommending a treatment). In recent years, however, these programs have become known as "expert systems." Some in the field, Clancey and Shortliffe (1984a), for example, say that this may be a generous characterization given the limitations of these programs. We discuss some of these limitations toward the end of this section. First, we describe several approaches to the design of expert systems.

Computer-assisted Diagnosis versus Expert Systems

Computer-assisted diagnosis (CAD) attempts to reach diagnoses by applying the formal methods of decision analysis discussed in Chapter 4. Several of the decision methods already mentioned in this book (Bayes' formula and utility theory) have been used for CAD with impressive results (see de Dombal, 1979, 1984a, 1984b; Politser, 1980; Rogers, Ryack, & Moeller, 1979; Shortliffe, 1980). The main virtues of these CAD systems are: (1) they can be run on desk-top computers (Bayesian inference can be expressed in a few lines of code), and (2) the techniques are well understood formally, and can be extended to any decision in which utility theory can be used to express values and in which probabilities may be estimated (Fox & Rector, 1982). Unfortunately, despite several successful demonstration systems (Pauker & Kassirer, 1981; Weiss, Kulikowski, & Safir, 1978), CAD technology has had little impact on routine clinical practice (Spielgelhalter & Knill-Jones, 1984; but see de Dombal, 1979, for an exception).

In an attempt to explain why CAD technology has not gained many adherents, it has been suggested that competence alone is not sufficient; clinical decision systems must also be acceptable (Fox, 1984). There are two ways of making decision systems acceptable. One is to make the formal methods better understood by doctors. Such understanding should convince more doctors of their potential (see Spielgelhalter & Knill-Jones, 1984, especially the discussion following the paper). Some problems involved in teaching doctors formal methods of decision analysis were covered in the preceding section of this chapter. From this discussion, it is fair to say that teaching such methods, and getting doctors to use them, are not easy tasks.

A second way to increase acceptability is to design CAD systems that "think" like doctors rather than mathematicians. In the last few years, expert systems have been gaining popularity as ways of making computer-assisted diagnoses and treatment recommendations. In contrast to the formal CAD systems, expert systems reason about clinical data using a set of logical rules that need not be mathematical. We use the term "expert systems" to refer to computer programs that reason by logical rules while "CAD systems" is reserved for those that apply mathematical decision theory to clinical judgments.

According to those who advocate a shift of approach toward expert systems (Fox, 1984, for example), there are two main problems with the traditional CAD approach. The first is the one already mentioned: physicians are neither familiar nor comfortable with the formal theories upon which the methods are based. The second problem is a practical one. A vast amount of data need to be stored to make a diagnostic system workable because almost every disease is linked with several indicants (symptoms, signs, and laboratory tests). Formal approaches require that each set of indicants be supported by epidemiological data (often with samples of several thousand patients). The cost and effort in constructing such data bases are substantial and there is a real concern that data (disease probabilities, for instance) collected from one population of patients may not generalize to other populations.

Formal methods also have difficulty taking into account a common occurrence in medical diagnosis—that disease indicants are themselves related. For example, a bronchitic patient who has a productive cough is also likely to have wheezes in the chest due to the nature of the illness. Illnesses may also be interrelated, and so too may test results. The number of such relationships is so large as to make many traditional decision analyses very complicated. Computer-assisted diagnosis systems based on decision trees, for example, may develop trees with hundreds, even thousands, of branches. To avoid this, many systems ignore interrelationships among signs, tests, and diseases. The result? Traditional CAD systems often impose an artificially simple model on diagnostic decision making.

Finally, perhaps the most important drawback to formal CAD methods is their focus on the decision point of diagnosis. Questions about how data are acquired and represented are not addressed (Clancey &

Shortliffe, 1984a). These are central issues to the developers of modern expert systems.

Expert Systems: Background

Because expert systems aim to encode expert knowledge, they are also referred to as knowledge-based systems. Knowledge-based systems are a subset of artificial intelligence (AI), which has as its goal the development of computer programs that can solve problems that require what most people refer to as "intelligence." This goal can be achieved through modeling the processes used by humans, but this is not strictly necessary. Some AI researchers are willing to consider a computer program intelligent if it can solve an "intellectual" problem by *any* method even if the method is not the one used by humans. Artificial intelligence has captured the interest of researchers in recent years, and rather more recently captured the imagination of computer companies and the media. Although some of the claims made for these systems are exaggerated, there are existing knowledge-based systems that interpret typed and spoken language, recognize visual images, and control robots and production lines. In medicine, knowledge-based programs control patient monitoring systems, x-ray and ultrasound equipment, and prosthetic devices (Clancey & Shortliffe, 1984a). Although they are interesting in their own right, our present concern is not with knowledge-based systems in general, but only with those used to assist, or train, doctors to make clinical decisions.

Expert Decision-Making Systems

Expert systems are one type of knowledge-based system. As Fox (1984, p. 304) wrote: "Expert systems are knowledge-based systems with two special features. First, they are primarily concerned with making decisions—as opposed to seeing, hearing etc. Second, they are interactive computer systems—not autonomous robots or process controllers." As their name suggests, expert systems address problems that would normally be solved by human specialists. It is because experts are characterized by extensive knowledge about a *narrow class* of problems that it is tenable to produce computer programs to handle these problems effectively.

Expert performance depends on expert knowledge. In any specialty there are two kinds of knowledge: public and private (Hayes-Roth, Waterman, & Lenat, 1983). Both types are made explicit in expert systems. Public knowledge includes published definitions, facts, and theories and can be thought of as "textbook" knowledge. However, expertise involves more than public knowledge. Experts also possess private knowledge

Table 5-2.   Examples of Knowledge Representation[a]

(a)   duodenal-ulcer *is-a-kind-of* peptic ulcer
duodenum *is-a-part-of* gi-system
ulceration *is-a-cause-of* bleeding
(b)   gastric-cancer is-associated-with weight-loss *(.7)*
cholecystitis is-associated-with severe-pain *(usually)*
oesophagitis is-*usually*-associated-with reflux
(c)   If: (1) An anti-inflammatory drug should be recommended for the patient,
(2) Oral drugs are suitable for the patient, and
(3) The patient is not suspected of having peptic ulcer
Then: It is definite (1.0) that the following is one of the recommendations
for pain:
Aspirin orally

[a] Reprinted from Fox (1984) with the permission of Elsevier Science Publishers.

that is not in the published literature. This latter type of knowledge consists largely of rules of thumb (heuristics) that enable the human expert to make educated guesses when necessary, to recognize promising approaches to problems, and to deal effectively with inexact or incomplete information. Elucidating and reproducing such knowledge is the central, and most difficult, task involved in building expert systems (Hayes-Roth et al., 1983).

Expert knowledge is usually represented in expert systems by a set of facts and rules (hundreds of each are needed to build a sophisticated system). Table 5-2, taken from Fox (1984), gives three examples. The first example (a) shows that facts can be represented as relationships between objects. If the relationship is not fully known, some measure of uncertainty may be used (b). The uncertainty measure may be a numerical probability or a qualitative judgement. The last example in Table 5-2 (c) shows a typical IF . . . THEN . . . rule for representing knowledge.

An important implication of representing knowledge in this way is that a system can be built incrementally, improved over time, and kept current. Moreover, because expert systems represent facts and heuristics explicitly, the user has no trouble following the system's logical steps. Many expert systems are specially designed to explain their logic to the user. The ability of an expert system to explain its "reasoning" (how it reached a recommendation) is its most important, if not its defining, feature.

In traditional CAD systems, knowledge is not explicit but embedded in the mathematical formulas, which are usually not available to the user. De Dombal (1979, 1984a, 1984b) argued that the fact that many doctors may not understand the basis for a CAD system's recommendation is not a sufficient reason to reject such systems. After all, most doctors have only a vague understanding of the technology underlying computer-assisted tomography, nuclear magnetic resonance, and other diagnostic procedures, yet these are generally accepted by most, if not all, physicians. De Dombal believes that doctors should treat the recommendations of CAD systems as if they were pathology or radiology reports. Of course, this requires that doctors have the same degree of faith in the value of the advice CAD systems offer as they have in radiological and pathological techniques. Thus far, such faith has not been widely available. Part of the problem is unfamiliarity. Most doctors have little knowledge of the rationale underlying decision analysis. Since traditional CAD systems were not designed as tutors, doctors are forced to either accept or reject their advice; they have no way of analyzing the reasoning behind the system's recommendations.

In contrast, the explanations offered by expert systems provide arguments for their recommendations in a way that can be evaluated by the physician. Examples of such explanations are shown in Tables 5-3 and 5-4 (taken from Davis, 1982), which show the initial and final parts of a sample dialogue with an expert system called MYCIN (Shortliffe, 1976). MYCIN was developed at Stanford University and is probably the best known clinical expert system. In the tables, the user input follows **; the italicized comments are not part of the dialogue.

MYCIN was designed as a consultant for making diagnoses and recommending treatment for bacterial infections. Typically, a patient showing signs of infection supplies a sample of blood or urine that is cultured to check for the presence of disease-causing bacteria. Although some evidence is available the same day, a period of 24–48 hours is usually required for the organisms to be positively identified. Often, treatment cannot wait for the definitive results, so the physician must base his/her diagnosis and treatment decision on information that is more readily available, such as the shape of the bacteria, whether they respond to oxygen, and so on. Other information typically available includes the patient's history (e.g., previous infections, other clinical evidence of infection, or factors that may predispose the patient to a particular type of bacterium) (Davis, 1982). Because of time constraints on beginning treatment, gaps in patient history, and the frequent impracticality of undertaking extensive tests before treatment, MYCIN must deal with incomplete information. It must also deal with inexact information, because many test results are qualitative rather than quantitative, sensitivities and specificities are less than perfect, and subjective impressions ("Has the patient responded to previous therapy?") form part of the data. Another source of inexactness is that the relationship between signs and diseases is not certain (see Table 5-2 section b).

Returning to Tables 5-3 and 5-4, we can see some helpful features of the MYCIN expert system. A user may respond UNKNOWN if information is missing (question 9, Table 5-3), ask for a question to be rephrased (question 13), or provide a measure of uncertainty (question

Table 5-3. Initial Part of a MYCIN Consultation[a]

PATIENT-1

1) Patient's name: (first-last)
** FRED SMITH
2) Sex:
** MALE
3) Age:
** 55
4) Have you been able to obtain positive cultures from a site at which Fred
   Smith has had an infection?
** YES

INFECTION-1

5) What is the infection?
** PRIMARY-BACTEREMIA
6) Please give the date and approximate time when signs or symptoms of the
   primary-bacteremia (INFECTION-1) first appeared. (mo/da/yr)
** MAY 5, 1975
The most recent positive culture associated with the primary-bacteremia (IN-
FECTION-1) will be referred to as:

CULTURE-1

7) From what site was the specimen for CULTURE-1 taken?
** BLODD
= BLOOD
8) Please give the date and time when this blood culture (CULTURE-1) was
   obtained. (mo/da/yr)
** MAY 9, 1975
The first significant organism from this blood culture (CULTURE-1) will be
referred to as:

ORGANISM-1

9) Enter the identity of ORGANISM-1:
** UNKNOWN
                    [typically the identity is not known and must be inferred]
10) Is ORGANISM-1 a rod or coccus (etc.):
** ROD
11) The gram stain of ORGANISM-1:
** GRAMNEG
12) Did ORGANISM-1 grow aerobically?
** YES (.8)
13) Is the patient's illness with ORGANISM-1 a hospital-acquired infection?
** ?
Was the infection with ORGANISM-1 acquired while the patient was hospital-
ized?
Expected responses are: YES NO
Enter HELP for list of options.
** Y
                    [More questions follow to gather sufficient information to
                        infer possible identities of the infecting organism]

---

[a] Reprinted from Davis (1982) with the permission of Westview Press.

Table 5-4. Final Part of a MYCIN Consultation[a]

My therapy recommendation will be based on the following probable infec-
tion(s) and potential causative organism(s):
INFECTION-1 is PRIMARY-BACTEREMIA

[possible identities]

⟨Item 1⟩ The identity of ORGANISM-1 may be
PSEUDOMONAS-AERUGINOSA
⟨Item 2⟩ The identity of ORGANISM-1 may be
KLEBSIELLA-PNEUMONIAE
⟨Item 3⟩ The identity of ORGANISM-1 may be E. COLI
⟨Item 4⟩ The identity of ORGANISM-1 may be ENTEROBACTER
⟨Item 6⟩ The identity of ORGANISM-1 may be PROTEUS-NON-MIRABILIS

   46) On a scale of 0 to 4, where higher numbers indicate increasing
       severity, how would you rate Fred Smith's degree of sickness?
  ** 3
   47) Does Fred Smith have a clinically significant allergic reaction to any
       antimicrobial agent?
  ** NO
   48) Fred Smith's weight in kilograms (or ⟨number⟩ POUNDS):
  ** 70

[note that 2 drugs cover for 6 potential organisms]

[Rec 1] My preferred therapy recommendation is as follows:
  In order to cover for Items ⟨1 2 3 5 6⟩:
    Give: GENTAMICIN
    Dose: 119 mg (1.7 mg/kg) q8h IV [or IM] for 10 days
    Comments: Modify dose in renal failure
  In order to cover for Item ⟨4⟩:
    Give: CLINDAMYCIN
    Dose: 595 mg (8.5 mg/kg) q6h IV [or MV] for 14 days
    Comments: If diarrhea or other GI symptoms develop, patient should
        be evaluated for possible pseudomembranous colitis.
  Do you wish to see the next choice therapy?
  ** Y   *[alternative choices are available]*
  Which, if any, of the above drugs do you wish eliminated from
  consideration?
  ** CLINDAMYCIN
[Rec 2] Next best therapy recommendation:
  In order to cover for Items ⟨2 3 4 5 6⟩:
    Give: CHLORAMPHENICOL
    Dose: 1 gm (15 mg/kg) q6h IV for 14 days
    Comments: Monitor patient's white count
  In order to cover for Item ⟨1⟩:
    Give: GENTAMICIN
    Dose: 119 mg (1.7 mg/kg) q8h IV [or MV] for 10 days
    Comments: Modify dose in renal failure

[a] Reprinted from Davis (1982) with the permission of Westview Press.

Table 5-5. Example of Consultation with ICRF Terminal Care System[a]

PATIENT-1

1) Name:
** FRED SMITH
2) What problems are troubling Fred Smith?
** DYSPNOEA
3) What is the severity of the dyspnoea?
** MILD
4) Does Fred Smith have bronchospasm?
** YES
5) Is Fred Smith taking any medication?
** NO
6) Does Fred Smith have a pleural effusion?
** NO
7) Does Fred Smith have anaemia?
** UNK
8) Does Fred Smith have a mediastinal tumour?
** NO

Advice for DYSPNOEA
 Steroids are the most effective treatment for bronchospasm (the long term
  effects are not important in terminal patients).
 Investigate the possibility of anaemia if its correction would improve Fred
  Smith's personal or family life.

General Advice for DYSPNOEA
 Oxygen is not recommended (because it does not usually ease the dyspnoea of
  terminal patients).

[a] Reprinted from Fox (1984) with his permission and the permission of Elsevier Science Publishers.

12). The system can even correct minor typing errors (question 7) so that those who lack keyboard skills are not handicapped.

An offshoot of MYCIN is EMYCIN (Essential MYCIN), which is an expert system with all of MYCIN's features but without any rules that commit it to a specific application. EMYCIN has been used to build expert systems in a number of other specialties. Table 5-5, for example, shows an example from Britain's Imperial Cancer Research Fund (ICRF) terminal care system (Fox, 1984). As may be seen, the terminal care system's method of explanation is usually to produce the rules that were used to generate its questions and recommendations. In Table 5-6, also from the terminal care system, the user was puzzled when he was asked if the patient has dyspepsia (indigestion). The command WHY produced the rule and the second WHY produced an explanation at the

Table 5-6.   The Explanation Facility of EMYCIN[a]

---

7)   Does Fred Smith have dyspepsia?

**   Why?

[i.e.,   WHY is it important to determine whether PATIENT-1 has dyspepsia?]

    [1.0]   This will aid in determining whether PATIENT-1 is suspected of having a peptic ulcer.

        If

           [1.1]   1)   Fred Smith has dyspepsia, or

                 2)   Fred Smith has evidence of gastro-intestinal haemorrhage

      then

        it is definite (1.0) that Fred Smith is suspected of having a peptic ulcer

[RULE020]

                                    [back to question 7 . . .]

    **   WHY?

[i.e.,   WHY is it important to determine whether PATIENT-1 is suspected of having peptic ulcer?]

[2.0]   . . . in order to determine the recommendations for pain.

        It has already been established that

[2.1]   an anti-inflammatory drug should be recommended for Fred Smith, and

[2.2]   oral drugs are suitable for Fred Smith

        Therefore, if

[2.3]   Fred Smith is not suspected of having a peptic ulcer then

        it is definite (1.0) that the following is one of the recommendations for pain: Aspirin orally

        [RULE079]

                                    [back to question 7 . . .]

    **   NO

---

[a] Reprinted from Fox (1984) with his permission and the permission of Elsevier Science Publishers.

next highest level (Fox, 1984). MYCIN's question-answering ability is shown in Table 5-7, where both private and public knowledge are given as explanations.

Well-known expert systems have been developed to diagnose and treat several conditions. The most famous systems include programs that diagnose and treat glaucoma (CASNET), assist with diagnosis in internal medicine (INTERNIST, now called CADUCEUS, which can diagnose over 600 diseases), interpret the clinical significance of signals from intensive care monitoring equipment and make recommendations (VM), diagnose respiratory conditions (PUFF), and assist in the management of chemotherapy treatment (ONCOCIN). The recommendations

Table 5-7. MYCIN's Question-Answering Capability[a]

(a) ** HOW DID YOU DECIDE THAT ORGANISM-1 MIGHT BE AN E. COLI?

I used RULE021 to conclude that the identity of ORGANISM-1 is e.coli. This gave a cumulative CF of (.47).

Then I used RULE084 to conclude that the identity of ORGANISM-1 is e.coli. This gave a cumulative CF of (.55).

Finally, I used RULE003 to conclude that the identity of ORGANISM-1 is e.coli. This gave a cumulative CF of (.74).

(b) ** DID YOU USE RULE 163 TO FIND OUT ANYTHING ABOUT ORGANISM-1?

RULE163 was tried in the context of ORGANISM-1, but it failed because it is not true that the patient has had a genito-urinary tract manipulative procedure (clause 3).

(c) ** DID RULE 116 TELL YOU ANYTHING ABOUT INFECTION-1?

No. RULE116 would be relevant to the primary-bacteremia when applied to ORGANISM-1.

But clause 2 ("the gram stain of the organism is not known") was already known to be false for ORGANISM-1, so the rule was never tried.

(d) ** WHY DIDN'T YOU CONSIDER STREPTOCOCCUS AS A POSSI-BILITY FOR ORGANISM-1?

The following rule could have been used to determine that the identity of ORGANISM-1 was streptococcus: RULE033

But clause 2 ("the morphology of the organism is coccus") was already known to be false for ORGANISM-1, so the rule was never tried.

(e) ** DO YOU RECOMMEND CLINDAMYCIN FOR BACTEROIDES?

Yes.

RULE060

If the identity of the organism is bacteroides

Then I recommend therapy be chosen from among the following: CHLORAMPHENICOL, CLINDAMYCIN, RIFAMPICIN, ERYTH-ROMYCIN, CARBENICILLIN, TETRACYCLINE, LINCOMYCIN

(f) ** IS BLOOD A STERILE SITE?

Yes, blood is one of those sites that are normally sterile.

(g) ** WHAT ARE THE ORGANISMS ASSOCIATED WITH THE GAS-TRO-INTESTINAL TRACT?

The likely pathogens associated with the gastro-intestinal tract are: EN-TEROCOCCUS, CLOSTRIDIUM-GANGRENE, BACTEROIDES, KLEBSIELLA, PSEUDOMONAS, E.COLI, ENTEROBACTER, PRO-TEUS.

[a] Reprinted from Davis (1982) with the permission of Westview Press.

of these systems compare favorably with those made by doctors (see Brachman et al., 1983; Clancey & Shortliffe, 1984b; Davis, 1982; Duda & Shortliffe, 1983; Fox, 1984; Hayes-Roth et al., 1983; Szolovits, 1982). A useful bibliography of expert systems and applications in a variety of domains can be found in Rychener (1985).

Another important offshoot of the development of knowledge-based expert systems in medicine is intelligent computerized instruction. In teaching, the verbosity of expert systems can prove a distinct advantage. For example, when expert systems are used to teach clinical skills to students, their ability to go through the chain of reasoning can help students to learn precisely where they may have made an error. An example of an expert system designed specifically to teach medical diagnostic skills is the GUIDON system (Clancey, Shortliffe, & Buchanan, 1979). Although computer-assisted instruction is hardly a new idea, most computerized courses are simply electronic versions of more traditional courses. The GUIDON system differs from traditional approaches to computerized instruction in its use of artificial intelligence techniques.

The GUIDON system uses a case method. The system engages the student in an interactive dialogue about patients suspected of having infections. The aim is to get the student to consider the relevant clinical and laboratory data necessary to diagnose the responsible organism. GUIDON's knowledge base is the MYCIN consultation system, including its entire set of 450 diagnostic rules about infections. GUIDON also includes 200 "tutorial" rules dealing with such matters as presenting information, answering student questions, and so on. Since the tutorial rules are independent of the knowledge base, the system is flexible enough to be used with knowledge bases other than MYCIN.

GUIDON does more than simply present problems and evaluate students' answers; the system also attempts to infer what the student has already learned from previous dialogues and adjusts its current dialogue accordingly. For example, if a student diagnoses a case correctly but GUIDON is unsure that the student actually knows the appropriate diagnostic rule, it will interrogate the student about his/her reasoning (see Table 5-8).

Although Guidon may be used with knowledge bases other than MYCIN's few of these exist and new ones take years to develop. GUIDON is also subject to the communication constraints inherent in any computerized system. For example, MYCIN only understands age given in precise years; it cannot handle references to "infants," "adolescents," or the "middle-aged" (Clancey et al., 1979). Nevertheless, there is much to admire in the GUIDON system and every reason to believe that the current surge of interest in expert systems will lead to further development of computerized tutors.

Table 5-8. GUIDON's Dialogue about a Student's Hypothesis[a]

What is the type of infection?
BACTERIAL
What facts about this case tell you that the type of infection is baterial?
PMNS
The per cent of PMN's in the CBC is not relevant for determining the type of infection.
PMNS IN THE CSF
CEREBRAL-FLUID GLUCOSE VALUE
PROTEIN OF THE CSF
You're right about the CSF protein, the percent of PMNs in the CSF and the CSF glucose value, however you should have mentioned the fact that meningitis is partially treated, the WBC from the CSF and the fact that the simultaneous blood glucose value is not known.
MYCIN rejected some possibilities you did not mention: What facts about this case tell you that the type of the infection is not viral?

[a] Adapted from Clancey et al. (1979).

Encoding Expertise

We have already seen how expert knowledge is represented in expert systems by the use of rules and statements. Now we turn to the problems of actually getting the knowledge from the expert so that the rules can be encoded. Knowledge elicitation is commonly acknowledged as the bottleneck in the development of expert systems (Hart, 1985). Fox, Myers, Greaves, and Pegram (1985) outlined several methods of acquiring knowledge from experts. Their preferred method was the analysis of "thinking-aloud" protocols. They considered more informal techniques, such as interviews with experts or panels of experts, followed by the formulation of decision rules by a "knowledge engineer" (computer programmer) as too time consuming and unreliable. Recently, expert system "shell" programs have become available. These programs interrogate the expert and automatically induce rules. Users of these programs are restricted to the type of rules and knowledge structures anticipated by the system designer.

In addition to the limitations of the various techniques, there are also some general difficulties with encoding expertise. One is that experts often find it difficult to verbalize their decision rules (Hart, 1985). According to Dreyfus and Dreyfus (1984), one of the first people to ask experts to reveal the secrets of their trades was Socrates. Among the experts whom Socrates quizzed was Euthyphro, a religious prophet and self-proclaimed expert at recognizing piety. Socrates asked "I want to know what is characteristic of piety to use as a standard whereby to judge your actions and those of other men." Instead of giving guidelines or rules, Euthyphro gave examples of situations in which men and gods had acted piously. Socrates could get no closer to a general rule for piety and concluded that perhaps experts had once known the rules by which they judge and act, but had simply forgotten them. The philosopher's role, he believed, was to help people rediscover these rules.

Rediscovering inference rules is not easy. With experience, a long chain of inferences that constitute reasoning for a decision may, to use a computing term, be "compiled" into a single simple rule (Kuipers & Kassirer, 1984). In everyday practice, expert doctors face many decisions in which they use "compiled" knowledge without bothering to go through all the inferences underlying that knowledge. In other words, they simply recognize the situation and know the appropriate response. In contrast, medical students and newly qualified doctors may have to struggle through the entire inference chain. If we think of the reasoning process as following a branching structure similar to a decision tree, then the novice must work along the branches of the tree to reach the logical conclusion while the expert skips many branches to arrive at the same point. Many expert judgments involve skipping over steps. Sometimes such judgments involve what Szolovits and Pauker (1978) called "categorical reasoning." A categorical judgment is one made without significant reservations: If the patient's serum sodium is less than 100 mEq/L, administer sodium supplements; if the patient complains of pain on urination, obtain a urine culture and consider the possibility of a urinary tract infection. As already pointed out, such judgments rely on compiled knowledge; the underlying inferences have not been traced in their entirety. Although categorical reasoning is easily encoded in expert systems, thereby speeding their response times, speed is gained at the expense of explanatory power (Brachman et al., 1983).

When experts are asked to elucidate the rules they use to make diagnoses they are, in effect, being asked to regress to the level of the beginner and recite rules that they no longer employ (Dreyfus & Dreyfus, 1984). It is too pessimistic a view, however, to say that experts cannot rediscover the rules they have compiled. Most seem able to recite these rules when necessary to explain their reasoning.

Another problem in encoding expertise relates to giving systems "common sense." Consider the following example of clinical "common sense" in a vignette presented by Szolovits (1982) which appeared originally in *The New Yorker*.

Mrs. Eloise Dobbs, 38, is married to a feed store owner and she comes to her physician, Dr. Elwood Schmidt, complaining of chest pain. The following dialogue ensues:
   "This whole side of my chest hurts, Elwood. It really hurts."
   "What about your heart—any irregular beats?"
   "I haven't noticed any. Elwood, I just want to feel good again."
   "That's a reasonable request. And I think it's very possible you will."

"But what do you think? Is it my heart? Is it my lungs?"

"Now you won't believe this—but I don't know. I do not know. But I wonder. Are you lifting any sacks down at the store?"

"I lift some. But only fifty pounds or so. And only for the woman customers."

"I think you'd better let your lady customers lift their own sacks. If I know those ladies, they can do it just as well as you can. Maybe better."

In this story, Dr. Schmidt used his knowledge of the patient's occupation and the practices of small-town stores, the weight of typical sacks of feed, and other similar knowledge along with his more formal understanding of the physiological basis of pain (that overexertion can exacerbate the underlying cause of pain but also can cause pain by itself, especially in older people) (Szolovits, 1982). Although it is possible that an expert system diagnostician might reach the same conclusion as Dr. Schmidt, it is unlikely that any present system would do so as quickly.

A potentially disconcerting characteristic of expert systems, related to their general lack of clinical common sense, is known as the "plateau and cliff" effect. Expert systems may perform very well in a well-defined application, but once they are asked to perform outside their limited domain, there is not a graceful decline, but rather a sudden and dramatic drop, in performance. To use a simple example, MYCIN may do very well at diagnosing meningitis, but have difficulty diagnosing a common cold. It may even have difficulty realizing that a patient is dead because it only interprets clinical information with respect to the diseases that it recognizes.

Although clearly a disadvantage, in practice an absence of common sense is not likely to be a great limitation to expert systems. Users realize that expert systems have well-defined domains, and do not expect them to perform tasks for which they were not designed. Medical specialties rely more on clinical information than the interpretation of everyday events for their medical significance. Moreover, the role of the expert system is to assist in diagnosis and treatment decisions, not act by itself in an environmental vacuum. The user is capable of recognizing the cliff effect and any gross oversight due to lack of common sense.

Another criticism of expert systems is that, because humans, even experts, are subject to error and limitations in decision making (many of these have been reported in this book) expert systems will also wind up encoding human failings. From this viewpoint, CAD systems are preferable because they rely on normative techniques not subject to human error (see Spiegelhalter & Knill-Jones, 1984; plus the following commentaries). Of course, not all situations can be represented by mathematical algorithms. In these situations, experts, by definition, are the best there is. Also, because expert systems can be built incrementally, errors (poor rules) can often be eliminated by incorporating the wisdom of several experts. Some critics appear to believe that expert systems should perform better than the experts on which they are based. Some of the data on "bootstrapping" presented in Chapter 3 also suggest that this should be the case. It is wrong, however, to expect such systems to be faultless. We agree with Szolovits (1982), who decried what he called the "super human" fallacy, the tendency for critics of expert systems to expect their performance to be faultless, or at least better than human experts, even in situations that will trip up the best human experts. We should also mention that, although they are not equivalent, expert systems do not necessarily preclude the use of formal approaches to decision making. An expert system can use a combination of knowledge-based and formal inference. At present, there is no evidence that one is superior to the other (Fox, 1980; Fox, Barber, & Bardhan, 1980).

Many recommendations for how to improve expert systems are really a response to the question: What can human experts do that expert systems cannot yet do? One thing an expert can do is make consultations in a relatively short time; expert systems tend to be verbose. Experts are also much more flexible in giving explanations. They can adapt them to suit the sophistication of the person receiving the explanation and can also summarize the reasons underlying a decision. Expert systems, on the other hand, use the long method of repeating all the rules they used (Alvey, 1983; Fox, Alvey, & Myers, 1983).

Finally, Hayes-Roth et al. (1983) provided three advantages for knowledge-based decision aids. The first is that many interesting and important problems originate in complex social or physical contexts, which generally resist precise description and rigorous analysis. Such problems do not have neat algorithmic solutions. (An example is the decision to perform cosmetic surgery.) A second, pragmatic reason, for preferring knowledge-based to formal decision methods is that human experts achieve outstanding performance because they are knowledgeable. Therefore, if computer programs contain and use this knowledge they too have the chance to achieve high levels of performance. The third reason for focusing on knowledge recognizes its intrinsic value. As Hayes-Roth et al. wrote:

Knowledge is a scarce resource whose refinement and reproduction creates wealth. Traditionally the transmission of knowledge from human expert to trainee has required education and internship years long. Extracting knowledge from humans and putting it in computable forms can greatly reduce the costs of knowledge reproduction and exploitation. At the same time the process of knowledge refinement can be speeded up by making private knowledge available for public test and evaluation. (1983, p. 5)

Summary

Traditional clinical training assumes that simply observing an expert at work is a sufficient method of gaining expertise. However, such observations are unsystematic and not always successful. Attempts to devise more efficient and more effective training methods were reviewed in this chapter. Indeed, one important reason for research in medical decision making is the development of new training methods.

Because evaluating teaching methods requires some measure of the skills being taught, we began the chapter with a discussion of measuring doctors' performance. Although several different measures have been developed, none is without some problem. On the whole, the more similar evaluation methods are to actual clinical practice the more valid and useful they are likely to be. Patient management problems, although they too are subject to some criticisms, are probably the best measures of clinical judgment presently available.

The last 10 years have seen a large expansion in the number of courses being offered in decision analysis by medical schools and postgraduate training programs. Although the students who complete these courses do appear to have learned a substantial amount about decision analysis, there is little evidence that they put this knowledge to work in their clinical practice. Moreover, some doctors appear to object to decision analysis as a patient management technique. Although these objections may be based on misconceptions about the nature of decision analysis, they cannot be ignored. Their existence poses a challenge for those who wish to increase the use of decision analysis in clinical situations.

Because it is hard for the busy clinician to find the time (or the data) required for decision analysis, some educators have favored teaching clinicians qualitative techniques to avoid judgment biases. Thus far, however, these teaching efforts have met with only limited success. Another, increasingly popular, teaching approach uses clinical algorithms to teach doctors proper management techniques. Algorithms are fairly easy to learn, and they do not appear to lead to rigidity and mindlessness, as some doctors feared, but they are clearly not a substitute for good decision-making skills. After all, knowing when to apply and not to apply algorithms is also a matter of clinical judgment.

Studies of experts in various fields, including medicine, have begun to clarify how their cognitive processes differ from those used by novices. It turns out that experts are not endowed with better memories or better perceptual skills. They also do not appear to be deeper thinkers. Instead, they perform better at *specific* tasks because their knowledge has been efficiently organized. Although it seems clear that expertise is learned from experience, the precise mechanism for learning in probabilistic situations remains unclear. It seems that the most efficient way to learn probabilistic relationships is by "lens model" feedback about the relationship between cue values and one's judgment.

The development of powerful computers, and the realization that computers can do more than simply calculate (they can also manipulate symbols), has led to the development of computerized "experts" (CAD and expert systems). Such experts have found a place in research laboratories and even a few clinics, but by and large clinicians have been slow to accept them. There are several possible reasons for this, one of which is that clinicians perceive the machines as "alien" because they think differently from humans. Knowledge-based systems that try to present their logic in human form may have a greater probability of acceptance. They also lend themselves to teaching and some are presently being used for this purpose.

Up to this point, we have been concerned mainly with cognitive factors in medical decision making. However, there is another large area of psychological research that is also relevant. This research deals with the interpersonal and social aspects of medical judgment. The effects of these factors on medical judgment are discussed in Chapter 6.

6

Interpersonal, Social, and Economic Factors in Medical Decision Making

> *Life is short, the Art long, Opportunity fleeting, Experiment treacherous, Judgment difficult. The physician must be ready, not only to do his duty himself, but also to secure the cooperation of the patient, of the attendants and the externals.*
>
> Hippocrates

As we have shown, clinical decision making involves the application of medical knowledge, the weighing of risks and benefits, and the estimation of probabilities and utilities. However, several important factors have been omitted from our discussions thus far; medical judgment is also subject to social, economic, and interpersonal influences. These include not only the cost of medical care but also the ethical strictures governing the medical profession, social norms, and the quality of the patient–doctor interaction. The present chapter is concerned with how these factors affect medical judgment and decision making. We begin with a discussion of interpersonal and social influences on medical care. This is followed by a look at how economic factors influence clinical judgment. The chapter concludes with an attempt to forecast future developments.

Interpersonal and Social Factors in Patient Care

Patient and Doctor Characteristics

Although most doctors, and patients, believe that medical judgment should be based solely on what is "best" for the particular patient, research suggests that extraneous variables such as patient personality, social class, and the like can also affect medical judgments (see Eisenberg, 1979, for a review). In this section, we describe some of the more important variables and their effects.

Social class

According to Eisenberg (1979), several investigators have found that a patient's social class affects not only the medical care he/she receives but also the diagnosis. For example, social class has been shown to be correlated with psychiatric diagnosis (lower social class patients are more likely to be diagnosed as suffering from a "character disorder"). In addition, members of lower social classes are more likely to receive organic treatment for psychological problems for which middle-class patients are treated with psychotherapy. Social class has also been found to be related to the number and type of operations patients receive. Although some researchers have tried to subdivide the social class variable into separate race, income, education, and occupation variables, this approach has met with only limited success. It seems that these factors are too strongly correlated to extricate their independent influences (see Eisenberg, 1979, for the appropriate references).

Sex and appearance

Although some writers have argued that women's complaints are more likely to be viewed as "psychogenic" than men's (Lennane & Lennane, 1973), others have viewed the patient's general appearance as more important (Duff & Hollingshead, 1968). Overweight patients, for example, are judged less likeable and more nervous than those of average weight. Alcoholics, drug addicts, the aged, the uneducated, the very poor, and anyone considered unimportant to society (the disabled, criminals, and so on) are also treated less favorably than more attractive and "productive" middle-class patients (see Eisenberg, 1979).

Physician background and beliefs

According to Eisenberg (1979), doctors in different specialties treat the same patients differently. Members of some specialties are more likely than others to view patients' complaints as psychogenic. Specialists also differ in how willing they are to resuscitate patients who have stopped breathing. Some resuscitate everyone, others make distinctions on the basis of health, age, and other variables. Physicians also differ in their general "styles." Interventionist physicians are more likely to advise immediate action for cases for which those oriented more toward health maintenance recommend a "wait-and-see" approach. The physician's relationship to his/her profession can also be an important determiner of behavior. Those in individual practice, with little opportunity to consult with their colleagues, tend to behave differently (more conservatively) than those in group practice. The behavior of other physicians in the community can exert a strong influence even on doctors in individual practice. This influence probably accounts for at least part of the regional differences found by surveys of medical practitioners (Hoey et al., 1982, for example).

The doctor–patient relationship

As is discussed later in this chapter, perhaps the most important determiner of the quality of patient care is the doctor–patient relationship (see Calnan, 1984). Doctors, like everyone else, find people that they cannot get along with for one reason or another, and it is inevitable that such conflicts will affect their relationship. The difficulty arises if such conflicts also affect the quality of patient care. Unfortunately, there do appear to be differences in the way "problem" and "good" patients are treated (see Groves, 1978). In addition to problems with certain patients (and doctors), there are also general problems associated with the doctor–patient relationship. Some of these problems derive from the uneven nature of the interaction. Szasz and Hollender (1956) described three types of interactions patients can have with their doctors: (1) the physician can be active and controlling while the patient is simply passive and accepting; (2) the physician offers guidance and attempts to get the patient's cooperation, and (3) the physician and the patient are equal and the physician's role is to help the patient to make his/her own decisions. Of course, the same physician can behave in each of these different ways depending on the situation and the patient. Patients may also behave differently depending on the particular problem. Researchers have found that even patients who take an active role in the doctor–patient relationship defer to medical authority when asked to make important decisions (Brien & Shanteau, 1982).

The research briefly described here indicates the importance of interpersonal characteristics in medical care. Several factors (social class, appearance, personality, and so on) have been found to affect clinical decisions, but all appear to exert their effect through the doctor–patient relationship. Although much has been written about how doctors do (and should) interact with their patients, most practicing clinicians give the matter little thought. Perhaps this is because strong traditions exist in this regard.

Traditional Views of the Doctor–Patient Interaction

In the traditional doctor–patient relationship, authority rests squarely with the doctor (Katz, 1984). Widely held authoritarian values, and the feeling that patients are not competent to make significant judgments about their own care, have led physicians to disregard their patients' preferences. To show that this tendency is not new, Katz quoted Hippocrates, who advised doctors to:

perform [these duties] calmly and adroitly, concealing most things from the patient while you are attending to him. Give necessary orders with cheerfulness and serenity, turning his attention away from what is being done to him; sometimes reprove sharply and emphatically, and sometimes comfort with solicitude and attention, revealing nothing of the patient's future or present condition. (Hippocrates, 1967, p. 297)

Modern views are similar. Katz quoted a "distinguished surgeon" writing on the topic of patient involvement in medical decision making:

There is no way that I can see that a patient can logically judge whether he should have a cardiac valve replacement or not, or when, or whether it is to be with a Starr valve, a Bjork-Shiley valve, a Magovern valve, a Hancock preserved porcine valve, etc. . . . The objection of some of the laymen concerned about the problem has been to what they call the "father knows best" authoritative, paternalistic attitude of physicians. In fact, if "father" didn't know best, he ought to retire from practice. (Katz, 1984, p. 27)

As Katz pointed out, the history of medicine has been largely a story of competition with other "healers" (homeopaths, for example). This struggle for dominance probably contributed to medicine's authoritarian stance, and the demand for blind obedience adopted by many doctors. It also led doctors to ignore the uncertainties inherent in medicine, or at least not to discuss these uncertainties with their patients. The implicit assumption was that patients who "trust" their doctors will follow their advice without question.

Recently, it has become clear that patients do not always do as their doctors request (see S. J. Cohen, 1979, Evans & Spelman, 1983, for example). Patients' failure to comply with doctors' orders cannot be explained by a single factor; it is possible, however, that a lack of trust may be an important contributing influence. The need for new laws requiring that patients give "informed consent" suggest that patients are not always willing to follow their doctors' advice purely on faith. Since even the best advice is valueless if patients elect to ignore it, it is important to learn exactly how interpersonal factors affect both patients and doctors. This section reviews research relevant to this topic.

Patient compliance

In the research literature, the degree of compliance has been defined as the correlation between a patient's behavior and medical advice. In practice, this has meant noting how faithfully patients take their medications, stick to diets, and follow other therapeutic regimens (Epstein & Cluss, 1982; Evans & Spelman, 1983). Most research studies on patient compliance have focused on errors of omission—the failure to take medications, do exercise, and so on. But noncompliant behavior may take other forms (overdoses, mistimings, and self-prescriptions).

Noncompliance with doctors' advice is a common, and serious, medical problem (Sackett & Haynes, 1976). According to Evans and Spelman (1983), nearly half of all patients do not take their medication as prescribed, and many stop taking it altogether as soon as they feel better (see also Davis, 1966; Kellaway & McCrae, 1975; Ley, 1976). Similar levels of noncompliance have been reported for patients prescribed special diets (Ley, 1976). Sackett and Snow (1979) reported that, on average, patients fail to keep half the appointments made for them by doctors. (They are a little better at keeping appointments they make for themselves.) One result of noncompliance may be ineffective treatment, which, in turn, may lead patients to mistrust their doctors' advice. (After all, the last treatment "didn't work.") Such patients are even less likely to comply in the future.

Noncompliance also makes it difficult for clinicians and researchers to interpret the results of clinical trials. For example, drugs may appear ineffective when the real problem is that patients are failing to take them correctly (Eraker, Kirscht, & Becker, 1984). Although the issue of patient compliance has received substantial attention in the medical literature, many doctors remain unaware of the size or importance of the problem (Davis, 1966) and few, if any doctors, can predict which patients will and will not comply with their advice (see references in Eraker et al., 1984, and Rothert, 1982).

Research on patient compliance requires some measure of how closely patients are following doctors' recommendations (Gordis, 1979 and Norell, 1984). The most obvious method is to note whether the recommended regimen has been effective. That is, if the patient recovers then he/she is assumed to have complied. The danger in this approach is that some patients will improve for reasons other than their treatment and their improvement will be incorrectly attributed to the doctor's advice. Eraker et al. (1984) gave the example of a hypertensive patient whose blood pressure is reduced by exercise, weight loss, or simply by a physician's reassurance. Focusing on outcome would lead researchers to the conclusion that the medicine prescribed by the doctor was solely responsible. Similarly, the lack of therapeutic effect can be taken as an indication that patients require a higher dosage when the real culprit is their failure to take the medication in the first place.

Various other techniques have been used to assess patient compliance; most fall into one of two categories: direct and indirect (Epstein & Cluss, 1982; Ley, 1982a; Pearson, 1982). The direct methods are those that do not depend on patient reports. Blood and urine assays to detect whether medicines have been taken fit in this category. So too does the examination of appointment registers to judge how often appointments are kept. Indirect methods rely on patient, physician, or observer reports, on pill counts (to see how many have been taken), or simply on observing outcomes to judge whether patients have complied with professional advice. Both direct and indirect techniques have their advantages and disadvantages. On the plus side, direct techniques are not prone to deception or forgetfulness, as indirect ones are. On the other hand, assays and other tests are expensive and inconvenient. The correlation between direct and indirect measures is not very high. Typically, more people are judged noncompliant by direct methods than by indirect ones (Ley, 1982b), but this may depend, in part, on the specific medication involved (Inui, Carter, Pecoraro, Pearlman, & Dohan, 1980).

Historically, research on patient compliance has been founded on the traditional view of the patient as a passive and obedient recipient of the doctor's advice. The noncomplying patient has been viewed as a defaulter, and the problem one of control (see Katz, 1984). Research emphasis has been placed on identifying groups of noncompliers on the basis of socioeconomic class, education, age, and sex. These efforts have met with little success; it seems that just about anyone can be a noncomplier given the right circumstances (Ley, 1979).

Another, more recent, research approach has looked for situational influences that may lead patients to ignore medical advice. A number of factors have been isolated. For example, one determiner of missed appointments is a time factor. The longer the interval between a referral and an appointment, the less likely the appointment is to be kept (Finnerty, Shaw, & Himmelsback, 1973; Glogo, 1973). Noncompliance with drug regimens has been found to be affected by several factors. Some patients are noncompliant because they find the therapy's side effects worse than the illness itself (Crome, Akehurst, & Keet, 1980). Family variables may be important for some patients (Doherty, Schrott, Metcalf & Iasiello-Vailas, 1983) while others simply do not like the inconvenience or complexity of a therapeutic regimen (Firestone, 1982; Gryfe & Gryfe, 1984). There are even a few people who fail to take medications because the safety caps on the bottles are too difficult for them to remove (Amdur, 1979). According to Ley (1982b), however, the most important predictor of compliance is the quality of the doctor–patient relationship.

Ley's view is supported by research reported by Wartman, Morlock, Malitz, and Palm (1983), who found that patients' ability to communicate with their doctor is related to the degree of compliance. In a similar manner, patient satisfaction with their consultation, with their doctor's communications, and with the care they received are all good predictors of their compliance (Haynes, Taylor, & Sackett, 1979). Memory tests have shown that satisfied patients also retain their doctor's advice better than dissatisfied ones (Ley, 1979). Korsch, Gozzi, and Francis (1968) summarize these findings as indicating that warmth, friendliness, and empathy for the patient's concerns by the doctor coupled with jargon-free explanations for any recommendations promotes both patient satisfaction *and* compliance.

It seems that, for most patients, compliance depends on the doctor–patient relationship and little else. There are a few exceptions, however.

Carr and Whittenbaugh (1968), for example, reported less compliance among psychiatric patients than among general medical patients, and Hertroij (1974) found a negative correlation between degree of disability and compliance. It is possible that the noncompliance found in these patients has its roots in the increased supervision their conditions require. In general, the longer the duration and complexity of treatment a patient needs, the greater the probability of noncompliance (Ley, 1982b).

Eraker et al. (1984) pointed out that there may be reasonable explanations of why a patient may fail to comply with medical advice. Patients are aware that physicians are sometimes wrong, that treatments sometimes fail, and that patients may improve without any treatment at all. Many patients are also aware that treatments are not without risk. Patients develop their own belief systems about illness and its treatment. These belief systems affect how they respond to treatment recommendations. For many years, researchers on patient compliance have conceptualized their efforts in terms of the Health Belief Model of patient behavior (Becker, 1976).

The Health Belief Model was first developed to predict compliance with prevention programs (stop smoking campaigns, for example). According to the model, the probability that a program will be followed is a function of the patient's perception of his/her susceptibility to the disease, the perceived severity of the disease if contracted, the efficacy of the recommended action, and the psychological, physical, and economic costs of the action. The model also stipulates that an internal or external cue (pain or reminders) must be present to trigger the appropriate behavior by making the individual aware of the health threat. Sociological, personality, and demographic variables are assumed to affect one or more aspects of the model (economic costs will be of greater concern to some patients than others, for example), but they are not direct influences on compliance. Over the years, the Health Belief Model has been altered to make it applicable to treatment compliance as well as prevention.

Most of the research on the Health Belief Model has been correlational, and many studies have been retrospective rather than prospective (Ley, 1982b). Because retrospective studies are vulnerable to the "overconfidence" bias described in Chapter 3, it is difficult to reach firm conclusions about the model's validity. One interesting prospective study conducted by Taylor, Sackett, Haynes, et al. (1979) on hypertensive patients found that the model did not predict compliance before the initiation of treatment but did predict compliance after treatment began. This finding suggests that the variables measured by the Health Belief Model are not so much predictors of compliance as correlates of it. That is, the beliefs and values measured by the model develop with compliance as the result of experience with the treatment.

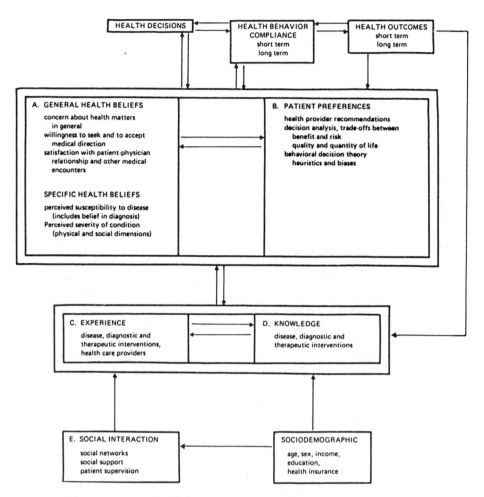

Figure 6-1   The Health Decision Model—a revision of the Health Belief Model that includes patient preferences and other decision theory constructs. Reprinted from Eraker et al. (1984) with the permission of the American College of Physicians and the Annals of Internal Medicine.

The Health Belief Model has recently been revised by Eraker et al. (1984) to make it more consistent with decision analysis and SEU theory. They call their model the Health Decision Model, and its general outline appears in Figure 6-1. As may be seen, the Health Decision Model views compliance as the result of a set of general health beliefs and an independent set of patient preferences. These beliefs and preferences are derived from experience and medical knowledge, both of which, in turn, depend on social factors. Feedback from previous decisions to comply also affect future decisions. Because no research has been conducted specifically on this new model, its predictive validity (its ability to predict who will comply) remains to be demonstrated.

Christensen-Szalanski and Northcraft (in press), like Eraker, et al. have also suggested a revision to the Health Belief Model. They pointed out that the model ignores the "time" dimension. For example, people may continue to smoke even though they realize the health benefits of stopping because the benefits are all in the future (and discounted) while the pleasures of smoking are immediate. They also emphasize the importance of previous experiences on health-related behavior. A patient who has already been induced to "invest" substantial time, money, and effort in a treatment program is less likely to quit than one who has made only a small commitment. The importance of previous events can be conceptualized in terms of the well-known "sunk costs' phenomenon (Arkes & Blumer, 1985) discussed in Chapter 4. Although they should not be considered, previous expenditures of money, time, and effort affect future behavior. The addition of the time dimension to the Health Belief Model permitted Christensen-Szalanski and Northcraft to explain behavior that is inexplicable by the model as originally formulated.

A variety of different techniques have been suggested to improve patient compliance. Simplifying therapeutic regimens (Fischer, 1980) is one obvious approach that does not require a great deal of effort. When this is impossible, some researchers favor educational strategies such as providing patients with written explanations of their treatment and written reminders (Hall, 1979; Morris & Halperin, 1979). Major educational programs designed to teach patients the rationale for their treatment have also been attempted (Ley, 1982; Sackett, Haynes, & Gibson, 1975). The most successful programs, however, are those that combine education with behavior modification (Dunbar et al., 1979). One particularly useful behavioral technique is contracting. Contracting refers to a process of specifying a target behavior and creating a formalized agreement to adhere to it. Hypertensive patients induced to agree to a contract were found to be more likely to comply with a treatment regimen than those simply given instructions to comply (Dunbar et al., 1979). Another behavioral technique, self-monitoring, in which patients are asked to keep careful records of their compliance to a therapeutic regime, has also been reported as improving compliance (Johnson & White, 1971; Maletsky, 1974). Unfortunately, the effects of many behavioral interventions have been transitory (Mahoney, 1974). Some research has shown that rewards and other motivators can maintain the benefits of behavioral programs for longer periods (Barber, 1976; Robbins, 1980) but patients must be motivated to comply in the first place. Some writers feel that this motivation can be supplied by supportive counseling (Kellaway, 1979, 1983). A number of additional ideas for improving patient compliance are reviewed by Eraker et al., 1984.

Table 6-1. Noncompliance by Professionals

Topic	Percent Not Complying[a]
Correct scoring of psychological tests	84–94
Warning patients of drug interactions	64–92
Giving adequate counseling about drug use	53–100
Prescribing the appropriate antibiotic	12–76
Attending refresher courses	44
Observing rules about issuing medicine	95

[a] The percentages represent the range of noncompliance found in several different studies. See Ley (1981) for the appropriate references.

Although the discussion has thus far focused on patients, it should be noted that clinicians may also fail to comply with their own professional standards and with the best advice on patient care. Ley (1981) reviewed the literature on what he called "professional non-compliance" and found substantial evidence for the hypothesis that noncompliance is not limited to patients. Ten percent of pharmacists make serious mistakes in giving patients directions for drug use, few note dangerous drug interactions for patients ordering several prescriptions, and many fill prescriptions that are clearly inappropriate for the particular patient. (See Ley's article for references for this and the following studies.) One study examined the content of preparations prepared specially by pharmacists. It found only 28 of 100 pharmacies provided the accurate ingredients (to within 5% of what was ordered) and only 20% gave adequate directions for the medicine's use. Only 5 of the 100 pharmacies managed to get both the ingredients and the directions correct. Incorrect prescriptions are also common. Doctors have been found to prescribe the wrong drugs and incorrect dosages of the correct drugs. Nurses who had been told to only prescribe drugs on the ward stocklist and only follow written orders were found to violate both rules. Table 6-1 summarizes Ley's findings.

Most of the research on how well patients adhere to therapeutic regimens has been devoted to studying why patients fail to "follow orders." As already noted, the idea that doctors give orders and patients follow them grows out of the history of medicine: doctors are the experts and patients are the recipients of their expertise. There is another, more modern view: patients should not be expected to comply with recommendations unless they have been involved in the decision making that produces them (Jonsen, 1979). To make sure that patients follow a treatment regimen, doctors must first discuss the regimen with them, make sure they understand its rationale, and give the patient the opportunity to consent. However, just how much information a patient requires to give "informed consent" is not entirely clear, nor is the exact role patients should play in medical decision making.

Patient involvement in decision making

Ever since ancient times, surgical patients have been required to consent to their operations, but their rights in this regard have traditionally been limited. Patients could refuse to undergo an operation, but they had no right to a detailed explanation of the operation's rationale (see Katz, 1984, for a historical review). It was not until the 1950s that courts began to assert that physicians have a duty to acquaint patients with the reasons for their therapeutic recommendations. Patients, it came to be believed, need to know the risks and benefits of any recommended actions as well as the available alternatives. The reason behind this belief, which eventually became legally codified in the doctrine of "informed consent," is that patients must have this information to make intelligent decisions affecting their own health. As Katz pointed out, once courts agreed that informed consent was desirable, they had to face the "staggering assignment" of deciding just what information must be communicated to patients. There are almost always a large number of potential facts available about any illness. Which of these should be given to patients, and how patients are supposed to use them, are questions the courts have thus far been unable to answer (Katz, 1984).

One thing seems clear—access to information, by itself, does not ensure good judgment. In earlier chapters, we noted the difficulties doctors have in handling excessive amounts of information; patients, of course, are even more likely to find the sheer amount of available data overwhelming. Cognitive overload may make patients *less* rather than more able to contribute to the decision-making process. A character in a novel stated what might be a representative reaction:

> It's not because my mind is made up that I don't want you to confuse me with any more facts. It's because my mind isn't made up. I already have more facts than I can cope with. (Brunner, 1975, p. 41)

So, if patient involvement in medical decision making is a worthwhile goal, and we believe it is, how can it best be accomplished? Some writers have said that what is needed is a more "open" and sharing relationship between patients and doctors (see Bursztajn et al., 1981, and Katz, 1984, for example). However, beyond providing patients with compassion, and appropriate information, there have been few *specific* suggestions made about the mechanism by which patient input can have a practical influence on medical decisions.

One possibility is to have patients exercise their rights as health care consumers. In most western nations, middle-class patients are free to choose their own doctors and, in some countries, hospitals as well. By exercising their choices with discretion, patients gain some degree of control over their health care; if they are not pleased with their treatment they can, and sometimes do, go elsewhere (see Brien, 1979, for a brief review of consumerist movements in medicine). However, shopping around for health care providers gives patients at best indirect control over medical decisions. It appears that, once patients choose a medical adviser, even active consumerists defer to medical expertise. In other words, having decided who their doctor is to be, people tend to follow his/her advice (Brien, Haverfield, & Shanteau, 1983; Brien & Shanteau, 1982).

Consumer movements in health care assume that patient desires, needs, and complaints must become part of the decision-making process. Unfortunately, it is not clear that the average person is equipped with the skills and traits necessary to play this role. Patients, to be fully involved in health care decision making, need to be able to interpret the information they are given and to place it in its appropriate context. For example, without some idea of what constitutes an acceptable risk–benefit ratio, many patients may be unduly concerned about rare treatment side effects.

Perhaps the best mechanism for giving patients a greater role in the decision-making process is to increase the use of decision analysis. Although it may sound strange, given the objections to formal decision making described in Chapter 4 (and by writers such as Bursztajn et al., 1981), decision analysis has been specially designed to permit meaningful patient input at the point in the decision-making process where it will have greatest impact—specifying utilities.

Decision analysis involves what Fischhoff (1979) called a "division of labor" between the physician and the patient. It is the physician who structures the problem, identifies the alternative actions and outcomes, and provides the relevant probabilities. All these tasks require clinical and scientific expertise. As the surgeon quoted earlier in this chapter correctly pointed out, only highly paid experts can be expected to know the difference between various cardiac valves (or other treatments), the likelihood of their success or failure, and so on. On the other hand, the patient is the only person qualified to judge the desirability of the various possible outcomes. Decision analysis permits both the doctor and patient to make contributions to the decision-making process that are commensurate with their individual roles and expertise. Decision analysis also makes clear exactly what information the patient requires—not technical details that require extensive medical training to understand but the expected outcomes of the various alternatives as they are likely to affect patients' longevity and life quality. The widespread use of decision analysis, coupled with easier and more acceptable methods of measuring utilities, seems to us the fairest and the easiest way of allowing patients to play a role in the medical decision-making process.

Economic Aspects of Medical Decisions

Medical decision making has thus far been viewed as largely a matter for doctors and their patients. However, the doctor–patient interaction does not take place in a social vacuum. It is one of many relationships that, together, constitute a modern society. Because they are human beings, the behavior of both doctors and patients is inevitably influenced by the social milieu in which they live and work. The ethical rules governing medical practice, cultural standards of proper behavior, and local customs all exert a powerful influence on what goes on in the clinic. We have mentioned several important social influences on clinical judgment in the preceding section (patients' social class and community standards, for example). We now wish to take a somewhat broader view and discuss how society-wide economic forces can affect medical practice.

Values and the Cost of Health Care

Health care is expensive. The United States currently spends over $1000 per person each year on health care. This represents more than 9% of the gross national product, and the amount continues to rise faster than the rate of inflation or economic growth (Cooper, 1983). There are several reasons usually offered for the high cost of health care: new technology is expensive, the aging population requires more medical attention than previous generations, doctors' fees are very high, and procedure-based reimbursement schemes (plus a fear of lawsuits) encourage doctors to perform more tests and procedures than are absolutely necessary (see the papers in Gay & Sax Jacobs, 1983, for more on each of these topics). Although they are not commonly listed as a reason for skyrocketing medical costs, it is arguable that public and professional attitudes toward health and illness are the most important reason for the current situation. Put simply, the high cost of health care simply mirrors widely held ideas of what constitutes desirable medical practice.

In Chapter 4, we described how the benefits, risks, and economic costs of large-scale medical programs (mass immunizations and screenings, for example) may be evaluated using cost–benefit and cost-effectiveness analysis. If the analysis is positive (marginal benefits are greater than costs, for example) and the resources are available, the project should proceed. Otherwise, the project should be shelved or revised. Although cost–benefit and cost-effectiveness analysis, like decision analysis in general, rests on a rational mathematical foundation, it does not reflect the way decisions are typically made in the clinic. When faced with a sick patient, doctors rarely calculate costs and benefits. Instead, they apply treatments until the treatments yield no additional payoffs. Similarly, doctors are likely to use any available diagnostic tool that promises to provide an increment in information about the patient, no matter how small the increment may be (routine electronic fetal monitoring, for example; Banta, 1983). As new diagnostic and treatment procedures are developed, the number of procedures and treatments a doctor can try before a patient can no longer be helped grows as well. The result—ever-increasing medical costs.

In a sense, this is what doctors and patients want—not higher costs but the feeling that "everything possible" has been done. If they consider them at all, most people feel that high costs are the price that must be paid for quality care. In any case, few patients wind up paying for medical care themselves; the burden is carried by the members of the patient's insurance fund or by society as a whole. Unfortunately, whether the money comes from private individuals, insurance companies, or governments, the total expenditure is the same. Because every dollar spent on health care leaves a dollar less to spend on something else, it is unimportant who pays the bill. The escalating cost of health care is a problem for everyone.

Medical Costs: A "Commons" Dilemma

The present health care system is an example of what Hardin (1968) called the "Tragedy of the Commons." In the example given by Hardin, each of 10 farmers owns one 1000-pound bull. All 10 bulls graze in a common pasture that produces just enough grass to sustain all the animals and reproduce itself each year. If one additional bull is introduced, the grass would be insufficient and the weight of *each* animal would be reduced to 900 pounds. Thus the introduction of the extra animal reduces the pasture's total "carrying capacity" from 10,000 pounds to 9900 pounds. Although the overall wealth of the commons has been reduced, any single individual who introduces an extra animal has increased his/her wealth from 1000 to 1800 pounds. This 800-pound gain is at the expense of the other farmers, who lose 100 pounds each.

It is important to realize that the tragedy of the commons is not the result of aberrant behavior. The farmer who introduces an extra bull is acting rationally according to the prevailing view of economic behavior. A community of free individuals, motivated by self-interest, all competing for goods and services, is what has made capitalism such a success. The farmer who introduces the extra bull is merely trying to maximize personal gain. Indeed, economic rationality demands that another animal be added, and another, without end. Of course, the other farmers, who are equally rational, reach the same conclusion. Before long, the common pasture is so overgrazed there is insufficient grass for any animals and they all die. The end result—neither grass nor meat for anyone.

This conflict between immediate personal gain and long-term loss to society as a whole has been called the "commons dilemma" because individuals acting logically to maximize their private gain (the very essence of the capitalist system) make the community as a whole poorer. The commons dilemma is not solely an agricultural problem; it occurs repeatedly in practically every area of social life. Standing at a crowded football match gives one a better view but keeps other spectators from seeing the game. If everyone decides to stand, no one is better off and many people will be unable to see at all. Similarly, but on a larger scale, building a polluting chemical plant on a clean river may produce short-term profits for the company's shareholders but will poison the river and create a large cleaning bill for generations to come.

Individual patients acting on their own self-interest will demand every treatment modern medicine has to offer, and doctors, many of whose incomes depend on the number of tests and procedures they perform, are likely to go along with them. The individual patient's gain, if any, is made at the expense of society as a whole. Insurance companies and governments can refuse to pay for certain procedures, but this will not affect those wealthy enough to pay their own medical costs. As long as the rich can buy any treatment they like, society is unlikely to deny access to health care to anyone else; we will find the money somewhere. If costs are ever to be contained, some way of changing the current medical system must be found, but what?

Cost Containment Procedures and Medical Decision Making

Several possible ways to contain medical costs have been suggested. Perhaps the most popular approach is education. Lectures, seminars, and discussions emphasizing the cost of care, the usefulness of laboratory tests, and suggestions for reducing expense (by using generic drugs, for example) all have the aim of making physicians aware of the economic impact of their decisions and of alternative strategies that might save money. Such educational programs have been shown to reduce costs, but their effect tends to be short-lived without continual reminders (Eisenberg & Williams, 1981).

Feedback to doctors about their behavior has also been suggested as a way to reduce costs (see Eisenberg & Williams, 1981, for a review). Feedback may be provided in a variety of ways. Physicians can be given copies of the bills sent to their hospitalized patients. In this way, doctors can become aware of what their recommendations cost. Doctors can also be told where they stand compared with other physicians (their percentile rank) as users of various tests and services. Chart audits and Professional Standards Review Organizations (PSROs) are also means of making physicians more aware of their own behavior. Although feedback has been found to produce small decreases in patient costs, the feedback itself is expensive to provide and the net gains may well be nil. Thus far, no feedback program has used rule-based (lens model) feedback as described in Chapter 5. It is possible that greater effects are achievable with more effective forms of feedback.

Financial rewards and penalties (fines, for instance) have also been advocated as ways to help contain costs. The idea is simple. If you do not want a farmer to introduce an extra animal to the commons, then make it illegal or expensive (by introducing a license fee) for him/her to do so. Not surprisingly, financial penalties (and rewards) have a similar motivating influence on doctors. Eisenberg and Williams (1981), in their review of cost-containment procedures, asserted that financial rewards and penalties are the most potent ways to get physicians to contain costs.

Free-market competition between different types of health care providers has also been suggested as a way to curb medical costs. The logic goes something like this. Physicians who practice in Health Maintenance Organizations (HMOs) stand to lose money by overservicing because their patients pay a standard yearly fee. Thus, HMO physicians will keep costs and fees down and serve as a brake on other physicians. To date, however, the existence of HMOs has not retarded the growth of medical costs, largely because of their small number and the relatively minor cost of medical insurance (not to mention free public hospital care). The problem is that HMOs are not competing in a completely free market. Their competition may be more costly, but since it is rarely the patient who pays, most do not care.

Instead of direct manipulations of financial incentives, some cost-containment programs have taken a regulatory approach. Thus, hospitals have restricted the number of tests a doctor can order each day, doctors have been made to fill out forms justifying each test they use, and approval has been required for certain treatments and procedures (Eisenberg & Williams, 1981, gave examples of each of these). It is possible to go even further and set standard fees based on patient diagnoses. This is more or less the system operating on some European countries (the United Kingdom, for instance), where government insurance schemes determine what they will pay for (and how much) and even the rich cannot buy additional services. The introduction of prospective payment systems in the United States is an attempt to accomplish much the same thing (Williams, 1985). Under a prospective payment system, hospitals are paid a standard, fixed amount for each case they admit according to the patient's diagnosis and regardless of how much it actually costs to treat the patient. There is no doubt that prospective payments based on diagnoses can reduce hospital costs, but there is always the possibility that such a system will encourage hospitals to "dump" expensive patients in favor of those they can treat more easily. Such a system is also fairly inflexible; doctors have little latitude to adjust their treatment to the specifics of the patient.

All cost-containment procedures reviewed here have some effect on physician behavior, but no single procedure represents a complete solution to the problem of escalating medical costs. The reason is that the commons dilemma transcends economics; it is an ethical rather than an economic issue. Patients expect that all possible measures will be taken to ensure their health; costs simply do not matter because they are shared among many people. Controlling costs requires a fundamental change in medical decision making, a shift in attitudes from "doing everything possible" to doing what is cost effective. Shifting attitudes is a psychological problem, one that requires an understanding of the psychology of medical decision making. Readers who have come this far in the book know that research in this area has just begun. In the next section, we take a look at where the field may be heading in the future.

Toward the Future

This book has presented a wide sampling of current psychological research and theory relevant to medical decision making. This final section represents an attempt to relate this work to longer term trends in psychology and medicine with the goal of predicting where future research and theory will head.

Theories Will Become More Explicitly Descriptive

Medical decision making is a hybrid field falling at the intersection of several disciplines: mathematical probability theory, game theory, economics, psychology, and, of course, the biological and health sciences. The present book has concentrated on psychological contributions, which, in historical terms, have come much later than those of other fields. Nevertheless, psychology's input has been crucial. Before the psychological study of judgment and decision making, it was generally believed that decision making could be understood solely in terms of normative theories. These theories assume that doctors (and everyone else) accept the axioms underlying such theories as subjective expected utility, and that, because they do accept these axioms, people will behave as the theories say they should. In essence, normative theories equate rationality with conforming to the theory, Those who fail to behave as the theory predicts are thought to be acting irrationally.

Although there is some controversy about the generalizability of some laboratory research findings to the clinic, psychological research has produced a substantial literature documenting important discrepancies between the predictions generated by normative theories and the behavior of decision makers in a variety of situations. Even when people are informed that their behavior violates the axioms of normative theories—even after the theories are explained to them—some people still fail to conform. To explain non-normative behavior, psychologists began to develop descriptive theories of decision making. These theories were not designed to prescribe how decision making *should* be done but rather to *describe* how it is actually done.

Initially, most psychological research was aimed at demonstrating that judgment is sometimes biased. The effect of heuristics and biases on medical decision making is now widely acknowledged, although the extent of this influence in the real world of the clinic, as opposed to the psychological laboratory, remains to be determined. Future research in this area will probably shift from demonstrating that biases exist to trying to determine when heuristics are most likely to be used and when they will be avoided. This means more research in clinical situations and less work using artificial judgment tasks.

Along with descriptive theories came a shift from studying judgment outcomes to studying the cognitive processes that give rise to them. The most tangible result of such efforts has been the development of expert systems based not simply on normative theories and formal mathematics but also on studies of experts' problem-solving techniques. It seems inevitable that future efforts at theory building will continue to follow the descriptive path. The result of such efforts is likely to be even more efficient expert systems. These systems will have obvious applications in training new doctors and as decision aids to practicing physicians. Because of the explicit nature of computer programs, such expert systems will also constitute precise descriptive theories of medical decision making.

Training Will Become the Focus of More Research

Because heuristics, biases, algorithms, and other judgment strategies must have been learned somehow, psychologists have become increasingly interested in how people develop strategies for decision making in probabilistic environments. Thus far, research in this area has focused on what can and cannot be learned and how well different types of feedback facilitate learning. In the future, this research is likely to focus more on studies of experts and the development of teaching strategies based on these studies. Expert systems will probably play an important role in this effort. In fact, developing expert systems based on the cognitive strategies of clinical experts is the first step in using such systems to train the next generation of clinicians. Because every training program needs some way to determine its effectiveness, greater efforts will be made to develop measures of medical decision-making skills. Ways to evaluate course effectiveness will also be necessary. In addition, research efforts will be directed to some of the basic measurement problems of the field, such as efficient ways to determine patient utilities. A practical method of measuring utilities is particularly important if decision analysis is ever to be accepted as a routine part of clinical practice.

Psychological Factors Will Become Part of Policy Making

The idea that choices are made as a function of probabilities and utilities dates at least as far back as von Neuman and Morgenstern's work in the 1940s. The idea constitutes the foundation of such techniques as cost–benefit and cost–effectiveness analysis. Yet, when it comes to making decisions about large-scale public programs, politicians often make their choice not on the basis of decision analysis but on what they believe the public wants (or is willing to accept). In democracies, there is a good reason to give the people what they want, provided it is clear just what this is. However, the public's desires are often unknown. What is required is some way of incorporating the personal attitudes of individuals into decisions that affect society as a whole. One possible way to do this has been proposed by Pauker, Pauker, and McNeil (1981), who provided an example in which prospective parents' attitudes about abortion, miscarriage, and birth defects are integrated into a decision analysis concerning whether to develop a screening program for neural tube defects.

Attempts to contain medical costs also offer substantial opportunities for research, particularly in the development of new patient management strategies (and more efficient algorithms) (see also Williams, 1985). As medicine becomes increasingly complex, many decisions are no longer made by a single clinician; they are made by a team. Unfortunately, most decision-analytic techniques do not easily lend themselves to group decisions. We cannot, for example, simply aggregate individual utilities into an overall group utility because the utility measures currently in use are relative, not absolute. There is clearly a need for more research on group decision making. New technology also presents an opportunity for future research. In the past, new technologies have been introduced before evidence for their cost effectiveness was available (see Banta, 1983). Millions of dollars have been spent on technologies that later proved useless.

Summary

Medical decision making is generally viewed as something that takes place in the privacy of the clinic. The doctor evaluates the relevant data and, based on his/her experience and professional judgment, maps out a patient management strategy. In this chapter, we tried to show that this view omits several important factors. Social and interpersonal variables such as social class can also play an important role in clinical judgment. The importance of interpersonal variables is particularly evident in studies of patient compliance, which reveal that the most important determinant of whether a patient follows a doctor's recommendations is the quality of the doctor–patient relationship. We also showed how cost considerations can have an important impact on patient management.

In the final section of the chapter, we described several important areas of psychological research that we believe will continue to develop. Although we have described those research areas we believe most likely to be pursued, it is entirely possible, even probable, that new research areas that we did not anticipate will also be developed. The psychology of medical decision making is a growing and important area of research for both doctors and psychologists. We look forward to further exciting developments in the years to come.

References

Abrams, H. L. (1981). Research in diagnostic radiology: A holistic perspective. *Clinical Radiology, 32,* 121–128.

Alcorn, F. S., & O'Donnell, E. (1969). The training of nonphysician personnel for use in a mammography program. *Cancer, 23,* 879–883.

Alcorn, F. S., O'Donnell, E., & Ackerman, L. V. (1971). The protocol and results of training nonradiologists to scan mammograms. *Radiology, 99,* 523–529.

Alfidi, R. J. (1971). Informed consent: A study of patient reaction. *Journal of the American Medical Association, 216,* 1325–1329.

Allais, M. (1953). Le comportement de l'homme rationnel devant le risque: Critique des postulats et axiomes de l'ecole americaine. *Econometrica, 21,* 503–546.

Allen, N. P., Wolf, F. M., Cassidy, J. T., Garrison, J. M., Davis, W. K., Maxim, B. R., & Dielman, T. E. (1984, April). *A factor analytic study of the structure of patient management problems.* Paper presented at the Annual Meeting of the American Educational Research Association, New Orleans.

Alvey, P. (1983, December). *The problems of designing a medical expert system.* Paper presented at the Proceedings of the Expert Systems Conference, Churchill College, Cambridge, England.

Amdur, M. A. (1979). Medication compliance in outpatient psychiatry. *Comprehensive Psychiatry, 20,* 339–346.

Anderson, N. H. (1972). Looking for configurality in clinical judgment. *Psychological Bulletin, 78,* 93–102.

Anderson, N. H. (1974). Information integration theory: A brief survey. In D. H. Krantz, R. C. Atkinson, R. O. Luce, & P. Suppes (Eds.), *Measurement, psychophysics and neural information processing* (Vol. 2). San Francisco: Freeman.

Anderson, N. H., & Shanteau, J. (1977). Weak inference with linear models. *Psychological Bulletin, 84,* 1155–1170.

Applegate, W. B. (1981). Decision theory for clinicians: Uses and misuses of clinical tests. *Southern Medical Journal, 74,* 468–473.

Arkes, H. R. (1981). Impediments to accurate clinical judgement and possible ways to minimize their impact. *Journal of Consulting and Clinical Psychology, 49,* 323–330.

Arkes, H. R., & Blumer, C. (1985). The psychology of sunk costs. *Organizational Behavior and Human Decision Processes, 35,* 2124–2140.

Arkes, H. R., & Harkness, A. R. (1980). The effect of making a diagnosis on subsequent recognition of symptoms. *Journal of Experimental Psychology: Human Learning and Memory, 6,* 568–575.

Arkes, H. R., Wortmann, R. L., Saville, P. D., & Harkness, A. R. (1981). Hindsight bias among physicians weighing the likelihood of diagnoses. *Journal of Applied Psychology, 66,* 252–254.

Aschenbrenner, K. M., & Kasubek, W. (1978). Challenging the Cushing syndrome: Multiattribute evaluation of cortisone drugs. *Organizational Behavior and Human Performance, 22,* 216–234.

Baida, P. (1984). 1884. *Atlantic, 269,* 15–16.

Balla, J. I. (1980). Logical thinking and the diagnostic process. *Methods of Information in Medicine, 19,* 88–92.

Banta, H. D. (1983). Some aphorisms concerning medical technology illustrated by specific case examples. In J. R. Gay & B. R. Sax Jacobs (Eds.), *The technology explosion in medical science: Implications for the health care industry and the public (1981–2001).* New York: SP Medical & Scientific Books.

Barber, B. (1976). Compassion in medicine: Toward new definitions and new institutions. *New England Journal of Medicine, 295,* 939–943.

Bar-Hillel, M. (1983). The base rate fallacy. In R. W. Scholz (Ed.), *Decision making under uncertainty.* Amsterdam: Elsevier.

Becker, M. H. (1976). Sociobehavioural determinants of compliance. In D. L. Sackett & R. B. Haynes (Eds.), *Compliance with therapeutic regimens.* Balitmore: Johns Hopkins University Press.

Bennett, M. J. (1980). *Heuristics and the weighting of base rate information in diagnostic tasks by nurses.* Unpublished thesis, Monash University.

Berbaum, K., Franken, E. A., & Smith, W. L. (1985). The effect of comparison films upon resident interpretation of pediatric chest radiographs. *Investigative Radiology, 20,* 124–128.

Berkeley, D., & Humphreys, P. (1982). Structuring decision problems and the 'bias heuristic'. *Acta Psychologica, 50,* 201–252.

Bernoulli, D. (1954). Exposition of a new theory on the measurement of risk. *Econometrica, 22,* 23–36. (Original work published 1738)

Berry, P. C. (1961). *Psychological study of decision making* (Technical Report NAV TRAD EVCEN 797). Port Washington, New York: US Naval Training Device Center.

Berwick, D. M., & Thibodeau, L. A. (1983). Receiver operating characteristic analysis of diagnostic skill. *Medical Care, 21,* 876–885.

Berwick, D. M., Fineberg, H. V., & Weinstein, M. C. (1981). When doctors meet numbers. *The American Journal of Medicine, 71,* 991–998.

Beyth-Marom, R., & Fischhoff, B. (1983). Diagnosticity and pseudodiagnosticity. *Journal of Personality and Social Psychology, 45,* 1185–1195.

Birnbaum, M. H. (1976). Intuitive numerical prediction. *American Journal of Psychology, 89,* 417–429.

Bishop, J., & Cicchetti, C. (1973). Some institutional and conceptual thoughts on the measurement of indirect and intangible benefits and costs. In H. M. Peskin & E. P. Seskin (Eds.), *Cost–benefit analysis and water pollution policy.* Washington, DC: The Urban Institute.

Bisseret, A., Redon, S., & Falzon, P. (1982). Computer-aided training for risky decision making. *International Review of Applied Psychology, 31,* 493–509.

Braakman, R., Gelpke, G. J., Habbema, J. D. F., Maas, A. I. R., & Minderhound, J. M. (1980). Systematic selection of prognostic features in patients with severe head injury. *Neurosurgery, 6,* 362–370.

Brachman, R. J., Amarel, S., Engelman, C., Engelmore, R. S., Feigenbaum, E. A., & Wilkins, D. E. (1983). What are expert systems? In F. Hayes-Roth, D. A. Waterman, & D. B. Lenat (Eds.), *Building expert systems.* Reading, MA: Addison-Wesley.

Brehmer, B. (1980). In one word: Not from experience. *Acta Psychologica, 45,* 223–241.

Brett, A. S. (1981). Hidden ethical issues in decision analysis. *New England Journal of Medicine, 305,* 1150–1152.

Brien, M. (1979). *Consumer involvement in health care evalution and decision making.* Unpublished doctoral dissertation, Kansas State University, Kansas.

Brien, M., Haverfield, N., & Shanteau, J. (1983). How Lamaze-prepared expectant parents select obstetricians. *Research in Nursing and Health, 6,* 143–150.

Brien, M., & Shanteau, J. (1982). *Patient involvement in health-care evaluation and decision making.* Paper presented at the Association for Computer Research Health Care Conference, Salt Lake City.

Broadbent, D. E. (1971). *Decision and stress.* London: Academic Press.

Brown, R. V., Kahr, A. S., & Peterson, C. (1974). *Decision analysis for the manager.* New York: Holt, Rinehart & Winston.

Brunner, J. (1975). *The shock wave rider.* New York: Ballantine Books.

Brunswick, E. (1952). The conceptual framework of psychology. In *International Encyclopedia of Unified Science. (Vol. 1, No. 10).* Chicago: University of Chicago Press.

Brunswick, E. (1956). *Perception and the representative design of experiments.* Berkeley: University of California Press.

Bryant, G. D., & Norman, G. R. (1980). Expressions of probability: Words and numbers. *New England Journal of Medicine, 302,* 411.

Bunker, J. P., Barnes, B. A., & Mosteller, F. (1977). *Costs risks and benefits of surgery.* New York: Oxford University Press.

Bursztajn, H., Feinbloom, R. I., Hamm, R. M., & Brodsky, A. (1981). *Medical choices, medical chances.* New York: Delacorte Press/Seymour Lawrence.

Bursztajn, H., & Hamm, R. M. (1979). Medical maxims: two views of science. *Yale Journal of Biology and Medicine, 52,* 483–486.

Bursztajn, H., & Hamm, R. M. (1982). The clinical utility of utility assessment. *Medical Decision Making, 2,* 161–165.

Bushyhead, J. B., & Christensen-Szalanski, J. J. J. (1981). Feedback and the illusion of validity in a medical clinic. *Medical Decision Making, 1,* 115–123.

Calnan, M. (1984). Clinical uncertainty: Is it a problem in the doctor–patient relationship? *Sociology of Health and Illness, 6,* 74–85.

Card, V. I., & Mooney, G. H. (1977). What is the monetary value of a human life? *British Medical Journal, 4,* 1622–1625.

Carmody, D. P. (1984). Lung tumour identification: Decision-making and comparison scanning. In A. G. Gale & F. Johnson (Eds.), *Theoretical and applied aspects of eye movement research.* B. V. North-Holland: Elsevier Science Publishers.

Carmody, D. P., Nodine, C. F., & Kundel, H. L. (1980a). An analysis of perceptual and cognitive factors in radiographic interpretation. *Perception, 9,* 339–344.

Carmody, D. P., Nodine, C. F., & Kundel, H. L. (1980b). Global and segmented search for lung nodules of different edge gradients. *Investigative Radiology, 15,* 224–233.

Carmody, D. P., Nodine, C. F., & Kundel, H. L. (1981). Finding lung nodules with and without comparative scanning. *Perception and Psychophysics, 29,* 594–598.

Carr, J. E., & Whittenbaugh, J. A. (1968). Volunteer and nonvolunteer characteristics in an outpatient population. *Journal of Abnormal Psychology, 73,* 16–17.

Cebul, R. D., Beck, L. H., Carroll, J. G., Eisenberg, J. M., Schwartz, J. S., Strasser, A. M., & Williams, S. V. A. (1984). A course in clinical decision making adaptable to diverse audiences. *Medical Decision Making, 4,* 285–296.

Chapman, L. J., & Chapman, J. P. (1969). Illusory correlation as an obstacle to the use of valid diagnostic signs. *Journal of Abnormal Psychology, 74,* 271–280.

Chase, W. G., & Chi, M. T. H. (1981). Cognitive skill: implications for spatial skill in large-scale environments. In J. H. Harvey (Ed.), *Cognition, social behavior and the environment.* Hillsdale NJ: Erlbaum.

Chase, W. G. & Simon, H. A. (1973a). The mind's eye in chess. In W. G. Chase (Ed.), *Visual information processing.* New York: Academic Press.

Chase, W. G., & Simon, H. A. (1973b). Perception in chess. *Cognitive Psychology, 4,* 55–81.

Chi, M. T. H., Feltovich, P. J., & Glaser, R. (1981). Categorization and representation of physics problems by experts and novices. *Cognitive Science, 5,* 121–152.

Chi, M. T. H., Glaser, R., & Rees, E. (1982). Expertise in problem solving. In R. Sternberg (Ed.), *Advances in the psychology of human intelligence* (Vol. 1). Hillsdale, NJ: Erlbaum.

Chikos, P. M., Figley, M. M., & Fisher, L. (1977). Visual assessment of total heart volume and specific chamber size from standard chest radiographs. *American Journal of Roentgenology, 128,* 375–380.

Christensen, E. F., Murry, R. C., Holland, K., Reynolds, J., Landay, M. J., & Moore, J. G. (1981). Effect of search time on perception. *Radiology, 138,* 361–365.

Christensen-Szalanski, J. J. J. (1984). Discount functions and the measurement of patient values: Women's decisions during childbirth. *Medical Decision Making, 4,* 41–48.

Christensen-Szalanski, J. J. J. (1985, August). *Toward an understanding of human judgment: Medical pills for psychological ills.* Paper presented at the 10th International Research Conference on Subjective Probability, Utility and Decision Making, Helsinki, Finland.

Christensen-Szalanski, J. J. J., Beck, D. E., Christensen-Szalanski, C. M., &

Koepsell, T. D. (1983). The effect of journal coverage on physicians' perception of risk. *Journal of Applied Psychology, 68,* 278–284.

Christensen-Szalanski, J. J. J., & Bushyhead, J. B. (1979). *Decision analysis as a descriptive model of physician decision-making* (Technical Report Vol-145). Washington DC: University of Washington, Department of Health Service Research.

Christensen-Szalanski, J. J. J., & Bushyhead, J. B. (1981). Physicians' use of probabilistic information in a real clinical setting. *Journal of Experimental Psychology, 7,* 928–935.

Christensen-Szalanski, J. J. J., & Bushyhead, J. B. (1983). Physician's misunderstanding of normal findings. *Medical Decision Making, 3,* 169–175.

Christensen-Szalanski, J. J. J., Diehr, P. H., Bushyhead, J. B., & Wood, R. W. (1982). Two studies of good clinical judgment. *Medical Decision Making, 2,* 275–284.

Christensen-Szalanski, J. J. J., Diehr, P. H., Wood, R. W., & Tompkins, R. K. (1982). Phased trial of a proven algorithm at a new primary care clinic. *American Journal of Public Health, 72,* 16–21.

Christensen-Szalanski, J. J. J., & Northcraft, G. B. (1985). Patient compliance behavior: The effects of time on patients' values of treatment regimes. *Social Science and Medicine (in press).*

Churchill, D. N., Lemon, B. C., & Torrance, G. W. (1984). A cost-effectiveness analysis of continuous ambulatory peritoneal dialysis and hospital renodialysis. *Medical Decision Making, 4,* 489–500.

Clancey, W. J., & Shortliffe, E. H. (1984a). Introduction: Medical artificial intelligence programs. In W. J. Clancey & E. H. Shortliffe (Eds.), *Readings in medical artificial intelligence: The first decade.* Boston, MA: Addison-Wesley.

Clancey, W. J., & Shortliffe, E. H. (Eds.). (1984b). *Readings in medical artificial intelligence: The first decade.* Boston, MA: Addison-Wesley.

Clancey, W. J., Shortliffe, E. H., & Buchanan, B. G. (1979). Intelligent computer-aided instruction for medical diagnosis. *Computer Applications in Medical Care, 3,* 175–183.

Cohen, J., & Hansel, C. E. M. (1956). *Risk and gambling: A study of subjective probability.* New York: Philosophical Library.

Cohen, L. J. (1979). On the psychology of prediction: Whose is the fallacy? *Cognition, 7,* 385–407.

Cohen, L. J. (1981). Can human irrationality be experimentally demonstrated? *The Behavioral and Brain Sciences, 4,* 317–370.

Cohen, S. J. (1979). *New directions in patient compliance.* Lexington, MA: Lexington Books.

Combs, B., & Slovic, P. (1979). Causes of death: Biased newspaper coverage and biased judgments. *Journalism Quarterly, 56,* 837–843.

Coombs, C. H. (1975). Portfolio theory and the measurement of risk. In M. F. Kaplan & S. Schwartz (Eds.), *Human judgment and decision processes in applied settings.* New York: Academic Press.

Coombs, C. H., & Huang, L. C. (1974). *Tests of the betweenness property of EU* (Technical Report Number 74-13). Ann Arbor: University of Michigan, Mathematical Psychology Program.

Cooper, T. (1983). The status of medical care: Where we are and where we are going. In J. R. Gay & B. J. Sax Jacobs (Eds.), *The technology explosion in medical science: Implications for the health care industry and the public (1981–2001)*. New York: SP Medical and Scientific Books.

Coppleson, L. W., Factor, R. M., Strum, S. B., Graff, P. W., & Rapaport, H. L. (1970). Observer disagreement in the classification and histology of Hodgkin's disease. *Journal of the National Cancer Institute, 45*, 731–740.

Crome, P., Akehurst, M., & Keet, J. (1980). Drug compliance in elderly hospital in-patients: Trial of the Dosett box. *Practitioner, 224*, 782–785.

Da Costa, J. M. (1864). *Medical diagnosis with special reference to practical medicine*. Philadelphia: Lippincott.

Davis, M. S. (1966). Variations in patients' compliance with doctors' orders: Analysis of congruence between survey responses and results of empirical investigations. *Journal of Medical Education, 41*, 1037–1048.

Davis, R. (1982). Consultation, knowledge acquisition, and instruction: A case study. In P. Szolovits (Ed.), *Artificial intelligence in medicine*. Boulder, CO: Westview.

Dawes, R. M. (1976). Shallow psychology. In J. S. Carroll & J. W. Payne (Eds.), *Cognition and social behavior*. Hillsdale, NJ: Erlbaum.

Dawes, R. M. (1977). Case-by-case versus rule-generated procedures for the allocation of scarce resources. In M. F. Kaplan & S. Schwartz (Eds.), *Human judgment and decision processes in applied settings*. New York: Academic Press.

Dawes, R. M. (1979). The robust beauty of improper linear models in decision making. *American Psychologist, 34*, 571–582.

Dawes, R. M., & Corrigan, B. (1974). Linear models in decision making. *Psychological Bulletin, 81*, 95–106.

De Dombal, F. T. (1979). Computers and the surgeon: A matter of decision. *Surgery Annual, 11*, 33–57.

De Dombal, F. T. (1984a). Computer based assistance for medical decision making. *Gastroenterology and Clinical Biology, 8*, 135–137.

De Dombal, F. T. (1984b). Information science, computers and medical decisions. *Acta Endoscopica, 14*(3), 201–206.

De Dombal, F. T., & Gremy, F. (Eds.). (1976). *Decision making and medical care: Can information science help?* Amsterdam: North-Holland.

de Groot, A. D. (1965). *Thought and choice in chess*. The Hague: Mouton.

de Groot, A. (1966). Perception and memory versus thought: Some old ideas and recent findings. In B. Kleinmuntz (Ed.), *Problem solving*. New York: Wiley.

De Smet, A. A., Fryback, D. G., & Thornbury, J. R. (1979). A second look at the utility of radiographic skull examination from trauma. *American Journal of Radiology, 132*, 95–99.

Deane, D. H., Hammond, K. R., & Summers, D. A. (1972). Acquisition and application of knowledge in complex inference tasks. *Journal of Experimental Psychology, 92*, 20–26.

Detmer, D. E., Fryback, D. G., & Gassner, K. (1978). Heuristics and biases in medical decision-making. *Journal of Medical Education, 53*, 682–683.

Diamond, G. A., & Forrester, J. S. (1983). Clinical trials and statistical verdicts: Probable grounds for appeal. *Annals of Internal Medicine, 98*, 385–394.

Diehr, P., Wood, R. W., Barr, V., Wolcott, B., Slay, L., & Tompkins, R. K. (1981). Acute headaches: Presenting symptoms and diagnostic rules to identify patients with tension and migraine headache. *Journal of Chronic Diseases, 34*, 147–158.

Dixon, R., & Lazlo, J. (1974). Utilization of clinical chemistry services by medical house staff. *Archives of Internal Medicine, 134,* 1064–1067.

Doherty, W. J., Schrott, H. G., Metcalf, L., & Iasiello-Vailas, L. (1983). Effect of spouse support and health beliefs on medication adherence. *The Journal of Family Practice, 17,* 837–841.

Doubilet, P. (1983). A mathematical approach to interpretation and selection of diagnostic tests. *Medical Decision Making, 3,* 177–195.

Dowie, J. (1984). *Professional judgment—a clinical odyssey* (A series of eleven films in progress). Milton Keynes, England: Open University.

Dowie, J. (1985). *The catch 22 of utility measurement* (unpublished). Milton Keynes, England: Open University.

Dreyfus, H., & Dreyfus, S. (1984). Mindless machines. *The Sciences* (Nov/Dec), 18–22.

Drummond, M. F. (1980). *Studies in economic appraisal in health care.* New York: Oxford University Press.

Duda, R. O., & Shortliffe, E. H. (1983). Expert systems research. *Science, 220,* 261–268.

Duff, R. S., & Hollingshead, A. B. (1968). *Sickness and society.* New York: Harper and Row.

Dunbar, J. M., Marshall, G. D., & Hovell, M. F. (1979). Behavioral strategies for improving compliance. In R. B. Haynes, D. W. Taylor, & D. L. Sackett (Eds.). *Compliance in health care.* Baltimore: Johns Hopkins University Press.

Durbridge, T. E., Edwards, F., Edwards, R. G., & Atkinson, M. (1976). Evaluation of benefits of screening tests done immediately on admission to hospital. *Clinical Chemistry, 22,* 968–971.

Ebbeson, E. B., & Konecni, V. J. (1980). On the external validity of decision making research: What do we know about decision in the real world? In T. S. Wallsten (Ed.), *Cognitive processes in choice and decision behavior.* Hillsdale, NJ: Erlbaum.

Eddy, D. M. (1980). *Screening for cancer: Theory, analysis and design.* Englewood Cliffs, NJ: Prentice Hall.

Eddy, D. M. (1982). Probabilistic reasoning in clinical medicine: Problems and opportunities. In D. Kahneman, P. Slovic, & A. Tversky (Eds.), *Judgement under uncertainty: Heuristics and biases.* Cambridge, England: Cambridge University Press.

Eddy, D. M. (1983). A mathematical model for timing repeated medical tests. *Medical Decision Making, 3,* 45–62.

Edwards, W. (1954). The theory of decision making. *Psychological Bulletin, 51,* 380–417.

Edwards, W. (1955). The prediction of decisions among bets. *Journal of Experimental Psychology, 50,* 201–214.

Edwards, W. (1983). Human cognitive capabilities, representativeness, and ground rules for research. In P. Humphreys, O. Svenson, & A. Vari (Eds.), *Analysing and aiding decision processes* (pp. 507–513). Amsterdam: North-Holland.

Edwards, W., Kiss, Y., Majone, G., & Toda, M. (1984). A panel discussion on 'What constitutes a good decision?' *Acta Psychologica, 56,* 5–28.

Edwards, W., Lindman, H., & Phillips, L. (1965). Emerging technologies for making decisions. In T. M. Newcomb (Ed.), *New directions in psychology* (Vol. 2). New York: Holt, Rinehart & Winston.

Einhorn, H. J. (1980). Learning from experience and suboptimal rules in decision making. In T. S. Wallsten (Ed.), *Cognitive processes in choice and decision behavior*. Hillsdale, NJ: Erlbaum.

Einhorn, H. J., & Hogarth, R. M. (1978). Confidence in judgement: Persistence of the illusion of validity. *Psychological Review, 85,* 395–416.

Einhorn, H. J., & Hogarth, R. M. (1981a). Behavioral decision theory: Processes of judgement and choice. *Annual Review of Psychology, 32,* 53–88.

Einhorn, H. J., & Hogarth, R. M. (1981b). Rationality and the sanctity of competence. *The Behavioral and Brain Sciences, 4,* 334–335.

Einhorn, H. J., & Hogarth, R. M. (1982). Prediction, diagnosis and causal thinking in forecasting. *Journal of Forecasting, 1,* 1–14.

Einhorn, H. J., & Hogarth, R. M. (1983). *A theory of diagnostic inference: Studying causality* (Technical Report Number 4). Chicago: University of Chicago Business School, Centre for Decision Research.

Eiseman, B., & Wotkyns, R. S. (Eds.). (1978). *Surgical Decision Making*. Philadelphia: Saunders.

Eisenberg, J. (1979). Sociologic influences on decision making by clinicians. *Annals of Internal Medicine, 90,* 957–964.

Eisenberg, J. M., & Nicklin, D. (1981). Uses of diagnostic services by physicians in community practice. *Medical Care, 19,* 297–309.

Eisenberg, J. M., & Williams, S. V. (1981). Cost containment and changing physician's practice behavior: Can the fox learn to guard the chicken coop? *Journal of the American Medical Association, 246,* 2195–2201.

Elinson, J., & Trussell, R. E. (1957). Some factors relating to degree of correspondence for diagnostic information obtained by household interviews and clinical examinations. *American Journal of Public Health, 47,* 311–321.

Elliot, D. L., Watts, W. J., & Reuler, J. B. (1983). Management of suspected temporal arteritis: A decision analysis. *Medical Decision Making, 3,* 63–68.

Elstein, A. S. (1976). Clinical judgment: Psychological research and medical practice. *Science, 194,* 696–700.

Elstein, A. S. (1981). Educational programs in medical decision making. *Medical Decision Making, 1,* 70–73.

Elstein, A. S. (1982). Decision making as educational subject matter. *Medical Decision Making, 2,* 1–5.

Elstein, A. S. (1983). Analytic methods and medical education. *Medical Decision Making, 3,* 279–284.

Elstein, A. S. (1984). *Symposium on teaching applications* (audio tape). Paper presented at the Judgment and Decision Making Meeting, San Antonio, Texas.

Elstein, A. S., & Bordage, G. (1979). Psychology of clinical reasoning. In G. Stone, F. Cohen, & N. Adler (Eds.), *Health Psychology: A Handbook*. San Francisco: Jossey-Bass.

Elstein, A. S., Holmes, M. M., Ravitch, M. M., Rovner, D. R., Holtzman, G. B., & Rothert, M. L. (1983). Medical decisions in perception: Applied research in cognitive psychology. *Perspectives in Biology and Medicine, 26,* 486–501.

Elstein, A. S., Rovner, D. R., Holzman, G. B., Ratvich, M. M., Rothert, M. L., & Holmes, M. M. (1982). Psychological approaches to medical decision making. *American Behavioral Scientist, 25,* 557–584.

Elstein, A. S., Rovner, D. R., & Rothert, M. L. (1982). A preclinical course in medical decision making. *Medical Decision Making, 2,* 207–216.

Elstein, A. S., Shulman, L. S., & Sprafka, S. A. (1978). *Medical problem solving: An analysis of clinical reasoning.* Cambridge, MA: Harvard University Press.

Epstein, L. H., & Cluss, P. A. (1982). A behavioral medicine perspective on adherence to long-term medical regimes. *Journal of Consulting and Clinical Psychology, 50,* 950–971.

Eraker, S. A., Kirscht, J. P., & Becker, M. (1984). Understanding and improving patient compliance. *Annals of Internal Medicine, 100,* 258–268.

Eraker, S. A., & Politser, P. (1982). How decisions are reached: Physician and patient. *Annals of Internal Medicine, 97,* 262–268.

Eraker, S. A., & Sox, H. C. (1981). Assessment of patients' preferences for therapeutic outcomes. *Medical Decision Making, 1,* 29–39.

Ericsson, K. A., & Simon, H. A. (1980). Verbal reports as data. *Psychological Review, 87,* 215–251.

Ericsson, K. A., & Simon, H. A. (1984). *Protocol analysis: Verbal reports as data.* Cambridge, MA: Massachusetts Institute of Technology.

Estes, W. K. (1980). Comments on directions and limitations of current efforts toward theories of decision making. In T. S. Wallsten (Ed.), *Cognitive processes in choice and decision behavior.* Hillsdale, NJ: Erlbaum.

Evans, L., & Spelman, M. (1983). The problem of noncompliance with drug therapy. *Drugs, 25,* 63–76.

Feltovich, P. J., Johnson, P. E., Moller, J. H., & Swanson, D. B. (1984). LCS: The role and development of medical knowledge in diagnostic expertise. In W. J. Clancey & E. H. Shortliffe (Eds.), *Readings in medical artificial intelligence: The first decade.* Reading, MA: Addison-Wesley.

Fidler, E. J. (1983). The reliability and validity of concurrent, retrospective, and interpretive verbal reports: An experimental study. In P. Humphreys, O. Svenson, & A. Vari (Eds.), *Analysing and aiding decision processes.* Amsterdam: North-Holland.

Fineberg, H. V. (1979). Clinical chemistries: The high cost of low cost diagnostic tests. In S. H. Altman & R. Blendon (Eds.), *Medical technology: The culprit behind health care costs* (US Department of Health, Education, and Welfare Publication Number PHS 79-3216). Washington DC: US Government Printing Office.

Fineberg, H. V. (1984). Doctors and decision analysis. *Medical Decision Making, 4,* 267–270.

Finnerty, F., Shaw, L., & Himmelsback, C. (1973). Hypertension in the inner city II: Detection and follow up. *Circulation, 47,* 76–78.

Firestone, P. (1982). Factors associated with children's adherence to stimulant medication. *American Journal of Orthopsychiatry, 52,* 447–457.

Fisch, H.-U., Hammond, K. R., Joyce, C. R. B., & O'Reilly, M. (1981). An experimental study of the clinical judgement of general physicians in evaluating and prescribing for depression. *British Journal of Psychiatry, 138,* 100–109.

Fischer, R. G. (1980). Compliance oriented prescribing: Simplifying drug regimens. *The Journal of Family Practice, 10,* 427–435.

Fischhoff, B. (1975). Hindsight ≠ foresight: The effect of outcome knowledge on judgment under uncertainty. *Journal of Experimental Psychology: Human Perception and Performance, 1,* 288–299.

Fischhoff, B. (1977). Cost benefit analysis and the art of motorcycle maintenance. *Policy Sciences, 8,* 177–202.

Fischhoff, B. (1979). Informed consent in societal risk–benefit decisions. *Technological Forecasting and Social Change, 12,* 347–357.

Fischhoff, B. (1980). *Informing people about the risks of oral contraception* (Technical Report Number 80-3). Eugene, OR: Decision Research.

Fischhoff, B. (1982a). Debiasing. In D. Kahneman, P. Slovic, & A Tversky (Eds.), *Judgment under uncertainty: Heuristics and biases.* Cambridge, England: Cambridge University Press.

Fischhoff, B. (1982b). For those condemned to study the past: Heuristics and biases in hindsight. In D. Kahneman, P. Slovic, & A. Tversky (Eds.), *Judgment under uncertainty: Heuristics and biases.* Cambridge, England: Cambridge University Press.

Fischhoff, B. (1983). Reconstructive criticism. In P. Humphreys, O. Svenson, & A. Vari (Eds.), *Analysing and aiding decision processes.* Amsterdam: North-Holland.

Fischhoff, B., & Bar-Hillel, M. (1984a). Diagnosticity and the base-rate effect. *Memory and Cognition, 12,* 402–410.

Fischhoff, B., & Bar-Hillel, M. (1984b). Focussing techniques: A shortcut to improving probability judgments. *Organizational Behavior and Human Performance, 34,* 175–194.

Fischhoff, B., & Beyth, R. (1975). I knew it would happen: Remembered probabilities of once-future things. *Organizational Behavior and Human Performance, 13,* 1–16.

Fischhoff, B., & Beyth-Marom, R. (1982). *Hypothesis testing from a Bayesian perspective* (Technical Report). Eugene, OR: Decision Research.

Fischhoff, B., Goitein, B., & Shapira, Z. (1979). The experienced utility of expected utility approaches. In N. Feather (Ed.) *Expectancy, incentive and action.* Hillsdale, NJ: Erlbaum.

Fischhoff, B., Lichtenstein, S., Slovic, P., Derby, S. L., & Keeney, R. L. (1981). *Acceptable risk.* Cambridge, England: Cambridge University Press.

Fischhoff, B., & MacGregor, D. (1980). *Judged lethality* (Technical Report Number 80-4). Eugene, OR: Decision Research.

Fischhoff, B., Slovic, P., & Lichtenstein, S. (1977). Knowing with certainty: The appropriateness of extreme confidence. *Journal of Experimental Psychology: Human Perception and Performance, 3,* 522–564.

Fischhoff, B., Slovic, P., & Lichtenstein, S. (1978). Fault trees: Sensitivity of estimated failure probabilities to problem representation. *Journal of Experimental Psychology: Human Perception and Performance, 4,* 330–344.

Fischhoff, B., Slovic, P., & Lichtenstein, S. (1980). Knowing what you want: Measuring labile values. In T. S. Wallsten (Ed.), *Cognitive processes in choice and decision behavior.* Hillsdale, NJ: Erlbaum.

Fischhoff, B., Slovic, P., Lichtenstein, S., Read, S., & Combs, B. (1978). How safe is safe enough? A psychometric study of attitudes toward technological risks and benefits. *Policy Sciences, 9,* 127–152.

Fischhoff, B., Watson, S. R., & Hope, C. (1984). Defining risk. *Policy Sciences, 17,* 123–139.

Forrest, J. V., & Freidman, P. J. (1981). Radiologic errors in patients with lung cancer. *The Western Journal of Medicine, 134,* 485–490.

Fox, J. (1980). Making decisions under the influence of memory. *Psychological Review, 87,* 190–211.

Fox, J. (1984). Formal and knowledge-based methods in decision technology. *Acta Psychologica, 56,* 303–331.

Fox, J., Avey, P., & Myers, C. (1983, December). *Decision technology and man–machine interaction: The PROPS package.* Paper presented at the Proceedings of The Expert Systems Conference, Churchill College, Cambridge, England.

Fox, J., Barber, D. C., & Bardhan, K. D. (1980). Alternatives to Bayes? A quantitative comparison with rule-based diagnostic inference. *Methods of Information in Medicine, 19,* 210–215.

Fox, J., Myers, C. D., Greaves, M. F., & Pegram, S. (1985). Knowledge acquisition for expert systems: Experience in leukemia diagnosis. *Methods of Information in Medicine, 24,* 65–72.

Fox, J., & Rector, A. (1982). Expert systems for primary medical care? *Automedica, 4,* 123–130.

Friedlander, M. L., & Phillips, S. D. (1984). Preventing anchoring errors in clinical judgment. *Journal of Consulting and Clinical Psychology, 52,* 366–371.

Friedlander, M. L., & Stockman, S. J. (1983). Anchoring and publicity effects in clinical judgment. *Journal of Clinical Psychology, 39,* 637–643.

Fryback, D. G. (1974a). *Bayes theorem and conditional nonindependence of data in a medical diagnostic task* (Technical Report Number 74-7). Ann Arbor: University of Michigan, Mathematical Psychology Program.

Fryback, D. G. (1974b). *Use of radiologists' subjective probability estimates in a medical decision making problem.* Unpublished doctoral dissertation (psychology), University of Michigan.

Fryback, D. G., & Thornbury, J. R. (1978). Informal use of decision theory to improve radiological patient management. *Radiology, 129,* 385–388.

Gaeth, G. J., & Shanteau, J. (1984). Reducing the influence of irrelevant information on experienced decision makers. *Organizational Behavior and Human Performance, 33,* 263–282.

Gale, A. G., Johnson, F., & Worthington, B. S. (1979). Psychology and radiology. In D. J. Osborne, M. M. Gruneberg, & J. R. Eiser (Eds.), *Research in Psychology and Medicine* (Vol. 2). London: Academic Press.

Gale, A. G., & Worthington, B. S. (1983). The utility of scanning strategies in radiology. In R. Groner, C. Manz, D. F. Fisher, & R. A. Monty (Eds.) *Eye movements and psychological functions: International views.* Hillsdale, NJ. LEA.

Galen, R. S., & Gambino, S. R. (1975). *Beyond normality: The predictive value and efficiency of medical diagnosis.* New York: Wiley.

Gardiner, P. C., & Edwards, W. (1975). Public values: Multiattribute-utility measurement for social decision making. In M. F. Kaplan & S. Schwartz (Eds.), *Human judgment and decision processes in applied settings.* New York: Academic Press.

Garland, L. H. (1959). Studies on the accuracy of diagnostic procedures. *American Journal of Roentgenology, 82,* 25–38.

Gay, J. R., & Sax Jacobs, B. J. (1983). (Eds.). *The technology explosion in medical science: Implications for the health care industry and the public (1981–2001).* New York: SP Medical and Scientific Books.

German, P. S., Klein, L. E., McPhee, S. J., & Smith, C. R. (1982). Knowledge of and compliance with drug regimes in the elderly. *Journal of the American Geriatrics Society, 30,* 568–569.

Glogo, P. H. (1973). Noncompliance—a dilemma. *Sight Saving Review, Spring,* 29–34.

Goin, J. E., Preston, D. F., Gallagher, J. H., & Wegst, A. V. (1983). Comparison of five digital scintigraphic display modes: An ROC curve analysis of detection performance. *Medical Decision Making, 3,* 215–228.

Goldberg, L. R. (1968). Simple models or simple processes? Some research on clinical judgments. *American Psychologist, 23,* 483–496.

Goldberg, L. R. (1970). Man versus model of man: a rationale, plus some evidence, for a method of improving on clinical inferences. *Psychological Bulletin, 73,* 422–432.

Goodenough, D. J. (1975). The use of ROC curves in testing the proficiency of individuals in classifying pneumoconiosis. *Radiology, 114,* 472–473.

Goodenough, D. J., Rossman, K., Lusted, L. B. (1972). Radiographic applications of signal detection theory. *Radiology, 105,* 199–200.

Goran, M. J., Williamson, J. W., & Gonella, J. S. (1973). The validity of PMPs. *Journal of Medical Education, 48,* 171–177.

Gordis, L. (1979). Conceptual and methodological problems in measuring patient compliance. In R. B. Haynes, D. W. Taylor, & D. L. Sackett (Eds.), *Compliance in health care.* Baltimore: Johns Hopkins University Press.

Gorry, G., & Barnett, G. (1968). Experience with a model of sequential diagnosis. *Computers and Biomedical Research, 1,* 490–507.

Gorry, G. A., Pauker, S. G., & Schwartz, W. B. (1978). The diagnostic importance of the normal finding. *New England Journal of Medicine, 298,* 486–489.

Gough, H. G. (1962). Clinical versus statistical prediction in psychology. In L. Postman (Ed.), *Psychology in the making: Histories of selected research problems.* New York: Knopf.

Gray, J. E., Taylor, K. W., & Hobbs, B. B. (1978). Detection accuracy in chest radiography. *American Journal of Roentgenology, 131,* 247–253.

Gray, R., Begg, C. B., & Greenes, R. A. (1984). Construction of receiver operating characteristic curves when disease verification is subject to selection bias. *Medical Decision Making, 4,* 151–164.

Greegor, D. J. (1969). Detection of colorectal cancers using Guaiac slides. *Cancer, 22,* 360–364.

Green, C. H. (1979, July). *Someone out there is trying to kill me: Acceptable risk as a problem in definition.* Paper presented at the International Conference on Environmental Psychology, Surrey, England.

Greenfield, S., Cretin, S., Worthman, L. G., & Dorey, F. (1982). The use of an ROC curve to express quality of care results. *Medical Decision Making, 2,* 23–32.

Greenfield, S., Komaroff, A. L., & Anderson, H. (1976). A headache protocol for nurses: Effectiveness and efficiency. *Archives of Internal Medicine, 136,* 1111–1116.

Gregg, E. C., Rao, P. S., & Friedell, H. L. (1976). An analysis of the value of additional diagnostic procedures. *Investigative Radiology, 11,* 249–257.

Groves, J. E. (1978). Taking care of the hateful patient. *New England Journal of Medicine, 298,* 883–887.

Gryfe, C. I., & Gryfe, B. M. (1984). Drug therapy of the aged: The problem of compliance and the roles of physicians and pharmacists. *Journal of the American Geriatrics Society, 32,* 301–307.

Guiss, L. W., & Kuenstler, P. (1960). A retrospective view of survey photofluoro-grams of persons with lung cancer. *Cancer, 13,* 91–95.

Habbema, J. D. F., & Hilden, J. (1981). The measurement of performance in probabilistic diagnosis IV. Utility considerations in therapeutics and prognos-tics. *Methods of Information in Medicine, 20,* 80–96.

Hall, R. (1979). Helping patients take their medicine. *Australian Family Physician, 8,* 1081–1085.

Hammond, K. R. (1971). Computer graphics as an aid to learning. *Science, 172,* 903–908.

Hammond, K. R. (1980). *The integration of research in judgment and decision theory.* Boulder, University of Colorado, Center for Research in Judgment and Pol-icy.

Hammond, K. R., & Boyle, P. J. R. (1971). Quasi-rationality, quarrels and new conceptions of feedback. *Bulletin of the British Psychological Society, 24,* 103–113.

Hammond, K. R., McClelland, G. H., & Mumpower, J. (1980). *Human Judgement and Decision Making.* New York: Praeger Publishers.

Hammond, K. R., Rohrbaugh, J., Mumpower, J., & Adelman, L. (1977). Social judgement theory: Applications in policy formation. In M. F. Kaplan & S. Schwartz (Eds.), *Human judgement and decision processes in applied settings.* New York: Academic.

Hardin, G. (1968). The tragedy of the commons. *Science, 162,* 1243–1248.

Hardin, G. (1972). *Exploring new ethics for survival: The voyage of spaceship Beagle.* New York: Viking Press.

Hart, A. (1985). The role of induction in knowledge elicitation. *Expert Systems, 2,* 24–28.

Harvey, A. M., Bordley, J., III., & Barondess, J. A. (1979). *Differential diagnosis: The interpretation of clinical evidence* (3rd ed.). Philadelphia: Saunders.

Hayes, J. R. (1982). Issues in protocol analysis. In G. R. Ungson & D. N. Braun-stein (Eds.), *Decision making: An interdisciplinary inquiry.* Boston: Kent.

Hayes-Roth, F., Waterman, D. A., & Lenat, D. B. (1983). An overview of expert systems. In F. Hayes-Roth, D. A. Waterman, & D. B. Lenat (Eds.), *Building expert systems.* Boston: Addison-Wesley.

Haynes, R. B., Sackett, D. L., & Tugwell, P. (1983). Problems in the handling of clinical and research evidence by medical practitioners. *Archives of Internal Medicine, 143,* 1971–1975.

Haynes, R. B., Taylor, D. W., & Sackett, D. L. (Eds.). (1979). *Compliance in health care.* Baltimore: Johns Hopkins University Press.

Hellerstein, D. (1984). The slow costly death of Mrs. K. *Harper's, 268,* 84–89.

Herman, P. G., Gerson, D. E., Hessel, S. J., Mayer, B. S., Watnick, M., Blesser, B., & Ozonoff, D. (1975). Disagreements in chest roentgen interpretation. *Chest, 68,* 278–282.

Herman, P. G., & Hessel, S. J. (1975). Accuracy and its relationship to experi-ence in the interpretation of chest radiographs. *Investigative Radiology, 10,* 62–67.

Hertroijs, A. (1974). A study of some factors affecting the attendance of patients in a leprosy control scheme. *International Journal of Leprosy, 42,* 419–427.

Hilden, J., Habbema, J. D. F., & Bjerregaard, B. (1978). The measurement of performance in probabilistic diagnosis III. Methods based on continuous functions of the diagnostic probabilities. *Methods of Information in Medicine, 17,* 238–246.

Hillard, A., Myles-Worsley, M., Johnston, W., & Baxter, B. (1985). The development of radiologic schemata through training and experience: A preliminary communication. *Investigative Radiology, 18,* 422–425.

Hippocrates (1967). *Decorum* (J. Jones, Trans.) Cambridge, MA: Harvard University Press.

Hoey, J., Eisenberg, J. M., Spitzer, W. O., & Thomas, D. (1982). Physician sensitivity to the price of diagnostic tests. *Medical Care, 20,* 302–307.

Hoffman, P. J. (1960). The paramorphic representation of clinical judgment. *Psychological Bulletin, 47,* 116–131.

Hoffman, P. J., Earle, T. C., & Slovic, P. (1981). Multidimensional functional learning (MFL) and some new conceptualizations of feedback. *Organizational Behavior and Human Performance, 27,* 75–102.

Hoffman, P. J., Slovic, P., & Rorer, L. G. (1968). An analysis of variance model for the assessment of configural cue utilization in clinical judgment. *Psychological Bulletin, 69,* 338–349.

Hogarth, R. M. (1980). Judgment, drug monitoring and decision aids. In W. H. W. Inman (Ed.), *Monitoring for drug safety.* Lancaster, England: MTP Press.

Holland, R. R. (1975). Decision tables. Their use for the presentation of clinical algorithms. *Journal of the American Medical Association, 233,* 455–457.

Holmes, M. M., Rovner, D. R., Elstein, A. S., Holzman, G. B., Rothert, M. L., & Ravitch, M. M. (1982). Factors affecting laboratory utilization in clinical practice. *Medical Decision Making, 2,* 471–482.

Holt, R. R. (1958). Clinical and statistical prediction: A reformulation and some new data. *Journal of Abnormal and Social Psychology, 56,* 1–12.

Holt, R. R. (1978). *Methods in clinical psychology: Prediction and research* (Vol. 2). New York: Plenum.

Howard, R. A. (1978). Life and death decision analysis. *Proceedings of the Second Lawrence Symposium on Systems and Decision Sciences, 2,* 271–277.

Hubbard, J. P. (1971). Objective evaluation of clinical competence. In J. P. Hubbard (Ed.), *Measuring Medical Evaluation.* Philadelphia: Lea & Febiger.

Illich, I. (1977). *Medical nemesis: The expropriation of health.* Harmondsworth, England: Penguin.

Ingelfinger, F. (1973). Algorithms anyone? *New England Journal of Medicine, 288,* 847–848.

Inui, T., Carter, W. B., Pecoraro, R. E., Pearlman, R. A., & Dohan, J. J. (1980). Variations in patient compliance with common long-term drugs. *Medical Care, 18,* 986–993.

Irwin, F. W. (1953). Stated expectations as functions of probability and desirability of outcomes. *Journal of Personality, 21,* 329–335.

Jennett, B. (1975). Predicting outcome after head injury. *Journal of the Royal College of Physicians, London, 9,* 231–237.

Johnson, E. J., & Tversky, A. (1984). Representations of perceptions of risks. *Journal of Experimental Psychology: General, 113,* 55–70.

Johnson, P. E., Hassebrock, F., Duran, A. S., & Moller, J. H. (1982). Multimethod study of clinical judgement. *Organizational Behavior and Human Performance, 30,* 201–230.

Johnson, P. E., Moller, J. H., & Bass, G. M. (1975). Analysis of expert diagnosis of a computer simulation of congenital heart disease. *Journal of Medical Education, 50,* 466–470.

Johnson, S. M. & White, G. (1971). Self-observation as an agent of behavioral change. *Behavior Therapy, 2,* 488–497.

Jonsen, A. R. (1979). Ethical issues in compliance. In R. B. Haynes, D. W. Taylor, & D. L. Scakett (Eds.). *Compliance in health care.* Baltimore: Johns Hopkins University Press.

Jungerman, H. (1983). Two camps of rationality. In R. W. Scholz (Ed.), *Decision making under uncertainty.* Amsterdam: Elsevier.

Kahneman, D., Slovic, P., & Tversky, A. (Eds.). (1982). *Judgment under uncertainty: Heuristics and biases.* Cambridge, England: Cambridge University Press.

Kahneman, D., & Tversky, A. (1972). Subjective probability: A judgment of representativeness. *Cognitive Psychology, 3,* 430–454.

Kahneman, D., & Tversky, A. (1973). On the psychology of prediction. *Psychological Review, 80,* 237–251.

Kahneman, D., & Tversky, A. (1979). Prospect theory. *American Economic Review, 47,* 263–291.

Kahneman, D., & Tversky, A. (1982a). Intuitive prediction: Biases and corrective procedures. In D. Kahneman, P. Slovic, & A. Tversky (Eds.), *Judgment under uncertainty: Heuristics and biases.* Cambridge, England: Cambridge University Press.

Kahneman, D., & Tversky, A. (1982b). On the study of statistical intuitions. *Cognition, 11,* 123–141.

Kahneman, D., & Tversky, A. (1982c). Variants of uncertainty. *Cognition, 11,* 143–157.

Kaplan, R. M. (1982). Human preference measurement for health decisions and the evaluation of long-term care. In R. L. Kane & R. A. Kane (Eds.), *Values and long-term care.* Lexington, MA: Lexington Books.

Kaplan, R. M., & Bush, J. W. (1982). Health-related quality of life measurement for evaluation research and policy analysis. *Health Psychology, 1*(1), 61–80.

Kaplan, R. M., & Ernst, J. A. (1983). Do category rating scales produce biased preference weights for a health index? *Medical Care, 21,* 193–207.

Kaplan, S., & Garrick, B. J. (1981). The quantitative definition of risk. *Risk Analysis, 1,* 11–27.

Kassirer, J. P. (1983). Adding insult to injury: Usurping patients' perogatives. *New England Journal of Medicine, 308,* 898–901.

Kassirer, J. P., & Gorry, G. A. (1978). Clinical problem solving: A behavioral analysis. *Annals of Internal Medicine, 89,* 245–255.

Katz, J. (1984). *The silent world of doctor and patient.* New York: Free Press.

Kaufman, C. L. (1983). Informed consent and patient decision making: Two decades of research. *Social Science and Medicine, 17,* 1617–1664.

Keeney, R., & Raiffa, H. (1976). *Decisions with multiple objectives: Preference and value trade offs.* New York: Wiley.

Keighly, M., Hoare, A., & Horrocks, J. (1976). A symptomatic discriminant to identify recurrent ulcers in patients with dyspepsia after gastric surgery. *Lancet, 2,* 278–279.

Kellaway, G. S. M. (1979). The effect of counselling on compliance-failure in patient drug therapy. *New Zealand Medical Journal, 89,* 161–165.

Kellaway, G. S. M. (1983). Compliance failure and counselling in paediatric drug therapy. *New Zealand Medical Journal, 96,* 207–209.

Kellaway, G. S. M., & McCrae, E. (1975). Non-compliance and errors of drug administration in patients discharged from acute general medical wards. *New Zealand Medical Journal, 81,* 508–512.

Kelman, S. (1980). *Improving doctor performance.* New York: Human Sciences Press.

Kenney, R. M. (1981). Between never and always. *New England Journal of Medicine, 305,* 1098–1099.

Keown, C., Slovic, P., & Lichtenstein, S. (1984). Attitudes of physicians, pharmacists and laypersons toward seriousness and need for disclosure of prescription drug side effects. *Health Psychology, 3,* 1–11.

Kepner, C. H., & Tregoe, B. B. (1965). *The rational manager: A systematic approach to problem solving and decision making.* New York: McGraw-Hill.

Kern, L., & Doherty, M. E. (1982). 'Pseudodiagnosticity' in an idealized medical problem solving environment. *Journal of Medical Education, 57,* 100–104.

King, L. S. (1982). *Medical thinking: A historical preface.* Princeton, NJ: Princeton University Press.

Klayman, J. (1984). Learning from feedback in probabilistic environments. *Acta Psychologica, 56,* 81–92.

Klein, K. & Pauker, S. G. (1981). Recurrent deep venous thrombosis in pregnancy. *Medical Decision Making, 1,* 181–202.

Klein, N. M. (1983). Utility and decision strategies: A second look at the rational decision maker. *Organizational Behavior and Human Performance, 31,* 1–25.

Kleinmuntz, B. (1984). The scientific study of clinical judgment in psychology and medicine. *Clinical Psychology Review, 4,* 111–126.

Kleinmuntz, D. N., & Kleinmuntz, B. (1981). Systems simulation decision strategies in simulated environments. *Behavioral Science, 26,* 294–305.

Kneppreth, N. P., Gustafson, D. H., Leifer, R. P., & Johnson, E. M. (1974). *Techniques for the assessment of worth* (Technical Report Number 254). Arlington, VA: Army Research Institute.

Komaroff, A. L. (1979). The variability and inaccuracy of medical data. *Proceedings of the IEEE, 67,* 1196–1207.

Komaroff, A. L. (1982). Algorithms and the "Art" of medicine. *American Journal of Public Health, 72,* 10–12.

Komaroff, A. L., Pass, T. M., & McCui, J. D. (1978). Management strategies for urinary and vaginal infections. *Archives of Internal Medicine, 138,* 1069–1073.

Koplan, J. P., Schoenbaum, S. C., Weinstein, M. C., & Fraser, D. W. (1979). Pertussis vaccine: An analysis of benefits, risks and costs. *New England Journal of Medicine, 301,* 906–911.

Korsch, B. M., Gozzi, E. K., & Francis, V. (1968). Gaps in doctor–patient communication: Doctor–patient interaction and patient satisfaction. *Pediatrics, 42,* 855–871.

Kozielecki, J. (1981). *Psychological decision theory.* Warsaw: PWN-Polish Scientific Publishers.

Krieg, A. F., Gambino, S. R., & Galen, R. S. (1975). Why are clinical laboratory tests performed? When are they valid? *Journal of the American Medical Association, 223*, 76–78.

Krischer, J. P., & Dixon, V. L. (1982). Constancy of subjective assessments and the stability of treatment preferences in team decision making. *Medical Decison Making, 2,* 197–208.

Kuipers, B., & Kassirer, J. P. (1984). Causal reasoning in medicine: Analysis of a protocol. *Cognitive Science, 8,* 363–385.

Kundel, H. L. (1974). Visual sampling and estimates of the location of information on chest films. *Investigative Radiology, 9,* 87–93.

Kundel, H. L. (1982). Disease prevalence and radiological decision making. *Investigative Radiology, 17,* 107–108.

Kundel, H. L., & La Follette, P. S. (1972). Visual search patterns and experience with radiological images. *Radiology, 103,* 523–528.

Kundel, H. L., & Nodine, C. F. (1975). Interpreting chest radiographs without visual search. *Radiology, 116,* 527–532.

Kundel, H. L., & Nodine, C. F. (1978). Studies of eye movements and visual search in radiology. In J. W. Senders, D. F. Fisher, & R. A. Monty (Eds.), *Eye movements and higher psychological functions.* Hillsdale, NJ: Erlbaum.

Kundel, H. L., & Nodine, C. F. (1983). A visual concept shapes image perception. *Radiology, 146,* 363–368.

Kundel, H. L., Nodine, C. F., & Carmody, D. (1978). Visual scanning, pattern recognition and decision-making in pulmonary nodule detection. *Investigative Radiology, 13,* 175–181.

Kundel, H. L., Nodine, C. F., & Toto, L. (1984). Eye movements and the detection of lung tumors in chest images. In A. G. Gale & F. Johnson (Eds.), *Theoretical and applied aspects of eye movement research.* Amsterdam: North-Holland.

Kundel, H. L., Revesz, G., Ziskin, M., & Shea, F. (1972). The image and its influence on quantitative radiological data. *Investigative Radiology, 7,* 187–198.

Kundel, H. L., & Wright, D. J. (1969). The influence of prior knowledge on visual search strategies during the viewing of chest radiographs. *Radiology, 93,* 315–320.

Kunreuther, H. (1976). Limited knowledge and insurance protection. *Public Policy, 24,* 227–261.

Larkin, J., McDermott, J., Simon, D. P., & Simon, H. A. (1980). Expert and novice performance in solving physics problems. *Science, 208,* 1335–1342.

Ledley, R. S., & Lusted, L. B. (1959). Reasoning foundations of medical diagnosis. *Science, 130,* 8–21.

Le Minor, M., Alperovitch, A., & Knill-Jones, R. P., (1982). Applying decision theory to medical decision making: Concept of regret and error of diagnosis. *Methods of Information in Medicine, 21,* 3–8.

Lennane, K. J., & Lennane, R. J. (1973). Alleged psychogenic disorders in women—a possible manifestation of sexual prejudice. *New England Journal of Medicine, 288,* 288–292.

Lesgold, A. M. (1984a). Acquiring expertise. In J. R. Anderson & S. M. Kosslyn (Eds.), *Tutorials in learning and memory: Essays in honor of Gordon Bower.* San Francisco: Freeman.

Lesgold, A. M. (1984b). Human skill in a computerized society: Complex skills and their acquisition. *Behavior Research Methods, Instruments, and Computers, 16,* 79–87.

Lesgold, A. M., Feltovich, P. J., Glaser, R., & Wang, Y. (1981). *The acquisition of perceptual diagnostic skill in radiology* (Technical Report Number PDS-1). Pittsburgh: University of Pittsburgh, Learning Research and Development Center.

Lewis, B. N., & Horabin, I. (1979). *Algorithms.* Englewood Cliffs, NJ: Educational Technology Publications.

Ley, P. (1976). Towards better doctor-patient communications. In A. E. Bennett (Ed.). *Communications between patients and doctors.* Oxford: Oxford University Press.

Ley, P. (1979). The psychology of compliance. In D. Oborne, M. M. Gruneberg, & J. R. Eiser (Eds.) *Research in psychology and medicine.* London: Academic Press.

Ley, P. (1981). Professional non-compliance: A neglected problem. *British Journal of Clinical Psychology, 20,* 151–154.

Ley, P. (1982a). Giving information to patients. In J. R. Eiser (Ed.), *Social psychology and behavioral medicine.* New York: Wiley.

Ley, P. (1982b). Satisfaction, compliance and communication. *British Journal of Clinical Psychology, 21,* 241–254.

Lichtenstein, S. C., Earle, T., & Slovic, P. (1975). Cue utilization in a numerical prediction task. *Journal of Experimental Psychology: Human Perception and Performance, 104,* 77–85.

Lichtenstein, S., & Slovic, P. (1971). Reversal of preferences between bids and choices in gambling decisions. *Journal of Experimental Psychology, 89,* 46–55.

Lichtenstein, S., Slovic, P., & Zinc, D. (1969). Effect of instruction in expected value on optimality of gambling decisions. *Journal of Experimental Psychology, 79,* 236–240.

Lilienfeld, A., & Graham, S. (1958). Validity of determining circumcision status by questionnaire as related to epidemiological studies of cancer of the cervix. *Journal of the National Cancer Institute, 21,* 713–770.

Lindley, D. V. (1975). The role of utility in decision making. *Journal of the Royal College of Physicians, London, 9,* 225–230.

Lindley, D. V. (1977). Costs and utilities. In A. Aykac & C. Brunat (Eds.), *New developments in the application of Bayesian methods.* Amsterdam: North-Holland.

Llewellyn-Thomas, H. A., Sutherland, H. J., Ciampi, A., Etezadi-Amoli, J., Boyd, N. F., & Till, J. E. (1984). The assessment of values in laryngeal cancer: Reliability of measurement methods. *Journal of Chronic Diseases, 37,* 283–291.

Llewellyn-Thomas, H., Sutherland, H. J., Tibshirani, R., Ciampi, A., Till, J. E., & Boyd, N. F. (1984). Describing health studies: Methodologic issues in obtaining values for health studies. *Medical Care, 22,* 543–552.

Lopes, L. L. (1982). *Toward a procedural theory of judgment* (Technical Report Number 17). Madison: Wisconsin Human Information Processing Program.

Lusted, L. B. (1968). *Introduction to medical decision making.* Springfield, IL: Thomas.

Lusted, L. B. (1977). *A study of the efficacy of diagnostic radiologic procedures* (Final report on diagnostic efficacy). Chicago: Efficacy Study Committee of the American College of Radiology.

Lusted, L. B. (1984). ROC recollected. *Medical Decision Making, 4,* 131–135.

MacCrimmon, K. R. (1968). Descriptive and normative implications of the decision-theory postulates. In K. Borch & J. Mossin (Eds.), *Risk and uncertainty.* New York: St. Martins.

MacCrimmon, K. R. (1973). An overview of multiple objective decision making. In J. L. Cochrane & M. Zeleny (Eds.), *Multiple criteria decision making.* Columbia: University of South Carolina Press.

MacCrimmon, K. R., & Larsson, S. (1976). Utility theory: Axioms vs 'paradoxes'. In M. Allais & O. Hagen (Eds.), *Expected utility and Allais' Paradox.* Dordrecht: Reidel.

MacDonald, C. (1977). Protocol-based computer reminders, the quality of care and the perfectability of man. *New England Journal of Medicine, 295,* 1351–1354.

Mahoney, M. J. (1974). *Cognition and behavior modification.* Boston: Ballinger.

Maletsky, B. M. (1974). Behavior recording at treatment: A brief note. *Behavior Therapy, 5,* 107–111.

Manu, P., & Schwartz, S. E. (1983). Patterns of diagnostic testing in the academic setting: The influence of medical attendings' subspecialty training. *Social Sciences and Medicine, 17,* 1339–1342.

Margolis, C. Z. (1983). Uses of clinical algorithms. *Journal of the American Medical Association, 249,* 627–632.

May, K. O. (1954). Transitivity, utility and aggregation in preference patterns. *Econometrica, 22,* 1–13.

McCarthy, W. H. (1966). An assessment of the influence of cueing items in objective examinations. *Journal of Medical Education, 41,* 263–266.

McGuire, C. H., Solomon, L. M., & Bashook, P. G. (1976). *Construction and use of written simulations.* New York: Psychological Corporation.

McNeil, B. J., & Hanley, J. A. (1984). Statistical approaches to the analysis of receiver operating characteristic (ROC) curves. *Medical Decision Making, 4,* 137–150.

McNeil, B. J., Pauker, S. G., Sox, H. E., & Tversky, A. (1982). On the elicitation of preferences for alternative therapies. *New England Journal of Medicine, 306,* 1259–1262.

McNeil, B. J., Weichselbaum, R., & Pauker, S. G. (1978). Fallacy of the 5 year survival rate in lung cancer. *New England Journal of Medicine, 299,* 1397–1401.

McNeil, B. J., Weichselbaum, R., & Pauker, S. G. (1981). Speech and survival: tradeoffs between quality and quantity of life in laryngeal cancer. *New England Journal of Medicine, 305,* 982–987.

Meade, T. W., Gardner, M. J., & Cannon, P. (1968). Observer variability in recording the peripheral pulses. *British Heart Journal, 30,* 661–665.

Medin, D. L., Alton, M. W., Edelson, S. M., & Freko, D. (1982). Correlated symptoms and simulated medical classification. *Journal of Experimental Psychology: Learning, Memory and Cognition, 8,* 37–50.

Meehl, P. E. (1954). *Clinical versus statistical prediction: A theoretical analysis and a review of the evidence.* Minneapolis: University of Minnesota Press.

Merrill, P. F. (1977). Algorithmic organization in teaching and learning: Literature and research in the USA. *Improving Human Performance Quarterly, 6,* 93–112.

Metz, C. E. (1978). Basic principles of ROC analysis. *Seminars in Nuclear Medicine, 8,* 283–298.

Metz, C. E., Starr, S. J., & Lusted, L. B. (1976a). Observer performance in detecting multiple radiographic signals. *Radiology, 121,* 337–347.

Metz, C. E., Starr, S. J., & Lusted, L. B. (1976b). Quantitative evaluation of visual detection performance in medicine: ROC analysis and determination of diagnostic benefit. In G. A. Hayes (Ed.), *Medical images*. London: Wiley.

Michie, D. (1982). *Introductory readings in expert systems*. New York: Gordon & Breach Scientific Publishers.

Miller, G. A. (1956). The magical number seven, plus or minus two: Some limits on the capacity for processing information. *Psychological Review, 63*, 81–97.

Miller, G. A., Galanter, E., & Pribram, K. A. (1960). *Plans and the structure of behavior*. New York: Holt, Rinehart & Winston.

Mishan, E. J. (1976). *Cost–benefit analysis*. New York: Praeger.

Morris, L. A. & Halperin, J. A. (1979). Effects of written drug information on patient knowledge and compliance: a literature review. *American Journal of Public Health, 69*, 47–52.

Moskowitz, H. (1974). Effects of problem representation and feedback on rational behavior in Allais and Morlat-type problems. *Decision Science, 5*, 225–242.

Murphy, A. H., & Winkler, R. L. (1974). Subjective probability forecasting in meterology: Some preliminary results. *Bulletin of the American Meterological Society, 55*, 1206–1216.

Murphy, A. H., & Winkler, R. L. (1977). Can weather forecasters formulate reliable probability forecasts of precipitation and temperature? *National Weather Digest, 2*, 2–9.

Nakao, M. A., & Axelrod, S. (1983). Numbers are better than words: Verbal specifications of frequency have no place in medicine. *The American Journal of Medicine, 74*, 1061–1065.

Neisser, U. (1976). *Cognition and reality*. San Francisco: Freeman.

Neuhauser, D., & Lewicki, A. M. (1975). What do we gain from the sixth stool Guaiac? *New England Journal of Medicine, 293*, 226–228.

Neutra, R., & Neff, R. (1975). Fetal death in eclampsia: II. The effect of nontherapeutic factors. *British Journal of Obstetrics and Gynecology, 82*, 390–396.

Newble, D. I., Hoare, J., & Baxter, A. (1982). Patient management problems: Issues of validity. *Medical Education, 16*, 137–142.

Newell, A., & Simon, H. A. (1972). *Human problem solving*. Englewood Cliffs, NJ: Prentice-Hall.

Nickerson, R. S., & Feerher, C. E. (1973). *Decision making and training: A review of theoretical and empirical studies of decison making and their implications for the training of decision makers* (Technical Report 73-c-0128-1). Orlando, FL: Naval Training and Equipment Center.

Nisbett, R. E., Krantz, D. H., Jepson, C., & Fong, G. T. (1982). Improving inductive inference. In D. Kahneman, P. Slovic, & A. Tversky (Eds.), *Judgment under uncertainty: Heuristics and biases*. Cambridge, England: Cambridge University Press.

Nisbett, R. E., Krantz, D. H., Jepson, C., & Kunda, Z. (1983). The use of statistical heuristics in everyday inductive reasoning. *Psychological Review, 90*, 339–363.

Nisbett, R. E., & Wilson, T. D. (1977). Telling more than we can know: Verbal report in mental processes. *Psychological Review, 84*, 231–259.

Nishiyama, H., Lewis, J. T., Ashare, A. B., & Saenger, E. L. (1975). Interpretation of radionuclide liver images: Do training and experience make a difference? *Journal of Nuclear Medicine, 16*(1), 11–16.

Norell, S. E. (1984). Methods in assessing drug compliance. *Acta Medica Scandinavica, 683,* 35–40.

Orient, J. M., Kettel, L. J., Sox, H. C., Sox, C. H., Berggren, H. J., Woods, A. H., Brown, B. W., & Lebowitz, M. (1983). The effects of algorithms on the cost and quality of patient care. *Medical Care, 21,* 157–167.

Oskamp, S. (1965). Overconfidence in case-study judgments. *Journal of Consulting Psychology, 29,* 261–265.

Palmer, R. H., Strain, R., Rothrock, J. K., & Hsu, L-N. (1983). Evaluation of operational failures in clinical decision making. *Medical Decision Making, 2,* 299–310.

Papandreou, A. G. (1953). An experimental test of an axiom in the theory of choice. *Econometrica, 21,* 477 (Abstract).

Parker, T. W., Kelsey, C. A., Moseley, R. D., Mettler, F. A., Garcia, J. F., & Briscoe, D. E. (1982). Directed versus free search for nodules in chest radiographs. *Investigative Radiology, 17,* 152–155.

Pauker, S. G. (1982). Prescriptive approaches to medical decision making. *American Behavioral Scientist, 25,* 507–522.

Pauker, S. G., Gorry, G. A., Kassirer, J. P., & Schwartz, W. B. (1976). Towards the simulation of clinical cognition: Taking the present illness by computer. *The American Journal of Medicine, 60,* 981–996.

Pauker, S. G., & Kassirer, J. P. (1975). Therapeutic decision making: A cost–benefit analysis. *New England Journal of Medicine, 293,* 229–234.

Pauker, S. G., & Kassirer, J. P. (1981). Clinical decision analysis by personal computer. *Archives of Internal Medicine, 141,* 1831–1837.

Pauker, S. G., Pauker, S. P., & McNeil, B. J. (1981). The effect of private attitudes on public policy. *Medical Decision Making, 1,* 103–114.

Payne, J. W. (1980). Information processing theory: Some concepts and methods applied to decision research. In T. S. Wallsten (Ed.), *Cognitive processes in choice and decision behavior.* Hillsdale, NJ: Erlbaum.

Payne, J. W. (1982). Contigent decision behavior. *Psychological Bulletin, 92,* 382–402.

Payne, J. W., & Braunstein, M. L. (1971). Preferences among gambles with equal underlying distributions. *Journal of Experimental Psychology, 87,* 13–18.

Pearson, R. M. (1982). Who is taking their tablets? *British Medical Journal, 285,* 757–758.

Peterson, C. R., & Beach, L. R. (1967). Man is an intuitive statistician. *Psychological Bulletin, 68,* 29–46.

Peterson, O., Andrews, L. P., Spain, R. S., & Greenberg, B. G. (1956). An analytical study of North Carolina general practice, 1953–1954. *Journal of Medical Education, 31* (Whole Pt. 2).

Phillips, L. D. (1983). A theoretical perspective on heuristics and biases in probabilistic thinking. In P. Humphreys, O. Svenson, & A. Vari (Eds.), *Analysing and aiding decision processes.* Amsterdam: North-Holland.

Phillips, L. D., & Edwards, W. (1966). Conservatism in a simple probability inference task. *Journal of Experimental Psychology, 72,* 346–357.

Piaget, J., & Inhelder, B. (1969). *The psychology of the child.* London: Routledge & Kegan Paul.

Pitz, G. F. (1980). The very guide of life: The use of probabilistic information for making decisions. In T. S. Wallsten (Ed.), *Cognitive processes in choice and decision behavior.* Hillsdale, NJ: Erlbaum.

Pitz, G. F., & Sachs, N. J. (1984). Judgment and decision: Theory and application. *Annual Review of Psychology, 35,* 139–163.

Plisken, J. S., & Pliskin, N. (1980). Decision analysis in clinical practice. *European Journal of Operational Research, 4,* 153–159.

Pliskin, N., & Taylor, A. K. (1977). General principles: Cost benefit and decision analysis. In J. P. Bunker, B. A. Barnes, & F. Mosteller (Eds.), *Costs, risks, and benefits of surgery.* New York: Oxford University Press.

Politser, P. (1980). Computer-based consultation for repeated diagnostic tests. In J. T. O'Neill (Ed.), *IEEE proceedings of the fourth annual symposium on computer applications in medical care.* Washington, DC: National Center for Health Sciences Research.

Politser, P. (1981). Decision analysis and clinical judgement: A re-evaluation. *Medical Decision Making, 1,* 361–389.

Politser, P. (1982). Reliability, decision rules, and the value of repeated tests. *Medical Decision Making, 2,* 47–69.

Quiggin, J. (1985). Subjective utility, anticipated utility, and the Allais paradox. *Organizational Behavior and Human Decision Processes, 35,* 94–101.

Raiffa, H. (1968). *Decision analysis: Introductory lectures on choices under uncertainty.* Boston: Addison-Wesley.

Rapoport, A., & Wallsten, T. S. (1972). Individual decision behavior. *Annual Review of Psychology, 23,* 131–175.

Rappoport, L., & Summers, D. A. (1973). *Human judgment and social interaction.* New York: Holt, Rinehart & Winston.

Read, L., Pass, T. M., & Komaroff, A. L. (1982). Diagnosis and treatment of dyspepsia: A cost-effectiveness analysis. *Medical Decision Making, 2,* 415–438.

Rhea, J. T., Potsaid, M. S., & DeLuca, S. A. (1979). Errors of interpretation as elicited by quality audit of an emergency radiology facility. *Radiology, 132,* 277–280.

Rhodes, A., McCue, J. D., Komaroff, A. L., & Pass, T. M. (1976). Protocol management of male genitourinary infections. *Journal of the American Venereal Disease Association, 2,* 23–30.

Robbins, J. A. (1980). Patient compliance. *Primary Care, 7,* 703–711.

Robertson, W. O. (1983). Quantifying the meaning of words. *Journal of the American Medical Association, 249,* 2631–2632.

Rogers, W., Ryack, B., & Moeller, G. (1979). Computer-aided medical diagnosis: Literature review. *International Journal of Biomedical Computing, 10,* 267–289.

Rossman, K., & Wiley, B. E. (1970). The central problem in the study of radiographic image quality. *Radiology, 96,* 113–118.

Rothert, M. L. (1982). Physicians' and patients' judgments of compliance with a hypertensive regimen. *Medical Decision Making, 2,* 179–196.

Runyan, J. W. (1975). *Primary care guide.* Hagerstown, MD: Harper & Row.

Rychener, M. D. (1985). Expert systems for engineering design. *Expert Systems, 2,* 30–44.

Sackett, D. L., & Haynes, R. B. (1976). *Compliance with therapeutic regimens.* Baltimore: Johns Hopkins University Press.

Sackett, D. L., Haynes, R. B., Gibson, E. S. (1975). Randomized clinical trial of strategies for improving medication compliance in primary hypertension. *Lancet, 1,* 1205–1207.

Sackett, D. L. & Snow, J. C. (1979). The magnitude of compliance and noncompliance. In R. B. Haynes, D. W. Taylor, & D. L. Sackett (Eds.). *Compliance in health care.* Baltimore: Johns Hopkins University Press.

Savage, L. J. (1954). *The foundations of statistics.* New York: Wiley.

Schiffmann, A., Cohen, S., Nowik, R., & Selinger, D. (1978). Initial diagnostic hypotheses: Factors which may distort physicians' judgment. *Organizational Behavior and Human Performance, 21,* 305–315.

Schlaifer, R. (1969). *Analysis of decisions under uncertainty.* New York: McGraw-Hill.

Schoemaker, P. J. H. (1982). The expected utility model: Its variants, purposes, evidence and limitations. *Journal of Economic Literature, 20,* 529–563.

Schreibner, M. H. (1963). The clinical history as a factor in roentgenogram interpretation. *Journal of the American Medical Association, 185,* 399–401.

Schrenk, L. P. (1969). Aiding the decision maker: A decision process model. *Ergonomics, 12,* 543–557.

Schwartz, W. B., Gorry, G. A., Kassirer, J. P., & Essig, A. (1973). Decision analysis and clinical judgment. *The American Journal of Medicine, 55,* 459–472.

Segall, H. N. (1966). The electrocardiogram and its interpretation: A study of reports by 20 physicians on a set of 100 electrocardiograms. *Canadian Medical Association Journal, 82,* 2–6.

Sehnert, K. W., & Eisenberg, H. (1975). *How to be your own doctor—sometimes.* New York: Grosset & Dunlap.

Seltzer, S. E., Doubilet, P. M., Sheriff, C. R., & Katz, J. M. (1984). Educational impact of faculty review on radiology residents' radiographic interpretations. *Investigative Radiology, 19,* 61–64.

Seltzer, S. E., Hessel, S. J., Herman, P. G., Swensson, R. G., & Sheriff, C. R. (1981). Resident film interpretations and staff review. *American Journal of Roentgenology, 137,* 129–133.

Shanteau, J. (1975). An information integration analysis of risky decision making. In M. F. Kaplan & S. Schwartz (Eds.), *Human judgment and decision processes in applied settings.* New York: Academic.

Shanteau, J. (1980). Training expert decision makers to ignore nondiagnostic information. In J. D. Schendel (Ed.), *Selected topics in behavioral science research.* Alexandria, VA: US Army Research Institute.

Shanteau, J., & Phelps, R. H. (1977). Judgment and swine: Approaches and issues in applied judgment analysis. In M. F. Kaplan & S. Schwartz (Eds.), *Human judgment and decision processes in applied settings.* New York: Academic.

Shanteau, J., Grier, M., Johnson, J., & Berner, E. (1981, October). *Improving decision making skills of nurses.* Paper presented at the Annual ORSA/TIMS Meeting, Houston, Texas.

Shaw, M. L. (1982). Attending to multiple sources of information: I. The integration of information in decision making. *Cognitive Psychology, 14,* 353–409.

Sheft, D. J., Jones, M. D., Brown, R. F., & Ross, S. E. (1970). Screening of chest roentgenograms by advanced roentgen technologists. *Radiology, 94,* 427–429.

Shiels, L. (1981). *The training of decision makers.* Unpublished BS(Hons) thesis, University of Western Australia, Perth, WA.

Shortliffe, E. H. (1976). *Computer-based medical consultations: MYCIN*. New York: Elsevier.

Shortliffe, E. H. (1980). Medical cybernetics: The challenges of clinical computing. In S. B. Ahmed (Ed.), *Cybernetics, technology and growth*. New York: Lexington Books.

Shugan, S. M. (1980). The cost of thinking. *Journal of Consumer Research, 7*, 99–111.

Simon, D. P., & Simon, H. A. (1978). Individual differences in solving physics problems. In R. Seigler (Ed.), *Children's thinking: What develops?* Hillsdale, NJ: Erlbaum.

Simon, H. A. (1957). *Models of man: Social and rational*. New York: Wiley.

Simon, H. A. (1978). Rationality as a process and product of thought. *The American Economic Review, 68*, 1–16.

Sisson, J. C., Schoomaker, E. B., & Ross, J. C. (1976). Clinical decision analysis: The hazard of using additional data. *Journal of the American Medical Association, 236*, 1259–1263.

Sjoberg, L. (1983). Value change and relapse following a decision to quit or reduce smoking. *Scandinavian Journal of Psychology, 24*, 137–148.

Skinner, B. F. (1938). *The behavior of organisms*. New York: Appleton-Century-Crofts.

Slovic, P. (1962). Convergent validation of risk-taking measures. *Journal of Abnormal and Social Psychology, 65*, 68–71.

Slovic, P. (1982). Toward understanding and improving decisions. In M. D. Dunnette & E. A. Fleishman (Eds.), *Human capability assessment (Human performance and productivity series, Vol. 1)*. Hillsdale, NJ: Erlbaum.

Slovic, P., Fischhoff, B., & Lichtenstein, S. (1977). Behavioral decision theory. *Annual Review of Psychology, 28*, 1–39.

Slovic, P., Fischhoff, B., & Lichtenstein, S. (1979). Rating the risks. *Environment, 21*, 14–20, 36–39.

Slovic, P., Fischhoff, B., & Lichtenstein, S. (1980). Informing people about risk. In L. Morris, M. Mazis, & B. Barofsky (Eds.), *Product labeling and health risks* (Banbury Report 6). Cold Spring Harbor: New York:

Slovic, P., Fischhoff, B., & Lichtenstein, S. (1981). Perceived risk: Psychological factors and social implications. *Proceedings of the Royal Society of London, A376*, 17–34.

Slovic, P., Fischhoff, B., & Lichtenstein, S. (1982a). Facts versus fears: Understanding perceived risk. In D. Kahneman, P. Slovic, & A. Tversky (Eds.), *Judgment under uncertainty: Heuristics and biases*. Cambridge, England: Cambridge University Press.

Slovic, P., Fischhoff, B., & Lichtenstein, S. (1982b). Why study risk perception? *Risk Analysis, 2*, 83–93.

Slovic, P., & Lichtenstein, S. (1971). Comparison of Bayesian and regression approaches to the study of information processing in judgement. *Organizational Behavior and Human Performance, 6*, 649–744.

Slovic, P., Rorer, L. G., & Hoffman, P. J. (1971). Analyzing the use of diagnostic signs. *Investigative Radiology, 6*, 18–26.

Slovic, P., & Tversky, A. (1974). Who accepts Savage's Axiom? *Behavioral Science, 19*, 368–373.

Smedslund, J. (1963). The concept of correlation in adults. *Scandinavian Journal of Psychology, 4,* 165–173.

Smith, M. J. (1967). *Error and variation in diagnostic radiology.* Springfield, IL: Thomas.

Snyder, R. E. (1966). Mammography: Contributions and limitations in the management of the breast. *Clinical Obstetrics and Gynecology, 9,* 207–220.

Sox, H. C., Sox, C. H., & Tompkins, R. K. (1973). The training of physicians assistants: The use of a clinical algorithm system in patient care, audit of performance and education. *New England Journal of Medicine, 288,* 818–824.

Spiegelhalter, D. J., & Knill-Jones, R. P. (1984). Statistical and knowledge-based approaches to clinical decision support systems, with an application in gastro-enterology. *Journal of the Royal Statistical Society, A147,* 35–77.

Starr, C. (1969). Social benefit versus technological risk. *Science, 165,* 1232–1238.

Starr, C., & Whipple, C. (1980). Risks of risk decisions. *Science, 208,* 1114–1119.

Starr, S. J., Metz, C. E., Lusted, L. B., & Goodenough, D. J. (1975). Visual detection and localization of radiographic images. *Radiology, 116,* 533–538.

Sutherland, H. J., Dunn, V., & Boyd, N. F. (1983). Measurement of values for states of health with linear analog scales. *Medical Decision Making, 3,* 477–487.

Sutherland, H. J., Llewellyn-Thomas, H., Boyd, N. F., & Till, J. E. (1982). Attitudes toward quality of survival: The concept of 'maximal endurable time'. *Medical Decision Making, 2,* 299–309.

Svenson, O. (1979). Process descriptions of decision making. *Organizational Behavior and Human Performance, 23,* 86–112.

Svenson, O. (1981). Are we all less risky and more skillful than our fellow drivers? *Acta Psychologica, 47,* 143–148.

Sweller, J., Mawer, R. F., & Ward, M. R. (1983). Development of expertise in mathematical problem solving. *Journal of Experimental Psychology: General, 112,* 639–661.

Swensson, R. G., Hessel, S. J., & Herman, P. G. (1977). Omissions in radiology: Faulty search or stringent reporting criteria? *Radiology, 123,* 563–567.

Swensson, R. G., Hessel, S. J., & Herman, P. G. (1982). Radiographic interpretation with and without search: Visual search aids the recognition of chest pathology. *Investigative Radiology, 17*(2), 145–151.

Swensson, R. G., Hessel, S. J., & Herman, P. G. (1985). The value of searching films without specific preconceptions. *Investigative Radiology, 20,* 100–107.

Swets, J. A. (1973). The receiver operating characteristic in psychology. *Science, 182,* 990–1000.

Swets, J. A. (1979). ROC analysis applied to the evaluation of medical imaging techniques. *Investigative Radiology, 14,* 109–121.

Swets, J. A., & Pickett, R. M. (1982). *Evaluation of diagnostic systems.* New York: Academic Press.

Szanawkski, K. (1980). Philosophy of decision making. *Acta Psychologica, 45,* 327–341.

Szasz, T. S. & Hollender, M. H. (1956). A contribution to the philosophy of medicine. The basic models of doctor–patient relationship. *Archives of Internal Medicine, 97,* 585–592.

Szolovits, P. (1982). Artificial intelligence and medicine. In P. Szolovits (Ed.), *Artificial intelligence in medicine.* Boulder, CO: Westview.

Szolovits, P., & Pauker, S. G. (1978). Categorical and probabilistic reasoning in medical diagnosis. *Artificial Intelligence, 11*, 115–144.

Taylor, D. W., Sackett, D. L., Haynes, R. B., Johnson, A. L., Gibson, E. S., & Roberts, R. S. (1979). Compliance with antihypertensive drug therapy. *Annals of the New York Academy of Sciences, 304*, 390–403.

Taylor, T. R., Aitchison, J., & McGirr, E. M. (1971). Doctors as decision-makers: A computer-assisted study of diagnosis as a cognitive skill. *British Medical Journal, 3*, 35–40.

Theodossi, A., Spiegelhalter, D. J., McFarlane, S. G., & Williams, R. (1984). Doctors' attitudes to risk in difficult clinical decisions: Application of decision analysis in hepatobiliary disease. *British Medical Journal, 289*, 213–216.

Thomas, L. (1979). Medical lessons from history. In L. Thomas (Ed.), *The medusa and the snail.* New York: Viking Press.

Thornbury, J. R., Fryback, D. G., & Edwards, W. (1975). Likelihood ratios as a measure of the diagnostic usefulness of excretory urogram information. *Radiology, 114*, 561–565.

Todd, F. J., & Hammond, K. R. (1965). Differential feedback in two multiple-cue probability learning tasks. *Behavioral Science, 10*, 429–435.

Toogood, J. H. (1980). What do we mean by usually? *Lancet, 1*, 1094.

Tuddenham, W. J. (1962). Visual search, image organization, and reader error in roentogen diagnosis. *Radiology, 78*, 694–704.

Turner, D. A. (1978). An intuitive approach to receiver operating characteristic curve analysis. *Journal of Nuclear Medicine, 19*, 213–220.

Turner, D. A., Ramachandran, P. C., & Ali, A. A. (1976). Brain scanning with the Anger multiplane tomographic scanner as a primary examination: Evaluation by the ROC method. *Radiology, 121*, 125–129.

Tversky, A. (1969). Intransitivity of preferences. *Psychological Review, 76*, 31–48.

Tversky, A., & Kahneman, D. (1971). Belief in the 'law of small numbers'. *Psychological Bulletin, 76*, 105–110.

Tversky, A., & Kahneman, D. (1973). Availability: A heuristic for judging frequency and probability. *Cognitive Psychology, 4*, 207–232.

Tversky, A., & Kahneman, D. (1974). Judgment under uncertainty: Heuristics and biases. *Science, 185*, 1124–1131.

Tversky, A., & Kahneman, D. (1981). The framing of decisions and the psychology of choice. *Science, 211*, 453–458.

Vertinsky, I., & Wong, E. (1975). Eliciting preferences and the construction of indifference maps: A comparative empirical evaluation of two measurement methodologies. *Socioeconomic Planning Sciences, 9*, 15–24.

Von Neumann, J., & Morgenstern, O. (1944). *Theory of games and economic behavior.* Princeton, NJ: Princeton University Press.

Vydareny, K. H., Harle, T. S., & Potchen, E. J. (1982). An algorithmic approach to the roentgenographic evaluation of head trauma: Medical and financial applications. *Investigative Radiology, 18*, 390–395.

Waddell, G., Main, C. J., & Morris, E. W. (1982). Normality and reliability in the clinical assessment of backache. *British Medical Journal, 284*, 1519–1523.

Wallsten, T. S. (1981). Physician and medical student bias in evaluating diagnostic information. *Medical Decision Making, 1*, 145–164.

Wallsten, T. S. (1983). The theoretical status of judgment heuristics. In R. W. Scholz (Ed.), *Decision making under uncertainty.* Amsterdam: North-Holland.

Wallsten, T. S., & Budescu, D. V. (1981). Additivity and nonadditivity in judging MMPI profiles. *Journal of Experimental Psychology: Human Perception and Performance, 7,* 1096–1109.

Warner, K., & Luce, B. (1982). *Cost–benefit and cost-effectiveness analysis in health care: Principles, practice, and potential.* Ann Arbor, MI: Health Administration Press.

Warren, R. M. (1970). Perceptual restoration of missing speech sounds. *Science, 167,* 393–395.

Wartman, S. A., Morlock, L. L., Malitz, F. E., & Palm, E. A. (1983). Patient understanding and satisfaction as predictors of compliance. *Medical Care, 21,* 886–891.

Weinstein, M. C. (1981). Economic assessments of medical practices and technologies. *Medical Decision Making, 1,* 309–330.

Weinstein, M. C., & Fineberg, H. V. (1980). *Clinical decision analysis.* Philadelphia: Saunders.

Weinstein, N. D. (1980). Unrealistic optimism about future life events. *Journal of Personality and Social Psychology, 39,* 806–810.

Weiss, S., Kulikowski, C. A., & Safir, A. (1978). Glaucoma consultation by computer. *Computers in Biology and Medicine, 8,* 25–40.

Wertman, B. G., Sostrin, S. V., Pavlova, Z., & Lundberg, G. D. (1980). Why do physicians order laboratory tests? A study of laboratory test request and use patterns. *Journal of the American Medical Association, 243,* 2080–2082.

Wildavsky, A. (1979). No risk is the highest risk of all. *American Scientist, 67,* 32–37.

Williams, S. V. (1985). The impact of DRG-based prospective payment on clinical decision making. *Medical Decision Making, 5,* 23–29.

Williamson, J. W. (1965). Assessing clinical judgment. *Journal of Medical Education, 40,* 180–186.

Wilson, W. J., Templeton, A. W., Turner, A. H., Jr., & Lodwick, G. S. (1965). Analysis and diagnosis of gastric ulcers. *Radiology, 85,* 1064–1073.

Wolf, F. M. (1984). Validity of patient management problems re-examined. *Medical Education, 18,* 222–225.

Wolf, F. M., Allen, N. P., Cassidy, J. T., Maxim, B. R., & Davis, W. K. (1983). Concurrent and criterion-referenced validity of patient management problems. *Proceedings of the Association of American Medical Colleges: Annual Conference on Research in Medical Education,* 115–121.

Wolf, F. M., Gruppen, L. D., & Billi, J. E. (1984, April). *The competing hypothesis heuristic, Bayesian thinking, and clinical decision making.* Paper presented at the American Education Research Association, New Orleans.

Wood, R. W., Tompkins, R. K., & Wolcott, B. W. (1980). An efficient strategy for managing acute respiratory illness in adults. *Annals of Internal Medicine, 93,* 757–763.

Woody, R. H. (1968). Interjudge reliability in clinical electroencephalography. *Journal of Clinical Psychology, 24,* 251–256.

Wortman, P. M. (1972). Medical diagnosis: An information processing approach. *Computers and Biomedical Research, 5,* 315–328.

Wright, G. (1984). *Behavioural decision theory.* Harmondsworth, England: Penguin.

Wright, H. J., Stanley, I. M., & Webster, J. (1983). The assessment of cognitive abilities in clinical medicine. *Medical Education, 17,* 31–38.

Wulff, H. R. (1981). How to make the best decision: Philosophical aspects of clinical decision theory. *Medical Decision Making, 1,* 277–283.

Yerushalmy, J. (1969). The statistical assessment of the variability in observer perception and description of roentgenographic pulmonary shadows. *Radiologic Clinics of North America, 7,* 381–392.

Zadeh, L. A. (1973). Outline of a new approach to the analysis of complex systems and decision processes. *IEEE Transactions on Systems, Man and Cybernetics, 3,* 28–44.

Author Index

Subject Index

R
723.5
S38
1986

Schwartz, Steven.

Medical thinking

$39.00

C_1 **106887**

R
723.5
S38
1986

Schwartz, Steven.

Medical thinking

$39.00

DATE	BORROWER'S NAME	

© THE BAKER & TAYLOR CO.